FRONTIERS OF INFECTIOUS DISEASES
NEW ANTIBACTERIAL STRATEGIES

4/92

FRONTIERS OF INFECTIOUS DISEASES

NEW ANTIBACTERIAL STRATEGIES

PROCEEDINGS OF AN INTERNATIONAL SYMPOSIUM
SPONSORED BY GLAXO RESEARCH,
BROCKET HALL, HERTFORDSHIRE
30 JUNE—3 JULY 1990

EDITED BY

HAROLD C. NEU

Professor of Medicine and Pharmacology
Division of Infectious Diseases
Columbia University
New York, USA

ORGANIZING COMMITTEE

K.P.W.J. McADAM	**S.R. NORRBY**	**P.K. PETERSON**	**H.C. NEU**	**J. VERHOEF**
London	Lund	Minneapolis	New York	Utrecht
United Kingdom	Sweden	USA	USA	Netherlands

CHURCHILL LIVINGSTONE
EDINBURGH LONDON MELBOURNE AND NEW YORK 1990

Distributed in the United States of America by Churchill
Livingstone Inc., 1560 Broadway, New York, N.Y.
10036, and by associated companies, branches and
representatives throughout the world.

First Edition 1990

ISBN 0-443-04448-1

British Library Cataloguing in Publication Data available

Library of Congress Cataloging-in-Publication Data available

Printed in Great Britain by Bell and Bain Ltd., Glasgow

Preface

This book provides the record of a meeting held at Brocket Hall, Hertfordshire, England between 30 June and 3 July, 1990. The meeting was the third in an ongoing series on Frontiers of Infectious Diseases and was devoted to New Strategies in Bacterial Infections. The proceedings are published within six months of the meeting so that the material will be up to date and provide readers with the current opinions of leaders in the field of infectious diseases. As in the previous two meetings, which dealt with virology (1988) and parasitology (1989), the focus was an attempt to integrate the latest advances at a molecular level with the important infectious disease entities.

The first presentation by myself addressed the unsolved problems that bacterial diseases present for the 1990s and beyond. Diseases such as meningitis, hospital-acquired pneumonia, sepsis, and diarrhoeal disease illustrate conditions in which there are major problems of mortality and morbidity in both developed and developing countries. Bacterial resistance of staphylococci, enterococci, Enterobacteriaceae, and other pathogens such as *Pseudomonas aeruginosa* and related species will also offer major challenges for the development of new antibacterial agents. Even more complex is how immunomodulators may be utilized in the treatment of bacterial infections, since even though we know much about the activity of these substances, the cost of this approach will far exceed that of current antimicrobial agents.

The first session of the meeting dealt with the problem of Borrelia infections. Lyme disease has been known by different names for many years in Europe, but only within the past decade has it become an illness of note in the United States. Gerold Stanek (Vienna, Austria) presented data on the epidemiology of Borrelia infections in central Europe during the last few years. While it is clear that the disease is increasingly recognized, its real incidence remains uncertain. It is inconceivable that there has been a suggested 1000-fold increase in some areas. Russell Johnson (Minneapolis, USA) reviewed the current knowledge of the structure of the Borrelia organism and the potential for vaccines, pointing out the problems in determining the antimicrobial susceptibility of Borrelia. The complexity of the serologic response to Borrelia was reviewed by Bettina Wilske (Munich, Germany), who referred to the many cross-reacting antigens that confound currently used serological tests. Where diagnosis can be made from the distinct clinical rash, serology is not required, but in the confusing neurological problems, serum serology may be negative, while the CSF serology, similar to syphilis, may be positive for years.

In the second session, Alf Lindberg (Stockholm, Sweden) provided a superb review of the polysaccharide vaccines needed for the 1990s. He pointed out the value of the conjugate vaccines which utilize not only B-cells but the T-dependent axis. Indeed, the discussions highlighted the great progress made with the Haemophilus conjugate vaccines, which may be of major importance in reducing Haemophilus meningitis, a disease with important morbidity. Myron Levine (Baltimore, USA) reviewed the status of vaccines for *Salmonella typhi*, where major progress has been made in the past decade, and an oral vaccine may now be truly possible. Many of the lessons learned from the Salmonella vaccine hopefully will be applied to other vaccines for enteric infections.

Session three focused on musocal surface interactions. The role of surface fimbriae of *Escherichia coli* in attachment to bladder and kidney as reviewed by Gary Schoolnik (Stanford, USA) has been well known for the past decade. The observations of Catharina Swanborg (Lund, Sweden) that chronically infected bacteriuric patients do not have adhering strains and that blocking p-adherence would not prevent renal scarring raises serious questions about the possibility of vaccination as a strategy to prevent pyelonephritis. Torkel Wadstrom (Lund, Sweden) then provided an excellent review of our knowledge of *E. coli* as a cause of diarrhoea, and the concept that the enteroadherent organisms alter the cytoskeleton of the intestinal cell offers further areas of investigation for this field.

Martin Blaser (Nashville, USA) provided a most compelling rationale for the role of *Helicobacter pyloi* in gastritis and duodenal ulcer. His model of the pathogenesis of the infection with its effect on gastrin secretion and possible ultimate role in gastric malignancy proved most provocative. Although Guido Tytgat (Amsterdam, The Netherlands) provided impressive responses to triple antimicrobial programs, we have yet to solve the problem of recurrence of this disease.

Session four, which centres on the subject of resistance began with Staffan Normark (St Louis, USA) proposing a most interesting new model to explain β-lactamase induction. A peptidoglycan fragment is generated which is transported across the cytoplasmic membrane to interact with ampR. Equally fascinating has been the appearance of new plasmid β-lactamases as discussed by Laurent Gutmann (Paris, France).

Quinolone antimicrobials have caught the interest of scientist and practitioner alike. As Mark Fisher (London, UK) pointed out, our understanding of the interaction of the fluoroquinolones with DNA gyrase and DNA is far from complete. Excellent work by his group has demonstrated that changes in tyrosine-122 of the DNA gyrase of *E. coli* explain resistance in clinical isolates. Analogous changes occur in *Staphylococcus aureus* clinical isolates which have become resistant. How to prevent clinical resistance remains unclear, but a better understanding of the molecular changes associated with resistance may aid us in developing new compounds. The problem of transport in resistance in bacteria was reviewed by Christopher Higgins (Oxford, UK), who pointed out the value of the TonB system as an uptake system for the periplasmic space. Current research is directed at use of catechol compounds to capitalize on accessory channels to introduce antibiotics into bacteria.

In the second plenary lecture, Keith McAdam (London, UK) provided a most up to date look at the important infection, leprosy. Modern advances in immunology and molecular biology offer ways to control the disease and to identify those individuals in whom early treatment may abate the illness.

Paul Tulkens (Brussels, Belgium) and William Craig (Wisconsin, USA) each then presented and provided an up to date discussion of the intracellular location of antibiotics. Tulkens rightly concluded that different locations in the phagocytic cell are needed for different pathogens, after which Irun Cohen (Rehovot, Israel) provided a most provocative article on the 65k dalton heat shock protein and its association with murine autoimmune disease.

Immunomodulators provided the subject for the sixth and final session of the meeting. The interleukins, now well characterized, unfortunately have not so far been manipulated successfully in infectious diseases as the review by Chris Henney (Seattle, USA) showed. We clearly have a long way to go before we can manipulate interleukins to our benefit in disease. In contrast, the colony stimulating factors, as reviewed by Don Metcalf (Melbourne, Australia), have proved extremely useful in a number of clinical situations, though while potential uses are many, the costs may prove prohibitive.

I would like to thank Glaxo Research for providing the funding of these meetings, and in particular, Richard Sykes, Grahaem Brown and Carolyn Bennet of Glaxo, without whose continued help the meeting would not run in the efficient manner that it has over the past three years. Finally, I thank Amanda Ryde of Churchill Livingstone, without whom these proceedings would never have seen the light of day.

H.C.N.
1990

List of participants

BARRET, Nicola, Communicable Disease Surveillance Centre, Public Health Laboratory Service, London, United Kingdom

BENACH, Jorge L, Department of Health, State University of New York, United States of America

BERNSTEIN, Robert, Rheumatism Research Centre, University of Manchester, United Kingdom

BLASER, Martin J, Department of Medicine, Vanderbilt University, Nashville, United States of America

COHEN, Irun R, Department of Cell Biology, The Weizmann Institute of Science, Rehovot, Israel

CRAIG, William A, William S. Middleton Memorial Veterans' Hospital, Wisconsin, United States of America

FISHER, L Mark, Department of Cellular and Molecular Sciences, University of London, United Kingdom

GUTTMANN, Laurent, Department of Medical Microbiology, St Joseph's Hospital, Paris, France

GUY, Edward, Public Health Laboratory, Southampton, United Kingdom

HENNEY, Christopher S, ICOS Corporation, Washington, United States of America

HIGGINS, Christopher F, Institute of Molecular Medicine, John Radcliffe Hospital, Oxford, United Kingdom

JOHNSON, Russell C, University of Minnesota, Minneapolis, United States of America

KAYE, Paul, Department of Tropical Hygiene, London School of Hygiene and Tropical Medicine, United Kingdom

KEUSCH, Gerald T, Division of Geographic Medicine and Infectious Diseases, New England Medical Centre Hospital, Massachusetts, United States of America

LAGRANGE, Phillipe H, Service Central de Microbiologie, Paris, France

LAMBERT, Peter A, Department of Microbiology, Aston University, Birmingham, United Kingdom

LEVINE, Myron M, Division of Infectious Diseases and Tropical Pediatrics, University of Maryland, United States of America

LINDBERG, Alf A, Karolinska Institute, Huddinge Hospital, Sweden

McADAM, Keith P W J, Department of Clinical Sciences, London School of Hygiene & Tropical Medicine, United Kingdom

MAKELA P Helena, National Public Health Institute, Helsinki, Finland

METCALF, Donald, The Walter and Eliza Hall Institute of Medical Research, Victoria, Australia

MOXON, E Richard, Department of Paediatrics, John Radcliffe Hospital, Oxford, United Kingdom

NEU, Harold C, Division of Infectious Diseases, Columbia University, New York, United States of America

NORMARK, Staffan, Department of Molecular Microbiology, Washington University School of Medicine, United States of America

NORRBY, S Ragnar, Department of Infectious Diseases, Lund University Hospital, Sweden

PETERSON, Phillip K, Department of Medicine, Hennepin County Medical Center, Minneapolis, United States of America

SCHOOLNIK, Gary K, Department of Medicine, Stanford University, California, United States of America

SVANBORG, Catharina, Department of Medical Microbiology, University of Lund, Sweden

STANEK, Gerold, Hygiene Institute, Vienna University, Austria

TULKENS, Paul M, International Institute of Cellular and Molecular Pathology, Université Catholique de Louvrain, Belgium

TYTGAT, Guido N J, Academic Medicine Centre, Amsterdam, The Netherlands

VERHOEF Jan, Department of Clinical Microbiology, University Hospital, Utrecht, The Netherlands

WADSTRÖM, Torkel, Department of Medical Microbiology, Lund University Hospital, Sweden

WIEDEMANN, Bert, Pharmazeutisch Mikrobiologie der Universitët Bonn, Germany

WILSKE, Bettina, Max von Pettenkofer Institut für Hygiene und Medizinische Mikrobiologie, Ludwig-Maximilians-Universität, Munich, Germany

Contents

Plenary Lecture 1
Chairman: S. R. Norrby

1. Bacterial diseases: unsolved problems
H. C. Neu

INTRODUCTION

Although there are many antimicrobial agents available in a large number of different classes to inhibit and kill bacteria, the problems of bacterial infections are not solved. There are two approaches that can be taken to examine problems of bacterial diseases: one organism directed and the other disease oriented. I have chosen to use both approaches.

There are unsolved problems in both diagnosis and therapy for a number of important infections.

MENINGITIS

The organisms causing meningitis in different age groups and clinical settings has been established by investigations over the past several decades (Meningitis Study Group 1987, 1989). Although there has been a shift from *Escherichia coli* to group B streptococci as the major cause of neonatal meningitis in developed nations, there has been minimal decrease in the incidence of neonatal meningitis. Furthermore, even though excellent antimicrobial agents are available, there has been minimal improvement in mortality and morbidity in recent years. The same arguments could be made for childhood meningitis in which *Haemophilus influenzae* and *Streptococcus pneumoniae* are the pathogens. Indeed in childhood meningitis with a decline in mortality there may be an increase in morbidity due to survival of children who would previously have died. Permanent neurological sequelae occur in 10 to 20% of survivors (Klein et al 1986). Among the elderly there is major morbidity and mortality in meningitis due to *Streptococcus pneumoniae*. Do we lack adequate antimicrobial agents? No. Do we lack agents that enter the cerebrospinal fluid or the brain? No. What is the problem? The problem centres around the body's inflammatory response to organisms or even to bacterial cell wall in the spinal fluid. Bacterial cell wall components bind to CNS endothelium and promote the response of leukocytes with the associated interleukin (IL-1) which stimulates tumour necrosis factor (TNF). Autoregulation of cerebral blood flow is lost, and there is resultant brain oedema with ultimate irreversible neurone damage. In effect it would appear

3

that effective antibiotics cause rapid destruction of bacteria with an inflammatory burst and associated brain tissue damage. Ideally an antimicrobial agent would penetrate the blood-brain barrier rapidly, halt proliferation of bacteria, kill the bacteria, but not release surface components which activate IL-1 and TNF. Choramphenicol immediately comes to mind as an agent, but chloramphenicol is bactericidal and lytic to the CNS pathogens.

Clinical trials of dexamethasone for treatment of meningitis in children and adults have reported a reduction in neurological sequelae for pneumococcal meningitis. There was a 13% mortality rate in patients receiving dexamethasone with antibiotics versus 41% for patients who received ampicillin plus chloramphenicol alone (Girgis et al 1989). A similar study of treatment of meningitis by Lebel et al (1988) showed an improvement in hearing loss and neurological sequelae only in children with *Haemophilus influenzae* meningitis. These studies cannot be translated to all forms of meningitis. Unfortunately, there is only a small time period that agents that blunt the host's response to bacteria can be administered to obtain optimal effects. But it would seem that to make significant progress in the treatment of bacterial meningitis attention will have to switch from the antibacterial agents which have been the focus of the late 1970s and early 1980s to agents modifying the inflammatory response. It is important to realize that mortality and morbidity in a disease which requires that patients have rapid access to healthcare will not change in many developing and even developed countries. Patients who are not seen or diagnosed until well into the course of meningitis will do poorly. The economic incentive to improve morbidity is great since neurological sequelae are extremely costly in the long term to the health care system.

HOSPITAL-ACQUIRED PNEUMONIA

Nosocomial pneumonia is the second most common cause of hospital-acquired infection (Horan et al 1986), and the leading cause of death from nosocomial infection (Gross et al 1980). Patients who are at highest risk for nosocomial pneumonia are the ventilated patients, some 7 to 10-fold above non-ventilated hospitalized patients (Horan et al 1986, Celis et al 1988). We know that colonization of the oropharynx with Gram-negative bacilli or staphylococci is necessary before pneumonia develops, and we know that many factors contribute to colonization of the oropharynx with Gram-negative bacteria. Gross et al (1980) reported that 60% of fatal nosocomial infections were due to pneumonia, and a more recent study by Craven et al (1986) showed that of 233 mechanically ventilated patients there was a 55% fatality rate for patients with pneumonia compared with 25% for patients without pneumonia.

We know that most cases of nosocomial pneumonia result from aspiration of bacteria from the oropharynx or the stomach into the tracheobronchial tree. We know that oropharyngeal colonization with bacteria has been associated with increasing severity of illness, longer duration of hospitalization, use of antibiotics, advanced age, intubation, and many other factors. None of these factors will be changed in the coming years. Indeed, there will be more elderly patients and those patients who are hospitalized will be more severely ill as more and more attempts are

4

made to treat less severe illness in the community thereby decreasing costs. Attempts to decrease the incidence of pneumonia in intubated patients by maintaining the pH in the stomach at higher levels by avoiding H_2 blockers have met with variable success since even in patients who did not receive H_2 blockers, 41% developed pneumonia (Daschner et al 1988). Also, a study by Driks et al (1987) showed a very low incidence of pneumonia in patients who received a H_2 blocker alone. Thus it seems likely, irrespective of what is ultimately found for H_2 blockers, that there will be many patients who develop pneumonia in the hospital.

The diagnosis of pneumonia in the hospitalized patient in the intensive care unit (ICU) is not a simple matter, and in spite of extensive study, it is often impossible to separate pneumonia of a bacterial aetiology from an acute respiratory distress lung picture.

The difficulty in making a diagnosis of pneumonia in ICUs and the frequency with which it occurs has caused a resurgence of interest in antibiotic prophylaxis in ICUs. Early studies of aerosolization of antibiotics such as polymyxin B into the trachea reduced pneumonia due to *Pseudomonas aeruginosa* but resulted in increased Gram-positive pneumonia and resistant Gram-negative bacilli (Feeley et al 1975). More recently both systemic and local antibiotic prophylaxis have been used in ICUs to prevent colonization of the oropharynx and gastrointestinal tract (Stoutenbeck et al 1986; Ledingham et al 1988). These studies have reported a major reduction in Gram-negative pneumonia compared with placebo groups, but have not resulted in a major reduction of the time patients spend in ICUs or in fatality rates. Although antimicrobial resistance is said not to have occurred in these studies, the time of observation has been short, and it is likely that it will be a problem.

Hospital-acquired pneumonia thus remains an unsolved problem in spite of the reduction in infection due to the mechanical devices and other equipment used on intubated patients. Preventive measures that decrease oropharyngeal colonization, methods to diagnose pneumonia more rapidly, and better methods to deliver antimicrobial agents to all parts of the lung are needed.

CYSTIC FIBROSIS

Respiratory infection in cystic fibrosis patients is another problem which has not been solved by the introduction of new antimicrobial agents. Each new antimicrobial agent with activity against *Pseudomonas aeruginosa* has been used since the late 1960s with the development of carbenicillin. Ureido-penicillins such as azlocillin and pipera-cillin, cephalosporins such as ceftazidime, the monobactam aztreonam, and the carbapenem imipenem have been used to treat acute bacterial respiratory exacerbations in these patients. However, with use, all of the aforementioned agents, aminoglycosides, the newly introduced quinolones, such as ciprofloxacin, become ineffective due to resistance of the *Pseudomonas* (Scully et al 1987). It has been impossible to clear the tracheobronchial tree of *Pseudomonas* in those patients who routinely have 10^8 to 10^{10} CFU per ml of sputum. Clinical studies have clarified that antibiotics do make a difference in the course of the cystic fibrosis patient. Thus, it is imperative to continue to find new antibacterial agents for these patients. This is no small task since the patients are not a major part of the population, and if drugs

5

are used to treat these patients early in the development of the drug, it can cast a shadow over a compound because of resistance development. It is necessary to develop novel ways to administer antimicrobial agents to the cystic fibrosis patient, and it is important to learn better ways to overcome *Pseudomonas aeruginosa*, about which I will comment more subsequently.

SEPSIS

In the past two years, there has been an enormous advance in our understanding of the pathogenic processes which occur during septicaemia. The organisms that cause sepsis and the sources of the bacteria have been delineated so that it is possible to suspect the aetiologic agent with a high degree of accuracy. We have excellent antibacterial agents which inhibit many, if not most of both community and hospital-acquired organisms. Methods to decrease bacteraemia have been developed by improved hospital infection control procedures. The haemodynamics and pathophysiological changes which occur in the heart, lung, and kidney have been described. We realize that there is activation of the kinin cascades, and that IL-1 and TNF are produced and that cardiac contractility diminishes and capillaries in the lung become excessively permeable. Nonetheless, there is still a significant mortality due to sepsis, and the question remains how can this be altered?

Studies utilizing polyclonal, and more recently monoclonal, antibodies of either murine or human origin have shown a protective value in selected septic patients. More studies are needed to establish the efficacy of this treatment before it becomes a general procedure for suspected sepsis. The costs of antibody administration will be significant, and it is necessary to delineate specifically those patients in whom such therapy is unequivocally beneficial.

Equally complex is how to adjust the production of IL-1 and TNF in the septic patient. Can specific antibodies be made to modulate finely the host's response to sepsis? Are there situations in which it would be reasonable to modify the production and activity of these cytokines knowing that there is the potential for sepsis? Could agents be developed that could be administered before surgery which by modulating cytokine activity would cause a major reduction in septic shock?

The area of sepsis is one for interface of antimicrobial agents and immune modulators if further progress is to be made in reducing the mortality of sepsis. Antimicrobial agents, if active against the infecting organism, result in very similar cure rates. The number of organisms resistant to all agents currently available or under study is quite small. Thus the problem of this bacterial infection is primarily one of altering the host so that defences do not run amok and kill the patient.

Recently it has become evident that colony-stimulating factors, such as GMCSF and GCSF, are important in providing adequate re-establishment of phagocytic cells that are critical to prevention of serious bacterial infection which occurs during neutropenia. How these agents are to be optimally used has not been established. It is not clear that deleterious effects will not occur in some situations. Can the agents be used in a way that will not result in proliferation of undesired clones of cells in the patients with malignancy? Sepsis in the neutropenic patient remains a serious problem; albeit to a lesser extent due to aerobic Gram-negative bacteria, but aggressive chemotherapy directed against the malignancies and the use of oral agents of the quinolone class to sterilize the intestine has caused the appearance of Gram-positive species such as the viridans streptococci. This has been particularly evident in the bone marrow transplant patients. Thus new bacterial pathogens are likely to appear in the markedly immunocompromised patient. Strategies for the use of antimicrobial agents in these populations will undergo continued change.

GASTROINTESTINAL PATHOGENS

The role of *Helicobacter pylori*, formerly *Campylobacter pylori*, in gastritis is being more and more firmly established (Blaser 1987, Rauws et al 1988, Chamberlain & Peura 1990). Challenge of humans with *Helicobacter* produces gastritis (Marshall et al 1985, Morris & Nicholson 1987). Recently it has been shown that there are intrafamilial clustering of *Helicobacter* infections (Drumm et al 1990). It is now possible to culture *Helicobacter* easily, to detect serum antibodies to the organism, and even to detect it rapidly by the (^{13}C) urea breath test (Booth et al 1989, Goodwin et al 1989, Graham et al 1988, Evans et al 1989). Unfortunately, so far no serotyping system exists to characterize *Helicobacter pylori* isolates well in order to understand better the epidemiology and transfer of the organism.

Medical therapy has been associated with clearing *Helicobacter pylori* from the gastrointestinal tract and with healing of inflammation in patients with duodenal ulcers (Rauws et al 1988, Chamberlain & Peura 1990). However, relapse is common, and there has been the development of resistance to antibiotics such as the quinolones. It is clear that agents more effective against *Helicobacter* are needed. The fact that bisumuth subcitrate combined with amoxycillin has been more effective than bismuth alone makes it unclear if the effect of the antibiotic is on the organism or on other commensals which potentiate the *Helicobacter*. Long-term studies with more careful analysis of whether there is recurrence, reinfection, or both, occur is necessary if progress in this disease is to be achieved.

Intestinal infections are a major problem in the developing world, and with an increase in world travel a problem seen in the developed nations as well. Antimicrobial approaches to diarrhoeal disease have met with success, but there has been the development of major resistance that is plasmid-mediated in *Shigella*, *Salmonella* and other enteric pathogens (Murray 1986). Systemic disease due to *Salmonella typhi*, a pathogen unique to man, is still a problem in many parts of the world. Vaccination logically seems a way to approach the problem of bacterial enteric infections, and there has been extensive work in the field of vaccines against typhoid, *Shigella* and cholera. Unfortunately problems remain. The cholera-inactivated oral vaccines have been well tolerated and protect older children and adults for at least three years. The inactivated vaccines require multiple doses and do not protect the very young children who are most likely to suffer the serious effects of fluid loss (Clemens et al 1990). Ideally, an attenuated strain of vaccine will ultimately be possible that will not cause side-effects as did the early recombinant vaccines. Currently clinical trials are in progress to see the effect of the CVD 103 single-dose vaccine in 2 to 4-year-old children.

Shigella in many parts of the world have become increasingly resistant to antimicrobials including trimethoprim. Studies are under way with the use of quinolones other than nalidixic acid, but these agents would be quite costly in developing countries, and there is the risk that when the agents are used on such a large scale that resistance will develop as it has with other species. Although oral attenuated *Shigella* vaccines have been studied since the 1960s, the vaccines had required multiple doses and occasionally reverted to wild-type. Work has progressed on a *Shigella flexneri* vaccine, but there are no vaccines for the organism that causes the most severe disease *Shigella dysenteriae* 1 which rapidly spreads through communities and shows the greatest resistance to antimicrobials. There is an obvious need for further work on this problem.

Enterotoxigenic *Escherichia coli* have been treated with many antimicrobials, and recently studies show that any of the new oral fluoroquinolones are effective. In endemic areas protection is the result of IgA antibody against a variety of strains that have different antigens. Thus, for a vaccine approach to be successful, it would be necessary to deliver the correct antigens to the intestine. Perhaps if one could develop a way to deliver easily the fimbriae antigens that are involved in colonization, antibody would develop and be continually restimulated by the exposures that occur in the developing world. The magnitude of the problem of enterotoxigenic *Escherichia coli* for the less developed countries is that diarrhoea in infants and young children often requires hospitalization and more expensive rehydration measures that tax the health care system of these countries.

Typhoid vaccine will be discussed in this volume by Levine. There has been great improvement in the treatment of typhoid with antimicrobial agents such as the quinolones (DuPont 1989, Murray 1989). Although there is resistance to ampicillin and chloramphenicol in many parts of the world, antibiotics are not a pressing problem. The problem for vaccines is that a vaccine should confer immunity after ingestion of a single oral dose, should be well tolerated, and should not revert to a pathogenic strain in the wild. These are possible goals that can be achieved with the current genetic manipulations possible with bacteria.

SEXUALLY TRANSMITTED DISEASES

Although there appears to be a continued increase in resistance of *Neisseria gonorrhoeae* to penicillin and tetracycline, and *Haemophilus ducreyi* has been found with increasing frequency, there are excellent antibiotics to treat these organisms. *Chlamydia trachomatis*, however, still is a problem since single-dose therapy is not possible, and the patient population that acquires this infection often is poorly compliant to take medication for a week. Thus, it would be useful to have new agents for *Chlamydia* and in particular agents which could easily be administered to pregnant women.

Syphilis has once again become a serious problem in many parts of the world where 'crack' use is common and HIV infection prevalent. In Africa and large cities in the United States, there has been a major increase in this disease. Although *Treponema pallidum* remains susceptible to penicillin, other agents are needed, particularly those which achieve good cerebrospinal fluid concentrations. Preliminary studies of ceftriaxone are encouraging, but we need more information about other agents, and agents that could be used orally would be of benefit.

FOREIGN BODY INFECTIONS

Increasingly medicine, paediatrics, and surgery have come to rely upon the use of temporary or permanent foreign devices that are intravascular or extravascular. Infection of these devices is common and extremely difficult to eradicate (Dickinson & Bisno 1989a,b). There has been use of antibiotic prophylaxis to reduce the incidence of infections and improvement in the manner in which devices are placed by attention to methods of infection control. Research is needed into how prosthetic materials could be made with lower affinity for pathogens and how one might incorporate antimicrobial agents into materials without altering biocompatibility or selecting resistant bacteria in the tissue environment in which devices are placed. It would also be reasonable to develop agents which could be taken 'for life' to suppress the regrowth of organisms in patients with infected prostheses who were not suitable candidates for further surgery. This could be evaluated in animal models of infection.

MICROORGANISMS

In addition to the disease entities that have been enumerated, there are a number of problems that focus on specific microorganisms.

Staphylococcus aureus was a major pathogen in the 1940s and 1950s, but in the 1960s it was largely replaced by the aerobic Gram-negative bacilli. In the 1960s, methicillin-resistant isolates of *Staphylococcus aureus* (MRSA) were encountered in Europe but rarely were a problem in the United States. Unfortunately, beginning in the later part of the 1970s, MRSA began to appear in United States hospitals, and by the end of the 1980s they were often a major nosocomial pathogen (Lockley et al 1982, Horan et al 1986, Wakefield et al 1987). Once MRSA enter a hospital they are difficult to eradicate, and they may account for 5 to 50% of nosocomial infections. Therapy has been with vancomycin which has some relative toxicities compared with other agents used to treat susceptible staphylococci. MRSA are costly to a hospital, since the patients require more complicated isolation procedures, and it is also difficult to transfer patients out of the hospital to extended care facilities since these facilities do not wish to receive such patients. Indeed extended care facilities are a source of MRSA-colonized patients. There has been some success in eradicating carriage of MRSA by use of oral co-trimoxazole, rifampin, and topical bacitracin, and although nasal carriage has ceased, other sites are not eradicated and recolonization is common (Roccaforte et al 1988). Indeed in some areas resistance of MRSA to rifampin is very high. Oral fluoroquinolones have been used to treat MRSA and to eradicate carriage with success. Unfortunately there have been reports of increasing resistance of MRSA to fluoroquinolones (Schaeffer 1989, Shalit et al 1989). Thus we may be faced with an organism that will be resistant to all agents except glycopeptides and peptolides. Could MRSA become resistant to vancomycin? It is unknown, but the appearance of plasmid resistance to vancomycin in enterococci and resistance in *Staphylococcus haemolyticus* is a major concern (Leclercq et al 1988, Al-Obeid et al 1990).

Coagulase-negative staphylococci are now recognized as major pathogens in hospitalized patients. Although the most common isolate is *Staphylococcus epidermidis*, *Staphylococcus haemolyticus* has been of particular concern since it can be resistant not only to all β-lactams but to vancomycin, macrolides, lincinoids, and fluoroquinolones. As previously noted, there will be increased use of indwelling intravenous lines which are associated with coagulase-negative staphylococci (Dickinson & Bisno 1989a). Coagulase-negative staphylococci also have gradually had the MICs increase to both teicoplanin and vancomycin (Moore & Speller 1988, Goldstein et al 1990). It is conceivable that increased use of vancomycin for MRSA and *Clostridium difficile* will further elevate the MICs into the resistant category. Finally, it is conceivable that resistance to vancomycin could be transferred to MRSA from coagulase-negative staphylococci.

Whether the enterococcus is an organism of importance has been an area of controversy (Moellering 1990). There is no question that enterococci cause endocarditis, but there are few such infections given the frequency of other diseases. Nosocomial infections due to the enterococcus are increasing. But the major problem with the enterococcus is its general resistance to antimicrobial agents. Most importantly, enterococci have recently acquired resistance to a number of the agents used to treat infections due to these organisms. Enterococci became resistant to streptomycin in the 1970s, but gentamicin resistance was uncommon. Recently 25% of enterococci from NNIS hospitals referring isolates to the Centers for Disease Control had high-level resistance to gentamicin (Neu et al in press). This means that in those clinical situations in which synergy is necessary to achieve a clinical cure such as endocarditis or the rare meningitis patient cannot be treated. β-lactamases also have been found in enterococcus of a type similar to the β-lactamase of *Staphylococcus aureus* (Murray & Medereski-Samoraj 1983). Since this was reported in 1983, β-lactamase producing enterococci have been found in many states throughout the United States. In Europe there is the appearance of plasmid coded genes that produce a 39 kDa protein that makes *Enterococcus faecalis* and *Enterococcus faecium* resistant to vancomycin and teicoplanin (Leclercq et al 1988, Al-Obeid et al 1990). These latter organisms have been found in France, Spain, Great Britain, Germany, and recently in the United States.

It has been shown that enterococci can be spread in the hospital by hand contact as occurs with MRSA enteric species (Chenowith & Schaberg, 1990). Enterococci will continue to be present in the hospital environment since many of the antibiotics used to treat complicated infections, i.e. cephalosporins, cause an increase of enterococci in the intestine. Enterococci harbour conjugative transposons and can transfer in the absence of a mobilizing plasmid. Thus one is concerned that resistance from these organisms will be transferred to other species such as haemolytic streptococci and *Streptococcus pneumoniae* (Clewell 1990).

At the moment, *Streptococcus pyogenes* are highly susceptible to many antibiotics, β-lactams, macrolides, and glycopeptides. But I am concerned that with the widespread use of some of the macrolides there may be increased resistance to these agents. Resistance has been noted in the United Kingdom (Phillips et al 1990). This could be a problem of concern since there has been a resurgence of rheumatic fever in a number of areas of the United States, and rheumatic fever still is a major illness in developing countries.

Resistance of *Streptococcus pneumoniae* to penicillin is a major problem in some countries (Pallares et al 1987). Penicillin-resistant *Streptococcus pneumoniae* have recently been discovered in Hong Kong (Yuen et al 1990). Vancomycin can be used as treatment, and relatively penicillin-resistant isolates are susceptible to aminothiazolyl cephalosporins, but this could change.

The problem of bacterial resistance to β-lactams and fluoroquinolones will be reviewed in detail in this volume. However, there is concern about the increasing resistance of *Escherichia coli* to co-trimoxazole, of resistance of *Klebsiella* species to β-lactams due to the new plasmid β-lactamases which are derivatives of the TEM enzyme (Phillippon et al 1989). *Enterobacter cloacae* clearly is a major problem for resistance. Although carbapenems inhibit *Enterobacter* and surprisingly resistance has not been a problem for aminoglycosides nor for the fluoroquinolones, it would be extremely useful to have other agents to treat infections due to this organism which colonizes many hospital units. In 1986 to 1988 it was the fifth most commonly encountered species causing nosocomial infections in ICU patients and in surgical wounds (Horan et al 1988).

Pseudomonas aeruginosa is an organism of major importance for many areas of the hospital. In 1986-88 it was the third most common cause of nosocomial urinary infection, first cause of nosocomial pneumonia, eighth cause of bacteraemia—a fall from fifth in 1984, and fifth cause of nosocomial surgical wounds. *Pseudomonas aeruginosa* was the most common pathogen (13.4%) infecting ICU patients. *Pseudomonas* has the ability readily to become resistant to many antibiotics. Loss of the D-2 protein makes it resistant to the carbapenems and penems (Gotoh & Nishino 1990), aminoglycoside-modifying enzymes makes it resistant to aminoglycosides, and alteration of porins and hyperproduction of β-lactamase produce resistance to penicillins and cephalosporins. A major concern has been the increase in resistance of *Pseudomonas* to fluoroquinolones which is a combination of altered DNA gyrase and changed permeability. The aspects of resistance to β-lactams and to fluoroquinolones are reviewed elsewhere in this volume. Research on mechanisms of transport and on the structural and genetic aspects of the β-lactamases and fluoroquinolones may provide insights into ways to overcome the resistance.

Xanthomonas maltophilia until recently was considered a minor commensal organism which rarely caused serious infection. This organism is highly resistant to most β-lactams because of a β-lactamase that is not inhibited by any of the current agents or by β-lactamase inhibitors. It has caused serious respiratory infection in the ICU setting. It has also been a problem as a cause of nosocomial wound and urinary tract infections and even has contaminated fluids to produce bacteraemia. With the exception of co-trimoxazole, most antibiotics are of little effect, and the use of carbapenems in ICUs may select for this organism since it produces a β-lactamase that hydrolyses imipenem and meropenem. Study of the enzymatic activity of this agent and of the transport of agents within *Xanthomonas* may lead to advances in finding agents for this organism.

An organism which has been brought to the fore with the AIDS epidemic is *Mycobacterium avium* (Greene et al 1982), but this organism has increasingly been recognized as a cause of pulmonary infection in individuals with chronic lung disease (Prince et al 1989). Drug therapy for non-immunocompromised patients with pulmonary *Mycobacterium avium* infection has an overall cure rate of approximately 50% (Iseman et al 1985). There are no adequate drug programmes for *Mycobacterium avium*. Research on this organism may also provide agents to treat

Mycobacterium tuberculosis since this organism has not vanished and resistance to isoniazid in New York in some areas is at 14%, and there is increasing resistance to rifampin and the other antituberculosis agents. The problems of tuberculosis in third world countries as well as in HIV patients make it certain that many people will be exposed to drug-resistant *Mycobacterium tuberculosis*.

Among the anaerobic species, it is interesting that resistance to agents such as clindamycin has increased, some anaerobic species will hydrolyse the β-lactamase stable compounds, including carbapenems and penems, and even metronidazole resistance has been noted in *Bacteroides* and *Clostridium* species. These are not major problems but are examples that there is a continually changing ecology of microorganisms, and that bacteria are very resourceful in being able to develop ways to survive the latest antimicrobial agent.

I have left *Borrelia burgdorferi*—the cause of Lyme disease—to the last. This organism has become the most 'in' organism in the United States. Indeed as I am writing this manuscript, I am called by a physician to ask whether I believe it is safe for him to buy a home in a wooded area north of New York since he has small children and the area has deer, mice, and ticks. Lyme is not HIV; is not tuberculosis; is not staphylococcal sepsis. But Lyme as a disease is a problem, since its sequelae are arthritis, neurological disease, chronic skin disease, and rarely cardiac disease. The problems that will be discussed in this volume are that we still do not have good diagnostic tools to be certain of the diagnosis, and the optimal preventive and curative therapy is not established (Steere 1989). Until the issue of reliable diagnosis is solved, much of the data on therapy are suspect. Long-term studies to follow treated individuals are needed to establish the true incidence of arthritis and neurological sequaleae after treatment.

SUMMARY

I have provided many problems associated with bacterial infections. Some of these problems may not be amenable to solution. There are some factors that will impact on the solutions. It is not easy to develop new antimicrobial agents. A disease such as mycobacterial infection requires multiple agents, long-term therapy, and to be most useful for the world must be inexpensive. There is little financial incentive to develop such agents. The uncommon organisms that I mentioned may in the long-term be too infrequent to provide an adequate financial return for the investment required to see a drug through the arduous registration track that exists in the United States and will also exist, I suspect, in a united Europe. Thus I see that progress will be slow. Bacteria will continue to be extremely important causes of morbidity and mortality in developed as well as developing nations. Vaccines, antimicrobial agents, and ultimately immunomodulators such as interleukins, interferon, and colony-stimulating factors will be important in the efforts to improve our prevention and treatment of bacterial infections.

REFERENCES

Al-Obeid S, Collatz E, Gutmann L 1990 Mechanism of resistance to vancomycin in *Enterococcus faecium* D366 and *Enterococcus faecalis* A256. Antimicrobial Agents and Chemotherapy 34: 252-256

Blaser M J 1987 Gastric Campylobacter-like organisms, gastritis, and peptic ulcer disease. Gastroenterology 93: 371-383

Booth L, Holdstock G, MacBride H et al 1989 Clinical importance of *Campylobacter pyloridis* and associated IgG and IgA antibody responses in patients undergoing upper gastrointestinal endoscopy. Journal of Clinical Pathology 39: 215-219

Celis R, Torres A, Gatell J M et al 1988 Nosocomial pneumonia. A multivariate analysis of risk and prognosis. Chest 93: 318-324

Chenowith C, Schaberg D 1990 The epidemiology of enterococci. European Journal of Clinical Microbiology and Infectious Diseases 9: 80-89

Clemens J D, Sack D A, Harris J R et al 1990 Field trial of oral cholera vaccines in Bangladesh: results from long-term follow up. Lancet 335: 270-273

Clewell DB 1990 Moveable genetic elements and antibiotic resistance in enterococci. European Journal of Clinical Microbiology and Infectious Diseases 9: 90-102

Chamberlain CE, Peura DA 1990 *Campylobacter* (Helicobacter) pylori: is peptic disease a bacterial infection? Archives of Internal Medicine 150: 951-955

Craven D E, Kunches L M, Kilmsky V et al 1986 Risk factors for pneumonia in patients receiving continuous mechanism ventilation. American Review of Respiratory Diseases 133: 792-796

Daschner F, Kapstein I, Engels I et al 1988 Stress ulcer prophylaxis and ventilation pneumonia. Prevention by antibacterial cytoprotective agents. Infection Control 9: 59-65

Dickinson G M, Bisno A L 1989a Infections associated with indwelling devices: concepts of pathogenesis; infections associated with intravascular devices. Antimicrobial Agents and Chemotherapy 33: 597-601

Dickinson G M, Bisno A L 1989b Infections associated with indwelling devices: infections related to extravascular devices. Antimicrobial Agents and Chemotherapy 33: 602-607

Driks M R, Craven D E, Celii B R et al 1987 Nosocomial pneumonia in intubated patients given sucralfate as compared with antacids or histamine type 2 blockers. New England Journal of Medicine 317: 1376-1382

Drumm B, Perez-Perez G I, Blaser M J, Sherman P M 1990 Intrafamily clustering of *Helicobacter pylori* infection. New England Journal of Medicine 322: 359-363

DuPont H L 1989 Quinolone antimicrobial agents in the management of bacterial enteric infections. In: Wolfson J S, Hooper D C (eds) Quinolone antimicrobial agents. American Society of Microbiology, Washington, DC pp 167-176

Evans D J Jr, Evans D G, Graham D Y, Klein P D 1989 A sensitive and specific serologic test for detection of *Campylobacter pylori* infection. Gastroenterology 96: 1004-1008

Freeley T W, duMoulin G C, Hedley-Whyte J et al 1975 Aerosol polymyxin and pneumonia in seriously ill patients. New England Journal of Medicine 293: 471-475

Girgis N I, Farid Z, Mikhail I S et al 1989 Dexamethazone treatment for bacterial meningitis in children and adults. Pediatric Infectious Diseases Journal 8: 849-851

Goldstein F W, Coutrot A, Sieffer A, Acar J F 1990 Percentages and distribution of teicoplanin- and vancomycin-resistant strains among coagulase-negative staphylococci. Antimicrobial Agents and Chemotherapy 34: 899-900

Goodwin C S, Binslow E, Peterson G et al 1987 Enzyme-linked immunosorbent assay for *Campylobacter pyloridis*: correlation with presence of *C. pyloridis* in gastric mucosa. Journal of Infectious Diseases 155: 488-494

Gotoh N, Nishino T 1990 Decrease of the susceptibility to low molecular weight β-lactam antibiotics in imipenem-resistant *Pseudomonas aeruginosa* mutants: role of outer membrane protein D2 in their diffusion. Journal of Antimicrobial Chemotherapy 25: 191-198

Graham D Y, Klein P D, Opekum A R, Boutton T W 1988 Effect of age on the frequency of active *Campylobacter pylori* infection diagnosed by the [^{13}C] urea breath test in normal subjects and patients with peptic ulcer disease. Journal of Infectious Diseases 157: 777-780

Greene J B, Sidhu G S, Lewin S et al 1982 *Mycobacterium avium-intracellulare* a cause of disseminated life-threatening infection in homosexuals and drug abusers. Annals of Internal Medicine 97: 539-546

Gross P A, Neu H C, Aswapokee P et al 1980 Deaths from nosocomial infection. Experience in a university hospital and community hospital. American Journal of Medicine 68: 219-223

Horan T C, White J W, Jarvis W R et al 1986 Nosocomial infection surveillance-1984. MMWR Surveillance Summary 35: 17SS-29SS

Horan T, Culver D, Jarvis W et al 1988 Pathogens causing nosocomial infections: preliminary data from the National Nosocomial Infections Surveillance System. Antimicrobic Newsletter 5: 65-68

13

Iseman M D, Corpe R F, O'Brien R J et al 1985 Disease due to *Mycobacterium avium-intracellulare*. Chest 87 (Suppl 2): 139S-149S

Klein J O, Feigen R D, McCracken G H Jr 1986 Report of the task force on the diagnosis and management of meningitis. Pediatrics 78: 959-982

Laebel M H, Freij B J, Syroglannopoulos G A et al 1988 Dexamethasone therapy for bacterial meningitis: results of two double-blind, placebo-controlled trials. New England Journal of Medicine 3: 964-971

Leclercq R, Derlot E, Duval J, Courvalin P 1988 Plasmid-mediated resistance to vancomycin and teicoplanin in *Enterococcus faecium*. New England Journal of Medicine 319: 157-161

Ledingham I, Alcock S R A J, Eastway A T et al 1988 Triple regimen of selective decontamination of the digestive tract, systemic cefotaxime, and microbiological surveillance for prevention of acquired infection in intensive care. Lancet i: 785-790

Locksley R M, Cohen M L, Quinn T C et al 1982 Multiple antibiotic resistant *Staphylococcus aureus*: introduction, transmission, and evolution of nosocomial infection. Annals of Internal Medicine 97: 317-324

Marshall B J, Armstrong J A, McGechie D B, Glancy R J 1985 Attempt to fulfil Koch's postulates for pyloric Campylobacter. Medical Journal of Australia 142: 436-449

Meningitis Study Group 1987 Report of a workshop: Pathophysiology of bacterial meningitis—implications for new management strategies. Pediatric Infectious Diseases Journal 6: 1143-1171

Meningitis Study Group 1989 Report of a second workshop: Pathophysiology of bacterial meningitis. Pediatric Infectious Diseases Journal 8: 899-933

Moellering R C Jr 1990 The enterococci: an enigma and a continuing therapeutic challenge. European Journal of Clinical Microbiology and Infectious Diseases 9: 73-74

Moore E P, Speller D C E 1988 In vitro teicoplanin resistance in coagulase-negative staphylococci from patients with endocarditis and from a cardiac surgery unit. Journal of Antimicrobial Chemotherapy 21: 417-424

Morris B J, Nicholson G 1987 Ingestion of *Campylobacter pyloridis* causes gastritis and raised fasting gastric pH. American Journal of Gastroenterology 82: 192-199

Murray B E 1986 Resistance of Shigella, Salmonella, and other selected enteric pathogens to antimicrobial agents. Reviews of Infectious Diseases 8: Sl72-Sl81

Murray B E 1989 Quinolones and the gastrointestinal tract. European Journal of Clinical Microbiology and Infectious Diseases 8: 1093-1102

Murray B E, Medereski-Samoraj B D 1983 Transferable beta-lactamase: a new mechanism for in vitro penicillin resistance in *Streptococcus faecalis*. Journal of Clinical Investigation 72: 1168-1171

Neu H C, Thornsberry C, Martone W J in press Enterococci in the United States. Reviews of Infectious Diseases

Pallares R, Gudiol F, Linares et al 1987 Risk factors and response to antibiotic therapy in adults with bacteremic pneumonia caused by penicillin-resistant pneumococci. New England Journal of Medicine 317: 18-22

Phillippon A, Labia R, Jacoby G 1989 Extended-spectrum beta-lactamases. Antimicrobial Agents and Chemotherapy 33: 1131-1136

Phillips G, Parratt D, Orange G V et al 1990 Erythromycin resistant *Streptococcus pyogenes*. Journal of Antimicrobial Chemotherapy 25: 723

Prince D S, Peterson D D, Steiner R M et al 1989 Infection with *Mycobacterium avium* complex in patients without predisposing conditions. New England Journal of Medicine 321: 863-868

Rauws E A J, Langenberg W, Houthoff H J et al 1988 *Campylobacter pyloridis*-associated chronic active antral gastritis. Gastroenterology 94: 33-40

Roccaforte J S, Bittner M J, Stumpf C A et al 1988 Attempts to eradicate methicillin-resistant *Staphyloccus aureus* colonization with the use of trimethoprim-sulfamethoxazole, rifampin, and bacitracin. American Journal of Infection Control 16: 141-146

Shalit I, Bergez S A, Gorea A, Frimerman M 1989 Widespread quinolone-resistance among methicillin-resistant *Staphylococcus aureus* isolates in a general hospital. Antimicrobial Agents and Chemotherapy 33: 593-594

Schaefler S 1989 Methicillin-resistant strains of *Staphylococcus aureus* resistant to quinolones. Journal of Clinical Microbiology 27: 335-336

Scully B E, Nakatomi M, Ores C et al 1987 Ciprofloxacin therapy in cystic fibrosis. American Journal of Medicine 82(4A):196-201

Steere A C 1989 Lyme disease. New England Journal of Medicine 321: 586-596

Stoutenbeck C P, van Saene H K F, Miranda D R et al 1986 Nosocomial gram-negative pneumonia in critically ill patients. A 3 year experience with novel therapeutic regimens. Intensive Care Medicine 12: 419-423

Tauber M G 1989 Brain edema, intracranial pressure and cerebral flow in bacterial meningitis. Pediatric Infectious Diseases Journal 8: 15-17

Wakefield D S, Pfaller M, Massanari R M et al 1987 Variation in methicillin-resistant *Staphylococcus aureus* occurrence by geographic location and hospital characteristics. Infection Control 8: 151-157

Yuen K Y, Sato W H, Hai Wt, Chau P Y 1990 Multiresistant *Streptococcus pneumoniae* in Hong Kong. Journal of Antimicrobial Chemotherapy 25: 721-722

Section I:
Borrelia

Chairman: P. K. Peterson

2. THE EPIDEMIOLOGY OF *Borrelia burgdorferi* INFECTIONS

G. Stanek

INTRODUCTION

Lyme borreliosis (or Lyme disease) may be designated as a systemic infectious disease which is caused by the bacterium *Borrelia burgdorferi*. During the course of the infection, disorders of the skin, the nervous system, the muscles, joints, the heart and other internal organs may manifest solely or simultaneously.

At least part of the Lyme borreliosis spectrum, e.g. erythema chronicum migrans (ECM) (Lipschütz 1913), acrodermatitis chronica atrophicans (Buchwald 1883), lymphadenosis benigna cutis (Bäferstedt 1943) and meningopolyneuritis Garin-Bujadoux-Bannwarth (MPN) (Garin & Bujadoux 1922, Bannwarth 1944) has been known in Europe for many decades although demonstration of the causative agent was made in only 1982.

In the USA, the observation of a clustering of cases of arthritis in children in 1975 led to the description of Lyme arthritis (Steere et al 1977). Subsequently, a disease complex was recognized which developed after a tick bite and manifests with an erythema migrans, constitutional symptoms, neurological disorders, arthralgias or frank arthritis. This enlarged spectrum was named Lyme disease (Steere et al 1977, Reik et al 1979). The discovery of spirochetal organisms in ixodid ticks (Burgdorfer et al 1982) and the cultivation of such spirochetes from blood (Benach et al 1983), and from skin lesions and cerebrospinal fluid (csf) of patients with Lyme disease (Steere et al 1983), substantiated the spirochetal aetiology of the multisystem disorder. In 1984 the spirochete was identified as a new borrelia species and named *Borrelia burgdorferi* (Johnson et al 1984), and following the 2nd International Symposium on Lyme disease and related disorders (Vienna 1985), the term Lyme borreliosis was agreed as a more specific term for this disease complex.

The aim of any epidemiological consideration of Lyme borreliosis is to describe the frequency of the disease with respect to its causative agent. This includes questions of the infection source, the infection route, and its target. All sites of existence of the causative agent are designated the infection-source, while the route includes any possibility of the agent spreading to its infection target, a susceptible human being.

Table 2.1

Typing system for *Borrelia burgdorferi* based on the reaction with the monoclonal antibodies H5332 and H3TS, which are directed against the OspA protein.

H5332	H3TS	Type
+	+	I
+	−	II
−	−	III

INFECTION SOURCE

European borrelia isolates differ from US isolates in molecular weights of major proteins and in reactivity with monoclonal antibodies raised against the outer surface proteins of *Borrelia burgdorferi* type strain B31. In addition, heterogeneity of European isolates has been described (Stanek et al 1985a, Wilske et al 1985). A typing system based on reactivity with monoclonal antibodies (H5332 and H3TS) to the outer surface protein (OspA) has been suggested (Barbour 1984) which allows differentiation of three types. Interestingly, North American isolates belong almost exclusively to type I, whereas European isolates belong to types I to III (Table 2.1). Although some degree of geographical distribution of types was apparent in Europe (Stanek et al 1990), there is currently no available technique to differentiate between pathogenic and non-pathogenic strains. In addition, nothing is known of the relationship between *B. burgdorferi* 'types' and their clinical manifestations.

In the USA, many different mammals, birds (Anderson 1989) and even reptiles (Lane 1989) have been recognized as reservoir hosts for *B. burgdorferi*. In the north east of the USA, the white-footed mouse and the white-tailed deer were found to be the most important reservoirs. However, in Europe no detailed studies have been undertaken so far on this aspect.

Borrelia multiply in the mid-gut of ticks engorged during attachment to their host, and are also found in the haemolymph and salivary glands of ticks (Monin et al 1989). Trans-stadial and trans-ovarial transmission of borrelia may also occur while the ticks themselves may also act as a borrelia reservoir (Stanek et al 1986a, Monin et al 1989).

INFECTION ROUTES

Vectors of *B. burgdorferi* include hard ticks of the genus *Ixodes* and other haemato-phagous arthropods. Most recently, soft ticks of the genus *Argas* (Stanek et al 1989a) were considered as vectors. Although the latter were identified as vectors in single cases, there is little known about their modes of ingestion, maintenance and, finally, their importance in transmitting the spirochetes (Krampitz et al 1989).

The tick species *Ixodes ricinus* is the most frequent vector among Eurasian ixodid ticks. This species occurs in an area covering south Scandinavia, the British Isles, central Europe, France, Spain, Portugal, Italy, the Balkans to the Caspian Sea and northern Iran (Fig. 2.1). Within this area are distinct geographic regions wherein ixodid ticks are additionally infected with the tick-borne encephalitis (TBE) virus. To the east, in Asian Russia, China and Japan, the species *I. persulcatus* is found while

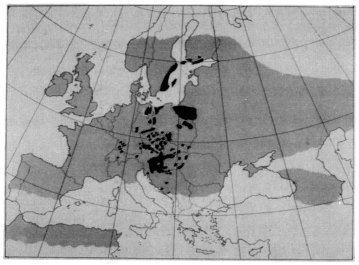

Figure 2.1
Distribution of the tick *Ixodes ricinus* in Europe (areas in dark grey). Black spots mark geographical areas where this tick is additionally infected with the tick-borne-encephalitis virus

in the USA, *I. dammini, I. scapularis* and *I. pacificus* populate the eastern and western states respectively (Anderson 1989, Burgdorfer 1989, Chenxu et al 1988, Kawabata et al 1987).

Frequency of infected tick populations
The frequency of ticks infected with *B. burgdorferi* has been studied in several European countries, including Austria, Czechoslovakia, southern Germany and Switzerland. Compared to the TBE virus, the frequency of borrelia-infected ticks is very high. In areas endemic for TBE, one tick in every thousand carries the virus, with 20% being infected with borrelia in natural habitat. A study from Bavaria shows that infection occurs more frequently in adult ticks (Wilske et al 1987). In Switzerland and Austria, infection rates are about 20%. (Table 2.2) (Aeschlimann et al 1986, Radda et al 1986). A recent study from the USSR showed average infection rates to be 34% (Korenberg et al 1989).

With the introduction of PCR for detecting the spirochete, values for borrelia infected ticks will probably change; for example, in parts of southern England, 60-80% of ixodid ticks have been seen as infected (Guy, personal communication).

Transmission of borrelia from ticks to humans is of the cyclic type. In contrast, tabanid flies or other haematophagous insects transmit the bacteria acyclically, in attempting to obtain an uninterrupted blood supply from their hosts.

Table 2.2 Percentage of *Ixodes*-ticks of Europe infected with *Borrelia burgdorferi*

Country	Mean	Range
Czechoslovakia (1985)	8.0	(3.0—20.0)
Austria (east) (1985)	20.0	(2.2—40.0)
Switzerland (1985)	20.0	(5.0—34.0)
FRG (Bavaria) (1987)	13.6	(0.0—33.8)
Czechoslovakia (1990)	20.0	(3.8—35.9)
Lithuania (Bunikis 1990)	27.0	(14.2—40.2)

Contact infection

Transmission of *B. burgdorferi* by contact infection has recently been described (Rockstroh et al 1989), in which erythema chronicum migrans developed from a scratch wound contaminated 5 days previously with manure. Examination of the manure by darkfield microscopy and silver staining revealed spirochetes, thus suggesting that *B. burgdorferi* might be transmitted by contact infection and perhaps also live outside an animal host.

The question of whether Lyme borreliosis can be transmitted by sexual contact has frequently been asked, but not yet answered.

TARGETS OF INFECTION

Lyme borreliosis in humans was reported as a systemic infection and divided into three stages by Steere et al (1986). More recently, Steere (1989) proposed a modified concept distinguishing between disseminated and chronic manifestations. From a clinical viewpoint, manifestations are either self-limited or chronic (Table 2.3). If not treated with antibiotics, some cases of erythema chronicum migrans may last for several months, but finally regress spontaneously. *B. burgdorferi* was cultivated repeatedly from skin biopsies of patients with erythema migrans and acrodermatitis, from csf and blood (Benach et al 1983, Preac-Mursic 1986, Stanek et al 1985). Single reports of spirochete isolation from a lymphocytoma (Asbrink 1989) and from an endomyocardial biopsy of a patient with longstanding cardiomyopathy (Stanek et al 1990) have been made. Other reported isolations were either in conjunction with erythema, or where patients had a history of a skin rash or a tick-bite and showed serum or csf antibodies to *B. burgdorferi*.

Table 2.3 Clinical manifestations of Lyme borreliosis arranged according to self-limited and chronic disorders

Organ systems	MANIFESTATIONS Self-limited	Chronic
Skin	Erythema chronicum migrans*, Borrelia lymphocytoma* Multiple anular erythema*, Urticaria	Acrodermatitis chronica atrophicans*, (circumscribed scleroderma)
Nervous system	Meningopolyneuritis* Garin-Bujadoux-Bannwarth, Meningitis*, Meningoencephalitis	Progressive meningoencephalitis, chronic myelitis, Peripheral neuropathies
Joints	Arthralgias, Brief attacks of arthritis	Intermittent oligo-arthritis, Symmetric polyarthritis, Chronic arthritis
Muscles	Myalgia, myositis	
Heart	Conduction disorders, Myopericarditis, pancarditis	Cardiomyopathy*
Eyes	Conjunctivitis, Iritis, panophthalmitis	
Respiratory tract	Pharyngitis, tracheobronchitis	
Liver	Acute hepatitis (SGOT)	
Lymphatic system	Regional or generalized lymphadenopathy	
Kidney	Microhaematuria, microproteinuria	

*Currently, *Borrelia burgdorferi* has been cultivated repeatedly from skin biopsies, blood, cerebrospinal fluid and singularly from endomyocardial biopsy.

Table 2.4 Age and sex distribution of patients with Lyme borreliosis in Austria*

Disorder	n	Age (years)		Sex ratio M/F
		Median	Range	
Arthritis	50	31	7—81	0.90
Erythema migrans	560	43	1—89	0.56
Meningopolyneuritis	720	45	1—83	1.09
Acrodermatitis	160	65	16—85	0.54
Carditis	13	56	37—71	13.0

*Registered at the Hygiene Institute of the University of Vienna (October 1984 to July 1985)

Age/sex characteristics
Lyme borreliosis occurs in both sexes and in all age groups. Data from Austria show skin manifestations to occur more in females, while neurological disorders occur more frequently in males (Table 2.4).

In terms of age distribution, acrodermatitis chronica atrophicans and joint manifestations peak at the ages of 65 and 30-50 years respectively (Stanek 1988). Other manifestations such as erythema migrans or meningopolyneuritis appear in all age groups.

Seasonal variations
A clear seasonal variation is seen in erythema migrans, which peaks in July (Fig. 2.2). Neurological cases also exhibit seasonal variations. In the period 1984 to 1986, peaks occurred in autumn, though in the period 1987-1988 (presumably due to an increased knowledge of Lyme borreliosis among physicians), minimal seasonal variation occurs in cases of neuroborreliosis registered.

Risk groups
Several studies are available on risk groups. An example is that of forestry workers who are regularly exposed to tick bites. Studies from Bavaria (Münchhoff et al 1986), Czechoslovakia (Pejcoch et al 1989) and England (Guy et al 1989) each refer to forestry workers who have never been ill with Lyme borreliosis, yet showed a

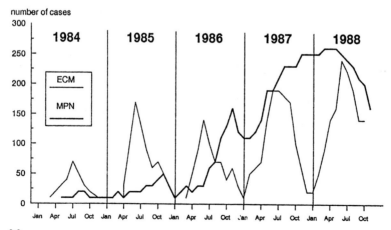

Figure 2.2
Seasonal distribution of cases of erythema migrans (ECM) and neurological manifestations (MPN) of Lyme borreliosis in Austria from 1984 to 1986

seropositive response of 14 to 48%. Whether these antibodies identify a latent infection is a matter of speculation.

Eestablishing and index of manifestation

How to establish an index of manifestation by studying persons exposed to the vectors of borreliosis remains a problem. A prospective study was performed in Austrian army recruits who were on outside duties for 3 months. Recruits were instructed to show each tick bite to the doctor, who immediately took a first blood sample. A subsequent sample was taken 6 weeks later and the recruit examined clinically. ECM was diagnosed in 4%; seroconversion was observed in 22% (Schmutzhard et al 1988). A similar study in a children's holiday camp indicated ECM in 2% and seroconversion in 13% (Paul et al 1989).

Lyme borreliosis is an endemic disease. Early studies of the condition showed that it occurs everywhere that ixodid ticks are living. In Europe, reports date back to the 1960s and early 1970s regarding the distribution of clinical features that today are recognized and proven. Interestingly, erythema migrans, lymphocytoma, acrodermatitis chronica atrophicans and meningopolyneuritis cases were considered as arbovirus infections (Müller & Schaltenbrand 1973), there being an awareness of the widespread distribution of some of the disorders, for example acrodermatitis and related neuropathies. In the light of the newly discovered agent, the former observations were confirmed and the clinical spectrum of disorders extended.

GEOGRAPHICAL CONSIDERATIONS

At the 2nd International Symposium on Lyme disease and related disorders (Vienna 1985) (Stanek et al 1986b) it became evident that Lyme disease is a health problem of the entire northern hemisphere. In Switzerland, the risk of becoming infected by ticks was shown to be limited by an altitude of approximately 1200 metres above sea level, a region where ticks do not exist (Fig. 2.3) (Aeschlimann et al 1986).

An update of Lyme borreliosis in 1987 revealed that the condition may also be present in regions of central and southern Africa (Stanek et al 1989b), while a recent

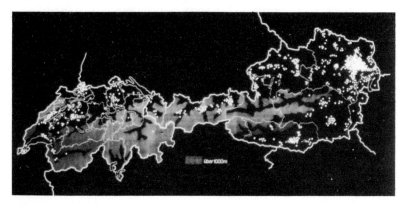

Figure 2.3
Erythema migrans cases in Switzerland and Austria according to the location of infection (Data obtained in 1985).

Table 2.5 Cases of *Borrelia burgdorferi* infections in Austria* in 1984

Disorder	Number patients	Percentage
Erythema migrans	273	70.1
Meningopolyneuritis	78	20.2
Acrodermatitis	28	7.1
Arthritis	7	1.8
Borrelia lymphpoytoma	3	0.8
Total	389	100.0

*Registered at the Hygiene Institute, University of Vienna

study from Russia describes a vast increase in areas populated by infected ticks which extended from European to Asian Russia, and to the Pacific coast (Dekonenko 1988, Korenberg 1988). Since the introduction of commercial tests in the serodiagnosis of Lyme borreliosis, accurate figures of the numbers of cases are difficult to obtain in any given country. The problem is two-fold: first, there is no organised reporting system; second, there is no widely-accepted case definition available.

Although there is a steady increase in the numbers of cases recorded, the distribution frequency of the various clinical manifestations appears almost constant. In 1984, 389 cases were identified in Austria (Table 2.5). Erythema migrans was seen most frequently, followed by meningopolyneuritis and acrodermatitis. Few cases of arthritis and borrelia lymphocytoma were reported. In 1985, we registered 1970 cases, an increase of over 400%. Erythema migrans and meningopolyneuritis were again the most frequently observed conditions (Table 2.6). In Slovenia, northern Yugoslavia, a 10-fold increase of registered cases was reported within a 3-year period (Table 2.7) (Strle et al 1990).

Figure 2.4 illustrates the increase in numbers of reported cases during 6 years in Austria and over 7 years in the USA. (USA figures were obtained from MMWR). The exponential increase may in fact be artefactual, due to an increased awareness by doctors and patients to recognize borrelia infections.

Table 2.6 Cases of *Borrelia burgerdorferi* infections in Austria* in 1985

Disorder	Number patients	Total	%
Skin manifestations		1,194	60.6
Erythema migrans	985		
Acrodermatitis	166		
Borrelia lymphocytoma	43		
Neurological manifestations		742	37.7
Meningopolyneuritis	218		
Polyradiculitis	192		
Meningitis	172		
Neuropathies	73		
Cranial nerve paresis	58		
Myelitis	28		
Joint manifestations		26	1.3
Arthritis	20		
Arthralgia	6		
Cardiological disorders		6	0.3
Myocarditis	6		
Other		2	0.1
Acute hepatitis	2		
Total		1,970	100.0

*Registered at the Hygiene Institute, University of Vienna

Number of Cases

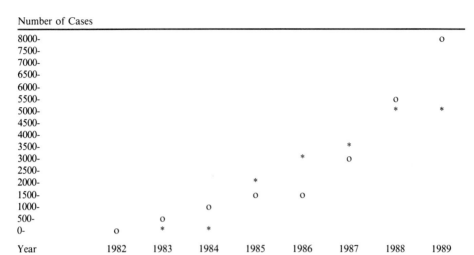

Fig. 2.4   Reported cases of Lyme borreliosis (o United States, 1982-1989, * Austria, 1983-1989)

In Austria, since 1988, 4000 to 5000 cases of Lyme borreliosis are registered each year. The annual incidence of Lyme borreliosis in central Europe is estimated as 0.1% of the total population. In the USA, Lyme borreliosis appears to have a focal distribution (Fig 2.5), the focality being first described in Connecticut, where communities separated by a river had vastly different incidences of disease.

There are very few complete, population-based studies on Lyme borreliosis. The incidence in New York was reported as being 11/100 000 (Birkhead et al 1990), though extrapolating this figure to the entire state population is misleading, since the disease is confined to a small area in the south (Smith et al 1988). In the endemic areas, therefore, the figure is much higher and similar to that in central Europe.

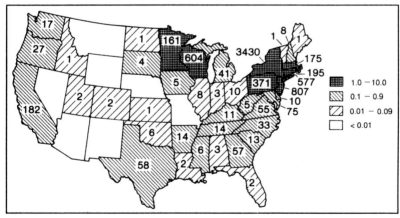

Figure 2.5 Number and average annual incidence rates of reported Lyme disease cases, per 100 000 population—United States, 1987-1988*

*Data for Oregon and California are for 1987 only.

Table 2.7 Lyme borreliosis in Slovenia: 1985-1988

Clinical manifestations	1985	1986	1987	1988	1985-88
Skin:—erythema migrans	4	138	189	517	848
—lymphocytoma		2	2	14	18
—ACA, scleroderma circ.			4	11	25	40
Neurologic:—early	6	84	104	134	328
—late		4	10	45	59
Cardiac (severe)		2	2	3	7
Joints		1	22	139	162
Others		10	21	99	130
Number of patients with LB	10	245	361	976	1592

CONCLUSIONS

Lyme borreliosis is recognized increasingly by doctors and serodiagnostic laboratories in Europe, the USA, and in other parts of the world. However, it is currently difficult to present conclusive epidemiological data. There are no widely-accepted case definitions for the very many clinical features that are due to, or reputed to be of, borrelial origin.

Clinical diagnosis of suggested cases of Lyme borreliosis requires confirmation by the demonstration of the aetiological agent and, moreover, by the demonstration of its causative role in the respective disorder.

Epidemiology of Lyme borreliosis cannot rely on serological results. Thus, the true incidence and prevalence of the condition cannot be determined before there are measures available which identify an actual infection.

REFERENCES

Aeschlimann A, Chamot E, Gigon F, Jeanneret J-P, Kesseler D, Walter Ch 1986 *B.burgdorferi* in Switzerland. Zentralblatt fur Bakteriologie, Mikrobiologie und Hygiene A263:450-458
Anderson J F 1989 Epizootiology of borrelia in ixodes tick vectors and reservoir hosts. Reviews of Infectious Diseases (Suppl 6): 1451-1459
Asbrink E 1989 Lymphadenosis benigna cutis solitaria—borrelia lymphocytoma in Sweden. Zentralblatt fur Bakteriologie (Suppl 19): 156-163
Bannwarth A 1944 Zur klinik und pathogenese der chronischen lymphozytären meningitis. Arch Psychiatr Nervenkr 117: 161
Barbour A G, Tessier S L, Hayes S F 1984 Variations in major surface proteins of Lyme disease spirochetes. Infection and Immunity 45: 94-100
Bäferstedt B 1943 Über Lymphadenosis benigna cutis. Eine klinische und pathologisch-anatomische Studie. PA Nordstedt & Söhne, Stockholm
Benach J L, Bosler E M, Hanrahan J P, et al 1983 Spirochetes isolated from the blood of two patients with Lyme disease. New England Journal of Medicine 308: 740-742
Birkhead G, Meldrum S, Heimberger T, Morse D 1990 Assessment of the completeness of Lyme disease surveillance reports using hospital records. IVth International Conference on Lyme Borreliosis, Stockholm
Buchwald A 1883 Ein Fall von diffuser idiopathischer hautatrophie. Arch Dermatol Syph 10: 553-556
Burgdorfer W, Barbour A G, Hayes S F, Benach J L, Grunwaldt E, Davis J P 1982 Lyme disease—a tick-borne spirochetosis? Science 216: 1317-1319
Burgdorfer W 1989 Borrelia burdorferi; its relationship to tick vectors. Zbl Bakt Suppl 18: 8-13
Chenxu A, W Yuxin, Z Yongguo et al 1988 Clinical manifestations and epidemiological characteristics of Lyme disease in Hailin county, Heilongjiang province, China. Ann NY Acad Scie 539: 302-313
Deknenko E P, Steere A C, Berardi V P, Kravchuk L N 1988 Lyme borreliosis in the Soviet Union. Journal of Infectious Diseases 158: 748-753
Garin C H, Bujadoux C H 1922 Paralysie par les tiques. Journale de Medecine de Lyon 71: 765-767
Guy E C, Martyn C N, Bateman D E, Heckels J E, Lawton N F 1989 Lyme disease prevalence and clinical importance of *Borrelia burgdorferi* specific IgG in forestry workers. Lancet i: 484-485

Johnson R C, Schmid G P, Hyde F W et al 1984 Borrelia burgdorferi sp.nov.: etiologic agent of Lyme disease. International Journal of Systemic Bacteriology 34: 496-497

Kawabata M, Baba S, K Iguchi et al 1987 Lyme disease in Japan and its possible transmitter the tick *Ixodes persulcatus*. J Infect Dis 156: 854

Korenberg I, Kovalevsky Y, Kovalevsky V et al 1988 Identifiication and primary results of treatment for the Lyme disease in the north-west of the USSR. Medical Parasitology 1: 45-48

Krampitz H E, S Bark 1989 Patterns of seasonal variation in the infestation of roe deer, *Capreolus capreolus* L. with borrelia infected *Ixodes ricinus* in northern Bavaria/ Zbl BaktSuppl 18: 21-25

Lane R, Lavoie P 1990 Lyme Borreliosis in California. Annals of the New York Academy of Science 539: 192-203

Lipschütz B 1913 Über eine seltene Erythemform (Erythema chronicum migrans). Arch Dermatol Syph 118: 349-356

MMWR 1989 Lyme Disease—United States, 1987 and 1988. MMWR 38 No 39: 668-672

Monin R, Gern L, Aeschlimann A 1989 A study of the different modes of transmission of *Borrelia burgdorferi* by *Ixodes ricinus*. Zentralblatt fur Bakteriologie (Suppl 18): 14-20

Müller WK, Schaltenbrand G (eds) 1973 Arboviruserkrankungen des Nervensystems in Europa. G Thieme Verlag, Stuttgart

Münchhoff P, Wilske B, Preac-Mursic V, Schierz G 1986 Antibodies against *Borrelia burgdorferi* in Bavarian forest workers. Zentralblatt für Bakteriologie, Mik robiologie und Hygiene A 263: 412-419

Paul H, Ackermann R, Gerth H J 1989 Infection and manifestation rate of European Lyme borreliosis in humans. Zentralblatt für Bakteriologie (Suppl 18): 44-49

Pejcoch M, Kralikova Z, Strnad P, Stanek G 1989 Prevalence of antibodies against *Borrelia burgdorferi* in forestry workers of south Moravia. Zentralblatt fur Bakteriologie (Suppl 18): 317-320

Preac-Mursic V, Wilske B, Schierz G 1986 European *Borrelia burgdorfen* isolated from humans and ticks. Zbl Bakt HygA: 112-18

Radda A, Burger I, Stanek G, Wewalka G 1986 Austrian hard ticks as vectors of *Borrelia burgdorferi*, overview. Zentalblatt fur Bakteriologie, Mikrobiologie und Hygiene A 263: 79-82

Reik L, Steere A C, Bartenhagen N H, Shope R E, Malawista S E 1979 Neurologic abnormalities of Lyme disease. Medicine 58: 281-294

Rockstroh T, Mochmann H P, Stanek G 1989 Lyme borreliosis by contact infection. Zentralblatt für Bakteriologie (Suppl 18): 40-41

Schmutzhard E, Stanek G, Pletschette M, et al 1988 Infections after tickbites. Tick-borne encephalitis and Lyme borreliosis—a prospective epidemiological study from Tyrol. Infection 16: 269-272

Smith P F, Benach J L, White D J, Stroup D F, Morse D L 1988 Occupational risk of Lyme disease in endemic areas of New York State. Ann NY Acad Scie 539: 289-301

Stanek G, Wewalka G, Groh V, Neumann R, Kristogeritisch W 1985a Differences between Lyme disease and European arthropod-borne infections. Lancet i 905-906

Stanek G, Wewalka G, Groh V, Neumann R 1985b Isolation of spirochetes from the skin of patients with erythema chronicum migrans in Austria. Zeutrallblatt für Baketeriologie, Mikrobiologie und Hygiene. A 260: 88-90

Stanek G, Burger I, Hirschl A et al 1986a Borrelia transfer by ticks during their life cycle. Zentralblatt für Bakteriologie Mikrobiologie und Hygiene A 263: 29-33

Stanek G, Flamm H, Barbour A G, Burgdorfer W (eds) 1986b Lyme Borreliosis. Gustav Fischer Verlag Stuttgart New York Zentralblatt für Bakteriologie, Mikrobiologie und Hygiene A 263

Stanek G, Pletschette M, Flamm H, et al 1988 European Lyme borreliosis. Annals of the New York Academy of Science 539: 274-282

Stanek G, Simeoni J 1989a Are pigeons' ticks transmitters of *Borrelia burgdorferi* to humans? A preliminary report. Zentralblatt fur Bakteriologie (Suppl 18): 42-43

Stanek G, Prinz A, Wewalka G, Hirschl A M, Kewbela-Ilunga 1989b Lyme borreliosis in central Africa. Zentralblatt fur Bakteriologie (Suppl 18): 77-81

Stanek G, Jurowitsch B, Köchl C, Burger I, Khanakha G 1990 Reactivity of European and American isolates of *Borrelia burgdorferi* with different monoclonal antibodies by means of a microimmunoblot technique. Zentralblatt fur Bakteriologie 278: 426-436

Stanek G, Klein J, Bittner R, Glogar D 1990 Isolation of *Borrelia burgdorferi* from the myocardium of patient with longstanding cardiomyopathy. New England Journal of Medicine 322: 249-252

Steere A C, Malawista S E, Snydman D R, et al 1977 Lyme athritis: an epidemic of oligoarticular arthritis in children and adults in three Connecticut communities. Arthritis and Rheumatism 20: 7-17

Steere A C, Grodzicki R L, Kornblatt A N et al 1983 The spirochetal etiology of Lyme disease. New England Journal of Medicine 308: 733-740

Steere A C, Bartenhagen N H, Craft J E, et al 1986 Clinical manifestations of Lyme disease. Zentralblatt fur Bakteriologie, Mikrobiologie und Hygiene A 263: 201-205

Steere A C 1989 Lyme disease. New England Journal of Medicine 321: 586-596

Strle F, Pejovnik-Pustinek A, Stanek G, Pleterski D, Rakar R 1989 Lyme Borreliosis in Slovenia in 1986. Zentralblatt fur Bakteriologie (Suppl 18): 50-54

Strle F, Cimperman J, Pejovnik A, Stanek G, Pleterski D, Jereb M, Ruzik E 1990 Lyme borreliosis in Slovenia: 1985-1988. IVth International Conference on Lyme Borreliosis, Stockholm

Wilske B, Preac-Mursic V, Schierz G 1985 Antigenic heterogeneity of European *Borelia burgdorferi* strains. Lancet i: 1099

Wilske B, Preac-Mursic V, Schierz G, Kühbeck R, Barbour A C, Kramer M 1988 Antigenic variability of *Borrelia burgdorferi*. Annals of the New York Academy of Science 539: 126-143

Discussion of paper presented by G. Stanek

Discussed by N. Barret
Reported by P. K. Peterson

The presentation by Stanek posed a number of pertinent questions regarding the epidemiology of Lyme borreliosis which I would like to reiterate. I would also like to raise several additional questions for consideration.

We should perhaps start with the question of case definition of Lyme disease. Can a diagnosis of Lyme disease be made purely on clinical grounds? This question will undoubtedly be addressed in Wilske's presentation of serological diagnosis of this infection. While Stanek showed a table containing a long list of clinical manifestations used in the case definition of Lyme disease, I am sure he would be the first to argue that this list is not exhaustive. Are the clinical manifestations similar in Europe and America? Initial reports seemed to indicate that the American disease differed from the European disease, but more recently, some case reviews of Lyme disease would seem to dispute this and indicate that there are more similarities on a clinical basis than were originally thought.

Stanek also pointed out the various animal reservoirs of infection—wild animals and domestic animals. But have all the animal reservoirs been identified and how important is each in any area? Also, the vectors of the infection have been discussed and the geographic areas harbouring the known vectors have been mapped out. How much bigger can these areas get?

We all know that treatment of Lyme borreliosis is generally successful. The infection is fairly amenable to treatment, but early diagnosis is obviously of prime importance. The prevention of infection also should be relatively simple, but who do we advise against the risks of infection?

To discuss the prevention of infection we must look at the risk factors. What are they? Should we be advising people not to go to, or to take precautions in, areas where the tick vectors or animal reservoirs are prevalent? Or should we be concerned primarily about areas where the ticks are known to be infected, or areas reporting endemic Lyme disease?

Finally, what about the incidence rates provided by Stanek? I return to my first question about case definition. If the diagnosis is inaccurate, or is being overlooked in certain areas, it is difficult to know if these figures are accurate. In Great Britain, we have been looking at the epidemiology in various ways. Epidemiology has been carried out with serological studies of Lyme disease; there have also been studies of erythema migrans reported by dermatologists. Currently, there is a study in progress looking at both the positive and negative serologies along with the clinical features to try to answer this question about Lyme disease.

In truth, we do not really know enough about the complete epidemiology of Lyme borreliosis. Although there might now be an epidemic of investigation in this field, I am not at all sure that this is a bad thing, since there are so many unanswered questions. As has been suggested recently, if it were not for AIDS, would not Lyme disease be described the 'new universal epidemic'?

3. Lyme borreliosis: host-parasite interactions, vaccines and antimicrobials

R. C. Johnson

INTRODUCTION

Currently, Lyme borreliosis is probably the leading vector-borne bacterial disease in the world. The aetiologic agent of this disease, *Borrelia burgdorferi*, is transmitted by the globally distributed ixodid ticks of the genus *Ixodes*. The spirochete is transferred to the host via infectious saliva of the feeding tick. Dissemination of the highly invasive spirochetes through the blood and lymph occurs early in the disease and acute abnormalities can develop in one or more of the major organ systems. The clinical manifestations of the disease are primarily observed in the skin, nervous system, heart, and joints. In addition to the acute form of the illness, a chronic disseminated infection may develop that can persist for years. Both the early and late manifestations of Lyme borreliosis can be correlated with the presence of low numbers of living spirochetes. Although patients appear to develop resistance to reinfection, this immunity may be *B. burgdorferi* strain specific. Clinical studies suggest that most patients respond satisfactorily to antimicrobial therapy, particularly if initiated early in the disease. However, long-term follow-up studies for determining the adequacy of treatment are needed. Evaluation of treatment for Lyme borreliosis is problematic because of the spirochete's latency and the intermittent pattern of exacerbations and remissions in the natural history of untreated infections. The lack of a laboratory test to judge treatment efficacy of Lyme borreliosis adds to the difficulties in the assessment of therapy for this disease. Presently the best measure for reducing the risk of contracting Lyme borreliosis is by personal protection measures such as the use of repellents, wearing protective clothing, and prompt removal of attached ticks. Controlling ticks over large areas by chemical, environmental, or biological methods has generally been ineffective or environmentally unacceptable. One of the most effective methods for preventing microbial diseases is by immunization. Vaccination of individuals and domestic animals at risk for contracting Lyme borreliosis could greatly reduce the morbidity associated with this spirochetosis. In this paper, the possible mechanisms of pathogenicity, appoaches for therapy, and the analysis of the immune response and the potential for a vaccine for Lyme borreliosis are addressed.

THE AETIOLOGIC AGENT

Borrelia burgdorferi is a slender (0.2-0.25 μm $\times$ 8-30 μm) helical bacterium that shares the same basic ultrastructural features present in other spirochetes. These features include a very fluid outer membrane that encloses the protoplasmic cylinder and 7 to 11 periplasmic flagella inserted subterminally and bipolarly in the protoplasmic cylinder. The outer membrane consists of 42% protein, 50% lipid and 4% carbohydrate (Coleman et al 1986). More than 100 polypeptides are present in the organism (Gill & Johnson in preparation) and several of these, such as polypeptides of apparent molecular weights of 31 and 34 kDa (Barbour et al 1983), and 22 kDa (Wilske et al 1986), are considered to be species specific. In contrast, the flagellin subunit of approximately 41 kDa, which is the first antigen recognized in patients, has significant amino acid homology with the flagellins of other spirochetes (Coleman & Benach 1989). The DNA organization of *B. burgdorferi* and other borreliae appears to be unique among the spirochetes and perhaps other bacteria as well. *Borrelia* were found to contain plasmids (Hyde & Johnson 1984). In addition to supercoiled plasmids, the borreliae contain linear plasmids, a form of DNA thought to be unique to eukaryotes (Barbour & Garon 1987, Plasterk et al 1985). As a result of in vitro cultivation, *Borrelia burgdorferi* will lose plasmids (Barbour 1988) as well as infectivity for hamsters (Johnson et al 1984a). Schwan et al (1988) observed that a recent tick isolate of *B. burgdorferi* contained nine plasmids, including seven linear plasmids ranging from 49 to 16 kilobases (kb) and two circular plasmids of 27 and 7.6 kb. Continuous cultivation in artificial medium resulted in the loss of a 7.6 kb circular plasmid and a 22 kb linear plasmid, in addition to a corresponding loss of infectivity for mice. The genome of several European and North American isolates of *B. burgdorferi* was examined using pulse-field gel electrophoresis (Baril et al 1989, Ferdows & Barbour 1989). These studies suggested that the chromosome of *B. burgdorferi* behaved as a eukaryotic linear chromosome of approximately 1000 kb. However, similar studies conducted at another laboratory concluded that *Borrelia* species contain a circular chromosome typical of prokaryotic organisms (Pernz et al in preparation). Fundamental differences in DNA methylation among members of the genus *Borrelia* were found to exist. The type species of the genus and causative agent of avian borreliosis, *B. anserina*, lacks an adenine methylation system, whereas this system was present in the relapsing fever borreliae *B. hermsii, B. turicatae, B. turicatae, B. parkeri,* and *B. duttonii,* and the putative agent of epizootic bovine abortion, *B. coriaceae.* Some heterogeneity in the presence of this system was observed with *B. burgdorferi.* The presence of a DNA methylation system was suggested in only 3 of 22 strains of this spirochete examined (Hughes & Johnson in preparation).

Borrelia burgdorferi is a relatively slow growing microaerophilic spirochete. In the culture medium developed by Kelly (1971) and modified by Stoenner et al (1982) and Barbour (1984), the organism divides every 12 to 24 h when incubated at 35°C. In contrast to *Treponema pallidum*, which will not survive more than one or two days at refrigeration temperatures, *B. burgdorferi* will survive for weeks to months at this temperature. The nutritional requirements for *B. burgdorferi* and other borreliae appear to be complex and they have the unusual requirement for Nacetylglucosamine (Kelly 1971). The spirochete can be readily isolated from ticks but generally is quite difficult to culture from patient specimens.

PATHOGENESIS OF LYME BORRELIOSIS

Lyme borreliosis can be characterized as a progressive, chronic infectious disease involving multiple organ systems. *Borrelia burgdorferi* is apparently transmitted to its host via the infectious saliva of the feeding tick (Ribeiro et al 1987, Zung et al 1989). An expanding annular erythematous rash, erythema migrans (EM), begins at the site of the tick bite within a few days to a month in 50 to 75% of patients. The infection is considered to be localized if the EM appears alone or in combination with minor constitutional symptoms. If the EM lesions are accompanied by extracutaneous signs and symptoms of major intensity, or if multiple EM occurs, Lyme borreliosis is considered to be disseminated. Patients with disseminated infections may progress to the chronic form of the disease. *Borrelia burgdorferi* is highly invasive. The spirochete interacts with and migrates through endothelial cell monolayers (Comstock & Thomas 1989) and will penetrate the central nervous system of rats within 24 h of injection (Garcia-Monco 1990). The spirochetaemia is of a low level, and there is a paucity of spirochetes in the infected organs. However, the disease manifestations, whether they be in the acute or chronic form of the illness, are associated with the presence of living spirochetes although they are few in number. The response of the disease to antimicrobial therapy supports this relationship.

Borrelia burgdorferi can elicit an inflammatory response which consists of mononuclear cells with the exception of the synovial fluid where granulocytes usually predominate. The most common histological pattern associated with the peripheral portion of EM is a superficial and deep perivascular and interstitial infiltrate composed mostly of lymphocytes but containing plasma cells (Berger et al 1983). Cardiac involvement is associated with an epi- and transmyocarditis with an interstitial infiltrate of lymphocytes and plasma cells. Lymphoplasmacellular infiltration is present in the meninges, ganglia, and peripheral nerves of patients manifesting the varying forms of meningopolyradiculitis. The arthritis is characterized by hypertrophic synovitis, frequently with fibrinaceous deposits and synovial vascular occlusion. The inflammatory cell infiltrate in the synovium consists of lymphocytes, plasma cells, mast cells, and macrophages. A similar cellular infiltrate is present in the chronic skin lesion, acrodermatitis chronica atrophicans (Duray & Steere 1988).

Since the pathology associated with Lyme borreliosis is caused by relatively few spirochetes there must be some mechanism for amplifying their pathogenicity. One possible mechanism would be the release of cytokines from the host cells by these organisms. *Borrelia burdgorferi* was found to induce the production of interleukin-1 (IL-1) when incubated with human monocytes (Habicht et al 1985) and cultured human synovial cells. The potent biological activity of IL-1 could be a major mechanism for the pathogenesis of Lyme borreliosis. The synovial fluids of Lyme borreliosis patients, in addition to IL-1, also contain tissue necrosis factor (Defosse & Johnson in preparation). The observation that *B. burgdorferi* will activate complement both in the absence and presence of antibody provides another potential mechanism of pathogenicity (Kochi & Johnson 1988). Through the activation of complement, chemotactic factors, mediators of inflammation and other biologically active substances are formed and could contribute to the inflammatory condition associated with this disease. Immune complexes (Hardin et al 1979) and autoimmune phenomena (Sigal & Tatum 1988, Aberer et al 1989) as mediators of injury in Lyme borreliosis have also been suggested. Studies with the severe combined immunodeficiency (scid) mouse have provided some insight concerning the role of cellular and humoral immune responses in the pathogenesis of Lyme borreliosis (Schaible et al 1989). These mice with severely impaired T-cell and B-cell functions develop a multisystemic disease with a preponderance for polyarthritis and carditis after inoculation with a low-passage tick isolate of *B. burgdorferi* but not with the high-passage tick isolate. The prominent and persistent arthritis as observed in *B. burgdorferi*-infected scid mice, which is not found in normal mice, is indicative of immunological control of the pathogenic activity of this spirochete. This is supported by studies in neonatal rats (Barthold et al 1988). The *B. burgdorferi*-induced arthritis in these rats decreased with the age of the animal correlating with the maturation of the immune system. This hypothesis is also supported by the induction of a more severe arthritis in irradiated hamsters infected with *B. burgdorferi* as compared with non-irradiated hamsters (Schmitz et al 1988). The possibility that arthritis, carditis, nephritis and hepatitis observed in the scid mice were elicited by inflammatory cell wall products of *B. burgdorferi* or were caused by circulating immune complexes or antigen-specific T-cells is unlikely, since inactivated spirochetes did not induce disease and the scid mice lacked mature lymphocytes. The presence of viable spirochetes in the synovium of these mice suggests a direct effect of the spirochete on the permeability of vessel walls and the underlying tissues. Another possibility is that the spirochetes may bind to and activate macrophages resulting in the release of various mediators of inflammation such as IL-1, interferon and tumour necrosis factor (Schaible et al 1989).

VACCINE FOR LYME BORRELIOSIS

One of the most effective methods for preventing microbial disease is by immunization. Vaccination of individuals and animals at risk for contracting Lyme borreliosis could greatly reduce the morbidity associated with this spirochetosis. This approach has been successful for a number of diseases, particularly when humoral immunity plays a major role in preventing infection. Since *B. burgdorferi* can be isolated from patients who have high levels of circulating antibodies, their protective value was questioned. We initially investigated the functional activity of anti- *B. burgdorferi* antibodies through the use of in vitro assays. We found that *B. burgdorferi* is resistant to the non-specific bactericidal activity of normal human serum (Kochi & Johnson 1988). This serum resistance of *B. burgdorferi* was of considerable interest since activation of complement by both the alternative and classical pathways did occur. The addition of human anti- *B. burgdorferi* IgG to normal human serum resulted in the rapid killing of the spirochete through the activation of complement by the classical pathway. We next examined the mechanism of serum resistance. It was determined that the bactericidal activity was not due to increasing the rate or the amount of complement deposition. We found that the effect of bactericidal IgG occurred at the C_5 step of the complement reaction. These results indicate that the effect of antibody in the killing process is to alter the outer membrane to allow increased membrane attack complex insertion (Kochi et al in preparation). Antibodies also act as opsonins. Although both opsonized and unopsonized *B. burgdorferi* are ingested by human polymorphonuclear cells and monocytes (Peterson et al 1984) and peritoneal exudate cells from rabbits and mice (Benach et al 1984), phagocytosis is enhanced by antibody, primarily mediated by the Fc receptor. These in vitro studies suggested that antibodies could have protective activity in the host. This possibility was explored by passive immunization studies using the hamster as the experimental animal. We had previously shown that hamsters were susceptible to infection with *B. burgdorferi* (Johnson et al 1984a) and the spirochete can be routinely isolated from the bladder, spleen and kidneys. For the passive immunization studies hamsters were injected subcutaneously with anti-*B. burgdorferi* antibodies and challenged by the intraperitoneal inoculation of the spirochete approximately 18 h later. Antibodies provided a high level of protection to experimental infection. As little as 0.01 ml of hyperimmune rabbit serum could provide immunity to infection (Johnson et al 1986a). If the passive immunization procedure were reversed, and the hamster infected and then administered antibodies, the results were very different. Antibodies administered one day after infection only provided 10% protection and no protection when administered on days three and seven post infection (Table 3.1). Thus, antibodies will prevent infection but have little if any anti-*B. burgdorferi* activity once the spirochetes are established in the host tissues (Johnson et al 1988). This observation provides an explanation for why it is possible to isolate the spirochete from patients with chronic Lyme borreliosis in spite of a high titre of serum antibodies. The results of our studies that antibodies can protect hamsters from experimental infection were recently confirmed and expanded by the experiments of Schmitz et al (1990). They prevented the development of arthritis in irradiated hamsters by the administration of hamster anti-*B. burgdorferi* antibodies prior to infection.

Although *B. burgdorferi* isolates from different geographical areas share many antigens, variations in protein antigens have been reported (Wilske et al 1986). We investigated the possibility that immunity to Lyme borreliosis could be strain-specific using the passive immunization assay. We chose as our test organisms *B. burgdorferi* isolates from Connecticut, California, and West Germany. These isolates are from diverse geographical areas and are transmitted by different species of *Ixodes*. Hamsters challenged with the same isolate for which they received antiserum were protected from infection. In contrast, antibodies to an isolate from one geographical area did not protect hamsters from infection by an isolate from a different

Table 3.1 Passive immunization of hamsters before and after experimental infection with *Borrelia burgdorferi*

Time of passive immunization	% Protection
18 h prior to infection	100
1 day after infection	10
3 days after infection	0
7 days after infection	0

Table 3.2 Vaccination of hamsters against experimental infection with *Borrelia burgdorferi*

Vaccine (μg dry weight of cells)	% Protection	
	Without adjuvant	With adjuvant*
Saline	0	0
5	0	25
10	20	100
25	60	100
50	80	100
75	80	80

* Adjuvant consists of monophosphoryl lipid A and trehalose dimycolate.

geographical area. However, a high level of cross-protection was observed among isolates from the same geographical area (Johnson et al 1988).

Since passive immunization provided hamsters with protection against experimental infection with *B. burgdorferi* we next investigated the effectiveness of vaccination (active immunization) for this purpose. Hamsters were vaccinated subcutaneously with a single dose of an inactivated whole cell preparation of a human spinal isolate and challenged 30 days later with the same isolate. Protection from experimental infection ranging from 86 to 100% was achieved by vaccination (Johnson et al 1986b). The immunogenicity of the Lyme disease vaccine was considerably less than that of vaccine preparations for another spirochetal disease, leptospirosis. In another study (Table 3.2) we found that the incorporation of an adjuvant containing monophosphoryl lipid A and trehalose dimycolate into the Lyme borreliosis vaccine increased its immunogenicity to that achieved with leptospiral vaccines (Johnson et al in preparation). Studies are needed to determine the feasibility of a polyvalent vaccine and to identify and isolate the components of *B. burgdorferi* that elicit the formation of protective antibodies.

ANTIMICROBIALS

Antimicrobials are effective in the treatment of Lyme borreliosis. However, the most efficacious antimicrobial agent, dosage, route of administration, and length of treatment have not been established. A major consideration in selecting an appropriate agent for the treatment of this disease is knowledge of the inherent antimicrobial susceptibility of *B. burgdorferi*. Unfortunately standard methods for determining the minimum inhibitory concentration and minimal bactericidal concentration (MBC) for slow-growing bacteria such as *B. burgdorferi* (generation time of 12–24 h) has not been established.

The in vitro susceptibility of *B. burgdorferi* to various antimicrobial agents has been reported for a number of human, animal, and tick isolates (Johnson et al 1984b, Berger et al 1985, Johnson et al 1987, Preac-Mursic et al 1987, Luft et al 1988, Preac-Mursic et al 1989, Johnson et al 1990). Although different protocols were used in these studies there was general agreement on the activity of most of the commonly used antimicrobials. Spirochetes were susceptible to the macrolides, tetracyclines, semisynthetic penicillins and the late second- and third-generation cephalosporins. *Borrelia burgdorferi* was only moderately sensitive to penicillin G and chloramphenicol and resistant to the aminoglycosides, trimethoprim-sulphamethoxazole, ciprofloxacin, and rifampicin. First-generation cephalosporins

Table 3.3 In vitro antimicrobial susceptibility of *Borrelia burgdorferi*

Antimicrobial agent *(n)*	Minimum bacteridical concentration (μg/ml)	
	Geometric mean	Range
Penicillin G (20)	17.5	3.2–51.2
Amoxycillin (15)	1.5	0.4–3.2
Cefotaxime (2)	0.5	0.5
Cefoxitin (1)	0.5	0.5
Ceftriaxone (17)	0.08	0.04–0.16
Tetracycline (22)	1.0	0.04–3.2
Doxycycline (16)	3.3	0.08–6.4
Erythromycin (19)	0.13	0.02–0.32
Azithromycin (20)	0.03	0.005–0.08
Ciprofloxicin (1)	4.0	4.0

The numbers in brackets refer to the testing frequency.

generally possessed a low level of anti-*B. burgdorferi* activity. We have used a macrodilution broth procedure to determine MBCs of these slow-growing spirochetes. This procedure incorporates the incubation of the spirochete with the antimicrobial agent for 3 weeks followed by transfer to medium without antimicrobials and an additional 3-week incubation period. Although the antimicrobial agents are inactivated early in the initial 3-week incubation period, we have found this prolonged incubation necessary because the MBCs of several antimicrobials required 2 weeks incubation to stabilize. The MBCs of a number of antimicrobials determined by this procedure are seen in Table 3.3. The in vivo susceptibility of *B. burgdorferi* to several of the antimicrobials was determined by the following procedure. Hamsters were infected 2 weeks prior to treatment which consisted of daily subcutaneous injections of one-fifth of the total dose for 5 days. Two weeks following the final day of treatment the hamsters were killed and the spleen, kidney and bladder cultured. The results of these studies are presented in Table 3.4 (Johnson et al 1987, Johnson et al 1990). Two considerations to keep in mind when comparing the efficacy of antimicrobial therapy of experimentally injected hamsters and Lyme borreliosis in humans are: in the hamster model we are assaying for the elimination of the spirochete from tissues, whereas in humans the adequacy of treatment is judged on the basis of resolution of signs and symptoms of the disease; and assessing the elimination of the spirochetes from the central nervous system of the hamster is not feasible. It is important in conducting antimicrobial assays in animals to include agents which have poor was well as good efficacy in the treatment of clinical Lyme borreliosis. In our hamster studies, therapy with tetracycline is significantly more effective than erythromycin. These results correlate

Table 3.4 In vivo antimicrobial susceptibility of *Borrelia burgdorferi*

Antimicrobial agent	50% Curative dose (mg/kg)
Penicillin G	> 197.5[1]
Amoxycillin	45.0[2]
Cefuroxime	28.6[2]
Ceftriaxone	24.0[1]
Tetracycline	28.0[1]
Tetracycline	15.6[3]
Doxycycline	36.5[2]
Erythromycin	235.2[1]
Erythromycin	122.2[3]
Azithromycin	3.7[3]

[1] Johnson et al 1987; [2] Johnson et al in preparation; [3] Johnson et al 1990.

well with the clinical experience (Steere et al 1980). However, penicillin G which has been used successfully to treat numerous cases of Lyme borreliosis manifests poor anti-*B. burgdorferi* activity in the hamster. Interestingly, some patients who have apparently failed to respond to penicillin G therapy have been successfully treated with ceftriaxone (Dattwyler et al 1988), an antimicrobial that possessed good activity in the hamster. The gerbil has been used by European investigators to evaluate the in vivo susceptibility of *B. burgdorferi* (Mursic et al 1987, Preac-Mursic et al 1989). Their results have been in general agreement with those obtained with the hamster. Amoxicillin, ceftriaxone, tetracycline, and azithromycin possessed good activity while penicillin G and erythromycin displayed a low level of activity. The results from the in vivo antimicrobial susceptibility method described appears to have a high predictive value for identifying agents for clinical trials.

Assessment of the adequacy of therapy for Lyme borreliosis is problematic. Identification of Lyme borreliosis patients with a high degree of certainty is often difficult except for early disease when erythema migrans is present. Problems are encountered in evaluating the patient's response to therapy due to the spirochete's latency and the intermittent pattern of exacerbations and remission in the natural history of untreated disease and the possibility of reinfection occurring. Therapy for Lyme borreliosis is an important area for future research activities.

SUMMARY

Lyme borreliosis is a world-wide evolving health problem. It is a complex multisystemic disease caused by the highly invasive spirochete, *B. burgdorferi*. The full spectrum of disease manifestations elicited in this infection continues to expand. Living spirochetes are associated with the pathology present in this illness. The mechanism of pathogenicity remains unknown but appears to be due to a direct effect of the spirochete on the host's cells or indirectly by interacting with mononuclear phagocytes leading to a release of mediators of inflammation. The inflammatory infiltrate consists of mononuclear cells with a predominance of lymphocytes. Antibodies play a critical role in immunity to Lyme borreliosis. They enhance phagocytosis and in the presence of complement will kill the spirochete. Immune serum will protect animals from experimental infection but appears to have a minimal effect on the spirochetes once they are established in host tissues. Vaccination as a method for preventing Lyme borreliosis appears to hold considerable promise. Presently the most effective measures to reduce the risk of Lyme borreliosis are efforts made by the individual to prevent tick bites and to locate and promptly remove attached ticks. Clinical studies suggest that the majority of patients respond satisfactorily to antimicrobial therapy with treatment failures most infrequently observed in patients with neurological involvement. The most effective antimicrobial, dose, route of administration and length of treatment are unknown and this is an important area for future research activities.

REFERENCES

Aberer E, Brunner C, Suchanek G, Klade H, Barbour A, Stanek G, Lassmann H 1989 Molecular mimicry and Lyme borreliosis: a shared antigenic determinant between *Borrelia burgdorferi* and human tissue. Annals of Neurology 26: 732-737

Barbour A G 1984 Isolation and cultivation of Lyme disease spirochetes. Yale Journal of Biology and Medicine 57: 521-525

Barbour A G 1988 Plasmid analysis of *Borrelia burgdorferi*, the Lyme disease agent. Journal of Clinical Microbiology 26: 475-478

Barbour A G, Garon C F 1987 Linear plasmids of the bacterium *Borrelia burgdorferi* have covalently closed ends. Science 237: 409-411

Barbour A G, Tessier S L, Tobd W J 1983 Lyme disease spirochetes and ixodid tick spirochetes share a common surface antigenic determinant defined by a monoclonal antibody. Infection and Immunity 41: 795-804.

Baril C, Richard C, Baranton G, Saint Giron I 1989 Linear chromosome of *Borrelia burgdorferi*. Research in Microbiology 140: 507-516

Barthold S W, Moody K W, Terwilliger G A, Duray P H, Jacoby R O, Steere A C 1988 Experimental Lyme arthritis in rats infected with *Borrelia burgdorferi*. Journal of Infectious Diseases 157: 842-846

Benach J L, Fleit H B, Habicht G S, Coleman J L, Bosler E M, Lane B P 1984 Interactions of phagocytes with the Lyme disease spirochete: Role of the Fc receptor. Journal of Infectious Diseases 150: 497-507

Berger B W, Clemmensen O J, Ackerman A B 1983 Lyme disease is a spirochetosis. American Journal of Dermatopathology 5: 111-124

Berger B W, Kaplan M H, Rothenberg I R, Barbour A G 1985 Isolation and characterization of the Lyme disease spirochete from the skin of patients with erythema chronicum migrans. Journal of the American Academy of Dermatology 13: 444-449

Coleman J L, Benach J L 1989 Identification and characterization of an endoflagellar antigen of *Borrelia burgdorferi*. Journal of Clinical Investigation 84: 322-331

Coleman J L, Benach J L, Beck G, Habicht G S 1986 Isolation of the outer envelope from *Borrelia burgdorferi*. Zentralblatt Fur Bakteriologie, Mikrobiologie, und Hygiene. Series A, Medical Microbiology, Infectious Diseases, Virology, Parasitology 23: 123-126

Comstock L E, Thomas D D 1989 Penetration of endothelial cell monolayers by *Borrelia burgdorferi*. Infection and Immunity 57: 1626-1628

Dattwyler R J, Halperin J J, Volkman D J, Luft B J 1988 Treatment of late Lyme borreliosis— randomized comparison of ceftriaxone and penicillin. Lancet i: 1191-1194

Duray P H, Steere A 1988 Clinical pathologic correlations of Lyme disease by stage. Annals of the New York Academy of Sciences 539: 65-79

Ferdows M S, Barbour A G 1989 Megabase-sized linear DNA in the bacterium *Borrelia burdorferi*, the Lyme disease agent. Proceedings of the National Academy of Sciences (USA) 86: 5969-5973

Garcia-Monco J C, Villar B F, Alen J C, Benach J L 1990 *Borrelia burgdorferi* in the central nervous system: Experimental and clinical evidence for early invasion. Journal of Infectious Diseases 161: 1187-1193

Habicht G S, Beck G, Benach J L, Coleman J L, Leichtling K D 1985 Lyme disease spirochetes induce human and murine interleukin 1 production. Journal of Immunology 134: 3147-3154

Hardin J A, Walker L C, Steere A C et al 1979 Circulating immune complexes in Lyme arthritis: Detection by the ^{125}I-Clq binding, Clq solid phase and Raji cell assays. Journal of Clinical Investigation 63: 468-477

Hyde F W, Johnson R C 1984 Genetic relationship of Lyme disease spirochetes to *Borrelia, Treponema,* and *Leptospira*. Journal of Clinical Microbiology 20: 151-154

Johnson R C, Marek N, Kodner C 1984a Infection of Syrian hamsters with Lyme disease spirochetes. Journal of Clinical Microbiology 20: 1099-1101

Johnson S E, Klein G C, Schmid G P, Feeley J C 1984b Susceptibility of the Lyme disease spirochete to seven antimicrobial agents. Yale Journal of Biology and Medicine 57: 549-553

Johnson R C, Kodner C, Russell M 1986a A passive immunization of hamsters against experimental infection with the Lyme disease spirochete. Infection and Immunity 53: 713-714

Johnson R C, Kodner C, Russell M 1986b Active Immunization of hamsters against experimental infection with *Borrelia burgdorferi*. Infection and Immunity 54: 897-898

Johnson R C, Kodner C, Russell M 1987 In vitro and in vivo susceptibility of the Lyme disease spirochete, *Borrelia burgdorferi*, to four antimicrobial agents. Antimicrobial Agents and Chemotherapy 31: 164-167

Johnson R C, Kodner C, Russell M, Duray P H 1988 Experimental infection of the hamster with *Borrelia burgdorferi*. Annals of the New York Academy of Sciences 539: 258-263

Johnson R C, Kodner C, Russell M, Girard D 1990 In vitro and in vivo susceptibility of *Borrelia burgdorferi* to azithromycin. Journal of Antimicrobial Chemotherapy 25 (Suppl A): 33-38

Kelly R 1971 Cultivation of *Borrelia hermsii*. Science 173: 443-444

Kochi S K, Johnson R C 1988 Role of immunoglobulin G in killing *Borrelia burgdorferi* by the classical component pathway. Infection and Immunity 56: 314-321

Luft B J, Volkman D J, Halperin J J, Dattwyler R J 1988 New chemotherapeutic approaches in the treatment of Lyme borreliosis. Annals of the New York Academy of Sciences 539: 352-361

Peterson P K, Clawson C C, Lee D A, Garlich D J, Quie P G, Johnson R C 1984 Human phagocyte interactions with the Lyme disease spirochete. Infection and Immunity 46: 608-611

Plasterk R H A, Simon M I, Barbour A G 1985 Transposition of structural genes to an expression sequence on a linear plasmid causes antigenic variation in the bacterium *Borrelia hermsii*. Nature (London) 318: 257-263

Preac-Mursic V P, Wilske B, Schierz G, Holmburger M, Süss E 1987 In vitro and in vivo susceptibility of *Borrelia burgdorferi*. European Journal of Clinical Microbiology 6: 424-426

Preac-Mursic V, Wilske B, Schlerz G, Süss E, Gross B 1989 Comparative antimicrobial activity of the new macrolides against *Borrelia burgdorferi*. European Journal of Clinical Microbiology and Infectious Diseases 8: 651-653

Ribeiro J M, Mather T N, Piesman J, Spielman A 1987 Dissemination and salivary delivery of Lyme disease spirochetes in vector ticks. Journal of Medical Entomology 24: 201-205

Schaible V E, Kramer M D, Museteanu C, Zimmer G, Mossman H, Simon M M 1989 The severe combined immunodeficiency (scid) mouse: a laboratory model for the analysis of Lyme arthritis and carditis. Journal of Experimental Medicine 170: 1427-1432

Schmitz J L, Schell R F, Hejka A, England D M, Konick L 1988 Induction of Lyme arthritis in LSH hamsters. Infection and Immunity 56: 2336-2341

Schmitz J L, Schell R, Hejka A G, England D M 1990 Passive immunization prevents induction of Lyme arthritis in LSH hamsters. Infection and Immunity 58: 144-148

Schwan T G, Burgdorfer W, Garon C F 1988 Changes in infectivity and plasmid profile of the Lyme disease spirochete *Borrelia burgdorferi*, as a result of in vitro cultivation. Infection and Immunity 56: 1831-1836

Sigal L, Tatum A 1988 Lyme disease patients' serum contains Igm antibodies to *Borrelia burgdorferi* that cross-react with neuronal antigens. Neurology 38: 1439-1442

Steere A C, Malawista S E, Newman J, Spieler P N, Bartenhagen N H 1980 Antibiotic therapy in Lyme disease: Annals of Internal Medicine 93: 1-8

Stoenner H G, Dodd T, Larson C 1982 Antigenic variation of *Borrelia hermsii*. Journal of Experimental Medicine 156: 1297-1311

Wilske B, Preac-Mursic V, Schierz G, Busch K V, 1986 Immunochemical and immunological analysis of European *Borrelia burgdorferi* strains. Zentralblatt Fur Bakteriologie, Microbologie, und Hygiene. Series A, Medical Microbiology, Infectious Diseases, Virology, Parasitology 263: 92-102

Zung J L, Lewengrub S, Rudzinska M A, Spielman A, Telford S R, Piesman J 1989 Fine structural evidence for the penetration of the Lyme disease spirochete *Borrelia burgdorferi* through the gut and salivary tissues of *Ixodes dammini*. Canadian Journal of Zoology 67: 1737-1748

Discussion of paper presented by R. C. Johnson

Discussed by J. L. Benach
Reported by P. K. Peterson

Although Johnson has covered the main areas of known pathogenesis of Lyme disease, mercifully he has left one to discuss.

Stanek referred to all the clinical manifestations of Lyme disease as probably non-specific. In fact they are, and much also of what Johnson showed is essentially non-specific. However, in our laboratory we have been trying to identify something very specific about Lyme disease, but have not yet been successful. However, I shall try to point out why this non-specificity may be very important to an eminently non-specific multi-organ disease.

If we cast our minds back to some of the platitudes given about syphilis in the early 1900s—for example 'to know syphilis is to know medicine', in addition to other statements made regarding this spirochetal infection—we are now clearly seeing something similar with Lyme disease.

First, I want to remind you of what Johnson said about the anatomy of this organism with respect to its outer coat. The outer envelope or membrane is very fluid; note too that the periplasmic flagella and the periplasmic space seldom come into contact with either the outer or external environments. Note too the peptidoglycan layer and the cell membrane.

Now let us look at the non-specificity of Lyme disease in itself. We know, for example, that there is extensive antibody cross-reactivity to the flagellin of Lyme disease, which presents as the antigen first recognised by IgM antibody and subsequently by IgG antibody. In many patients, this is the only antigen that is recognized. In others with advancing illness, however, alternative antigens begin to be recognized, but the flagellin, with an approximate molecular weight of 41 000 dalton, is ubiquitous and remains reactive for most, if not all, of the infection.

We know that approximately 25% of the normal population has antibodies to this flagellin—not a difficult concept when we consider the molecule itself. It has now been sequenced by a German group, who showed the carboxy and amino termini of the molecule to have extensive homology with the flagellin of other spirochetes. However there is also a variable region in the centre of the molecule that is often species specific.

Man normally produces antibodies to the flagellin directed at the fraction comprising 30–40 amino acids at the amino terminus end. The antibodies produced to the flagellin of *Borrelia burgdorferi* are precisely those that are least variable and most conserved among other spirochetes, and perhaps other bacteria.

There are indications, provided by a group at Yale, that Lyme disease patients produce antibodies to cardiolipid. There are indications also that antibodies or monoclonal antibodies directed to the flagellin bind neuronal components. In our own laboratory we have found that by injecting complete Freund's adjuvant into a mouse and testing its serum against *B. burgdorferi* by Western blot, there are numerous bands, some of which are homologous.

Continuing on the theme of the non-specificity of the host response in Lyme disease, we know from the early studies of Steere et al that spontaneous production of collagenase and PGE^2 can occur in synoviocytes from Lyme arthritic patients in culture. We know from the group at Stoneybrook and from our laboratory that macrophages incubated with *B. burgdorferi* can produce large amounts of interleukin-1 (IL-1); synoviocytes have the same ability. Also there is a lipopolysaccharide (LPS, whose chemical structure seems to be disputed) that induces polyclonal B-cell activation in laboratory animals. We also know from our Austrian colleagues that patients with Lyme disease produce antibodies to myelin. In our laboratory we have shown that such antibodies can be further defined as being against myelin basic protein, a finding confirmed by a group in Germany. In this case, not only B-cell responses but T-cell responses directed to myelin basic protein have been shown.

Lastly, this organism can, and does, adhere to virtually every eukaryotic cell with which it comes in contact. Consider its natural history. We see, for example, that the organism must adhere to the midgut epithelium of a tick, the cells of which are unlike anything seen in vertebrate biology. In the midgut is a phagocytic cell that ingests very large particles of both haematin and degraded erythrocytic membranes. The midgut epithelium consists of perhaps six to eight cells of this type, highly phagocytic, that can ingest almost anything of peptide or proteinaceous nature. Yet the organisms can, and often do, remain on the surface of the phagocytic cells. How Borrelia prevent themselves being ingested is uncanny, but we do know that they can pass either through or between the cells, eventually to invade the tick systemically.

We then take the organism from the tick to the vertebrate where we know—again from work in our laboratory—that they bind to epithelial cell lines. We also know that they adhere to endothelium, bind to glial cells, to primary rat brain cultures, and also to fibroblasts derived from the synovium. So there is a rather large array of cells to which the organism will bind and adhere.

In line with Johnson's comments, the organism has a very fluid outer membrane and seems almost to have a 'head'. The attachment at one end is particularly prominent and the fact that the organism can pass through spaces between midgut epithelial cells in the tick at least makes us think in terms of its having some self-propelled directional movement that is rare among the bacteria. We see much the same thing in the way the spirochete passes openings in an endothelial cell monolayer, for example a human umbilical cord monolayer.

My final point concerns the interaction of spirochetes with primary rat brain cultures. We carried out this work in order to understand some aspects of the neuropathogenesis of this disease. Stage one in our investigation showed that several strains of *B. burgdorferi* injected intravenously into rats crossed the blood-brain barrier in approximately 24 hours; invasion of the brain does no apparent damage to these animals. After this time they appear in the cerebrospinal fluid, followed by a minor pleiocytosis, with disappearance of both spirochetes and cells in about one week.

However, in vitro studies with rat brain cultures showed that these organisms tend to adhere to the glia. The spirochetes attach to the surface of oligodendrocytes. Again, the glycolipid outer surface component of *B. burgdorferi* seems very specific for oligodendrocytes. The organism's affinity for galactocerebroside—I might add a non-specific affinity—cannot be inhibited. But we do know that despite this non-specific affinity for an outer surface glycolipid, the organism can damage the brain cell in a manner that we do not quite, as yet, understand. Studies of oligodendrocytes in a primary rat brain culture have demonstrated extensive blebbing following adherence of *B. burgdorferi* to these cells.

Let me add that even though we have looked—with a battery of monoclonal antibodies—we have not found an adhesin in *B. burgdorferi* for any of the variety of cells to which it adheres. For that matter, because there are so many different types of cells to which it may adhere, we doubt there is a specific receptor which mediates binding, that is, a saturable, inhibitable and reversible receptor in *B. burgdorferi*. On the other hand, we have found a high non-specific capacity to bind to a large variety of cells, and in the case of oligodendrocytes not only to bind to the cell but also to at least damage it in a way that we feel is irreversible.

4. Immunodominant proteins of *Borrelia burgdorferi*: implications for improving serodiagnosis of Lyme borreliosis

B. Wilske, V. Preac Mursic, R. Fuchs, H. Bruckbauer,
A. Hofmann, G. Zumstein, S. Jauris, E. Soutschek,
M. Motz

INTRODUCTION

Due to the fact that Lyme borreliosis (LB) is a multisystem disorder which can imitate many other disorders involving the skin, the nervous system, the joints and the heart, highly sensitive and specific microbiological diagnostic tools are an urgent need for differential diagnostic purposes. Such methods should also be easy to perform, because high numbers of specimens need usually to be tested. Direct detection of the aetiological agent *Borrelia burgdorferi* (Burgdorfer et al 1982, Johnson et al 1984) by staining methods or cultivation (Duray et al 1985, Preac-Mursic et al 1986) is time consuming and laborious. Suitable specimens from patients (often material from biopsies is needed) are difficult to obtain and due to the low numbers of borreliae in tissues or body fluids the organism is often not detectable. The use of the polymerase chain reaction (PCR) may increase sensitivity of direct detection (Rosa & Schwan 1989, Malloy et al 1990) but will, however, not solve the difficulties obtaining suitable specimens from humans.

Therefore, as in syphilis, the most widely used method for microbiological diagnosis is serology. Unlike in syphilis the aetiological agent is antigenically heterogenous. This will imply that a suitable antigen should contain common epitopes of various isolates. Additionally these epitopes should be recognized by the patients' antibodies and should not cross-react with other bacteria.

This paper summarizes studies on:

1 Antigenic analysis of *B. burgdorferi*
2 Westernblot analysis of the antibody pattern in different stages of the disease
3 Analysis of *B. burgdorferi* for cross-reactive proteins
4 Use of selected immunodominant proteins as antigens in LB serology

The suitability of the Westernblot for serodiagnosis will also be discussed.

ANTIGENIC ANALYSIS OF *B. burgdorferi* ISOLATES

B. burgdorferi has been isolated from different biological sources as human specimens from wildlife and domestic animals and from ixodid ticks (Benach et al,

Steere et al 1983, Preac-Mursic et al 1986, Anderson et al 1988, 1989). Mostly samples are from skin and cerobrospinal fluid (CSF) and very rarely from other tissues and body fluids. Isolates were obtained from many geographical regions of Europe, North America and some strains have been isolated in Asia.

SDS-PAGE analysis

Analysis of SDS lysates from whole *B. burgdorferi* cells show certain characteristics in Coomassie blue-stained SDS-PAGE (Fig 4.1a). All strains so far analyzed have two major proteins, p60 and p41, with constant molecular weights (MW). P60 was described as a broadly cross-reacting antigen by Hansen et al (1988a). P41 represents the subunit of the *B. burgdorferi* endoflagellum (Barbour & Schrumpf 1986). Genes encoding *B. burgdorgeri* flagellum proteins have recently been cloned and sequenced (Gassmann et al 1989, Wallich et al 1990). The other group of major proteins is represented by three proteins with variable MW in the 20—36 KDa range.

Two such proteins, OspA (31-32 kDa) and OspB (34-36 kDa), were shown to be outer surface proteins of *B. burgdorferi* (Barbour et al 1983, 1984) usually present in North American isolates. About 50% of European isolates have an additional abundant protein in the 20 kDa range which we have designated 'pC' (Wilske et al 1986a). Major proteins in the 20kDa range have been rarely seen in cultures from North American isolates (Bissett & Hill 1987). In European isolates (especially those from ticks) a major OspB is often absent. In contrast, the OspA is present in nearly all cultured isolates. The few exceptions do have a major pC component. Considerable variations in the amount of OspA, OspB on the one side and pC on the other side have been observed in subcultured isolates (Wilske et al 1986a, Bissett & Hill 1987, Wilske et al 1988a, Karlsson et al 1990) (see also Fig 4.1b). It is unclear whether such variations occur also during infection in the host. It should be

Borrelia burgdorferi Isolates from Patients (n = 20)
SDS PAGE of Whole Cell Lysates (Coomassieblue Stain)

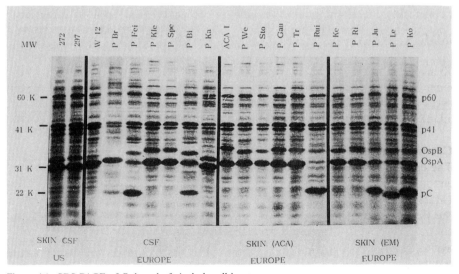

Figure 4.1a SDS PAGE of *B. burgdorferi* whole cell lysates

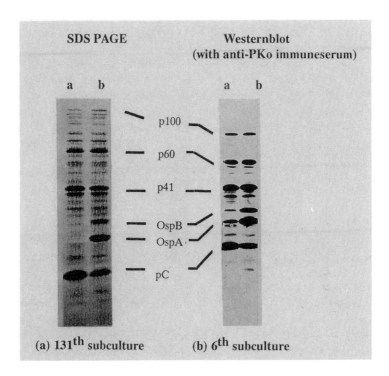

SDS PAGE

a   b

p100
p60
p41
OspB
OspA
pC

Westernblot
(with anti-PKo immuneserum)

a   b

(a) 131th subculture   (b) 6th subculture

Figure 4.1b Quantitative Changes of OspA, OspB and pC in 2 Subcultures
of Skin Isolate PKo

considered that the loss of certain antigens and the occurrence of new antigens may help the spirochete to escape host defence.

IMMUNOLOGICAL CHARACTERIZATION OF *B. burgdorferi*

To investigate questions of taxonomy, pathogenesis, immune prophylaxis or improvement of serodiagnosis, immunological characterization of *B. burgdorferi* antigens is necessary. In this respect both common and variable epitopes of the various proteins are of interest.

Common epitopes
The endoflagellae of borreliae (including relapsing fever borreliae) have common epitopes recognized by a monoclonal antibody (Mab H9724) (Barbour et al 1986). Until now, a Mab which is reactive with *B. burgdorferi*-specific common epitopes of the flagellum and nonreactive with relapsing fever borreliae, is not available. In contrast, *B. burgdorferi*-specific common epitopes are recognized by certain Mab against the OspA and against a 100kDa range protein (Wilske et al, unpublished results).

As shown in Fig. 4.1b an immune serum against *B. burgdorferi* is reactive with a

49

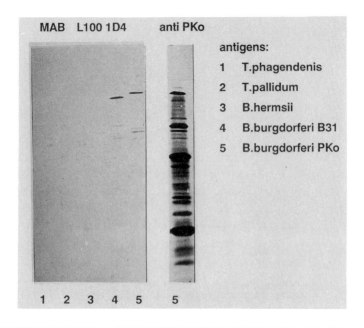

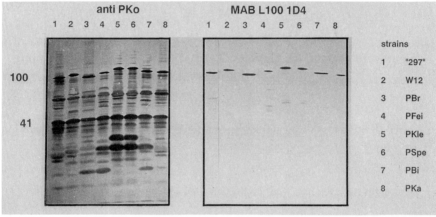

Figure 4.2 Reactivity of monoclonal antibody (L100 1D4) with a 100kDa range protein of *B. burgdorfei* (Westernblot); anti PKO = rabbit immune serum against *B. burgdorferei* (strain PKO)

100kDa band not visible as major band in the SDS-PAGE. This protein (p100) is reactive with a Mab (L100 1D4) (Fig. 4.2). This antibody detects common *B. burgdorferi*-specific epitopes of a 100kDa range protein and was reactive also in more than 50 *B. burgdorferi* isolates (except two tick isolates from Europe) and non-reactive in relapsing fever borreliae (Wilske et al unpublished results).

Figure 4.3a shows that the seven serotypes previously described by us (Wiske et al 1988a) were all reactive with a Mab against OspA (L321F11); in contrast, relapsing fever borrelia, treponemes and other unrelated bacteria were non-reactive. Meanwhile this antibody was tested with a panel of more than 50 *B. burgdorferi* isolates including 11 European and 3 American strains which were negative with the

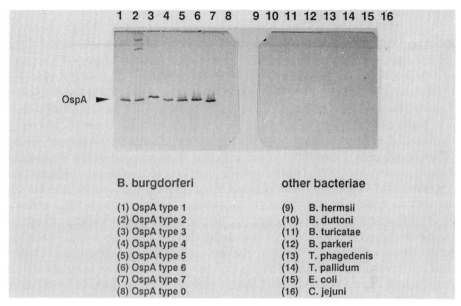

	1	2	3	4	5	6	7	8	9	10	11	12	13	14	15	16

OspA ▶

B. burgdorferi
(1) OspA type 1
(2) OspA type 2
(3) OspA type 3
(4) OspA type 4
(5) OspA type 5
(6) OspA type 6
(7) OspA type 7
(8) OspA type 0

other bacteriae
(9) B. hermsii
(10) B. duttoni
(11) B. turicatae
(12) B. parkeri
(13) T. phagedenis
(14) T. pallidum
(15) E. coli
(16) C. jejuni

Reactivity of monoclonal antibody (L32 1F11) with OspA

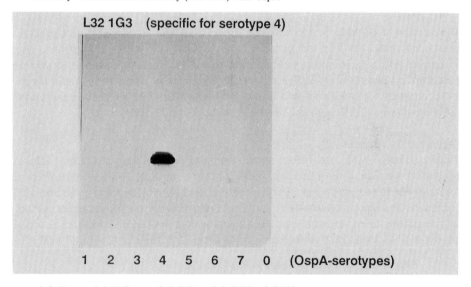

L32 1G3 (specific for serotype 4)

1	2	3	4	5	6	7	0	(OspA-serotypes)

(1) B31; (2) PGau; (3) PBr; (4) PBl (5) W12;
(6) TN; (7) T25; (0) PKo; OspA neg.

(b) Reactivity of monoclonal antibody (L32 1G3) with OspA

Figure 4.3 Common and serotype-specific epitopes of OspA

most widely-used Mab H5332. With the exception of four OspA negative strains all isolates were reactive; these four strains, however, were reactive with Mab L100 1D4 (against p100). Additionally, common epitopes of the pC component of isolates from patients were detected with a Mab L22 1F8. However, the pC components of several tick isolates were non-reactive (Wilske et al, unpublished results).

OspA and OspB components

By reaction with a Mab, antigenic heterogeneity has been demonstrated for OspA and OspB (Barbour & Schrumpf 1986, Wilske et al 1986a). Based on differences in the reactivity of OspA and OspB with monoclonal and polyclonal antibodies, seven serotypes have been described (Wilske et al 1988a). Meanwhile the serotyping system was based on the reactivity of OspA with a panel of eight Mab (Wilske et al unpublished results). Table 4.1 shows the distribution of the various serotypes among North American and European isolates and Fig 4.3b an example for the reactivity of a serotype-specific Mab. In North America, type 1 is predominant in the panel that has been tested, in Europe type 2 is predominant. With few exceptions skin isolates are serotype 2, whereas CSF- and tick-isolates from Europe are more heterogenous. These differences allow speculations on differences in the organotropism of the various serotypes. Finally, it cannot be excluded that the spirochetes which infect the hosts differ antigenically from the spirochetes in the tissue, or from those cultured from the host tissue. Antigenic changes of the OspB were seen to occur at low frequency in cloned cultures on *B. burgdorferi* (Bundoc & Barbour 1989). It is possible that similar changes occur in vivo with higher frequency.

Other proteins

By reaction with Mab it can also be shown that the *B. burgdorferi* flagellum-associated protein p41 is antigenically heterogenous (Fig 4.4a). A European skin isolate has p41 specific epitopes not detected in the American type strain B31 (Wilske et al unpublished results). A comparable heterogeneity is also demonstrable for the pC components (Fig 4.4b) of two strains (PKo and PBi). These strains express a pC component which differs in the reactivity with Mab L22 1F10.

Crossreactive proteins

To investigate possible cross-reactions of *B. burgdorferi* proteins with other bacterial proteins, heterologous immune sera raised against a panel of 15 other bacteria were reacted with *B. burgdorferi* antigens in the Westernblot (for examples, see Fig. 4.5). Except in a few instances, reactivity could be totally absorbed by the bacteria used for immunization. Even very unrelated bacteria induced cross-reacting antibodies. Many cross-reactions were directed to bands from 60 to 75 kDa respectively. The 60 kDa

Table 4.1 Distribution of *B. burgdorferi* OspA serotypes

OspA type	US	tick	Europe skin	CSF	total
1	7	2	1	1	11
2	—	2	18	2	22
3	—	1	—	1	2
4	—	—	1	2	3
5	—	—	—	2	2
6	—	6	1	—	7
7	—	1	—	—	1
X[1]	3	2	—	—	5
0[2]	—	1	1	2	4
Total	10	15	22	10	57

[1] other than type 1-7; [2] OspA negative

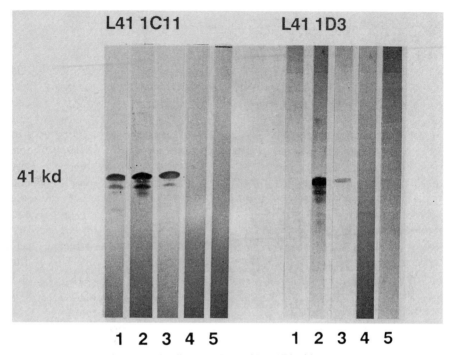

(a) Reactivity of monoclonal antibodies L41 1C11 and L41 1D3 with p41

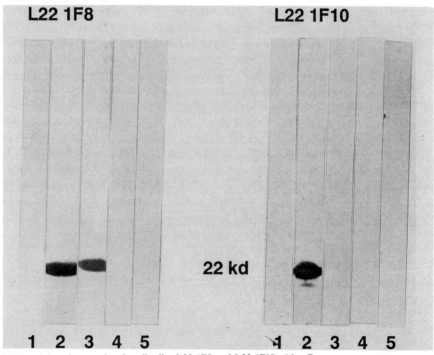

(b) Reactivity of monoclonal antibodies L22 1F8 and L22 1F10 with pC

Figure 4.4 Common and serotype-specific epitopes of the flagellum (p41) (a) and the pC-component (b) Strains: (1) *B. burgdorferi*, B31; (2) *B. burgdorferi*, PKo; (3) *B. burgdorferi*, PBi; (4) *B. hermsii*; (5) *T. phagedenis*.

c

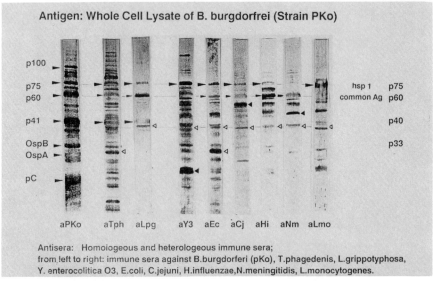

Antigen: Whole Cell Lysate of B. burgdorfrei (Strain PKo)

p100
p75
p60
p41
OspB
OspA
pC

hsp 1   p75
common Ag p60
p40
p33

aPKo aTph aLpg aY3 aEc aCj aHi aNm aLmo

Antisera: Homologeous and heterologeous immune sera;
from left to right: immune sera against B.burgdorferi (pKo), T.phagedenis, L.grippotyphosa,
Y. enterocolitica O3, E.coli, C.jejuni, H.influenzae,N.meningitidis, L.monocytogenes.

Figure 4.5 Crossreactive proteins of *B. burgdorferi* demonstrated by Westernblot with immune sera to unrelated bacteria

band represents the so-called common antigen, while the 75 kDa band might represent the heat shock protein 1 described by Cluss & Boothby (1990). The lowest number of reactions was seen with OspA (non-reactive) and p100 (only reactive with immune serum against *Borrelia hermsii*). Only three sera were reactive with p41 and pC (however, cross-reactivity was observed outside the genus *Borrelia*). Broadly cross-reacting bands may be close to more specific bands (i.e. p40 close to p41 or p33 close to OspA). Such bands may be mistaken for more specific bands in the immunoblot when a crude ultrasonicate is used as antigen (Bruckbauer et al unpublished results).

According to these findings OspA, p100, p41 and pC seem to be the most suitable antigens for serodiagnosis. However, the suitability of p41 is a controversial point. Enrichment of flagellae or the use of isolated flagellae as antigen has been described as increasing the sensitivity and specificity of antibody detection, especially in early disease (Coleman & Benach 1987, Hansen et al 1988a). However, in the immunoblot the p41 band is also often reactive with sera from healthy controls. An explanation for unspecificity may be provided by the fact that the amino- and carboxyterminal portions of the *B. burgdorferi* encoding genes have considerable sequence similarities (> 50%) with flagella encoding genes of unrelated bacteria (i.e. *Bacillus subtilis* and *Salmonella typhimurium* (Wallich et al 1990).

HUMORAL IMMUNE RESPONSE (ANTIBODY PATTERN IN DIFFERENT STAGES OF THE DISEASE)

The immunodominant proteins of the early antibody response in Lyme borreliosis are p41 and pC (Karlsson et al 1988, Wilske et al 1986a, 1989a). For IgM antibodies no obvious differences were detected in the reactivity of the p41 from different strains. Reactivity with the pC component mainly depends on whether a major pC is present or not in the test antigen (Fig 4.6). In patients with erythema migrans, more sera are

NEUROBORRELIOSIS, STAGE 2 (n = 3)

(IgM Westernblot with 5 Strains)

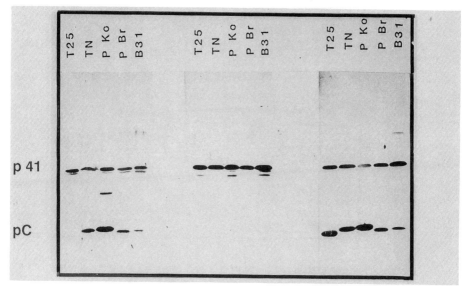

NEUROBORRELIOSIS, STAGE 2 (n = 3)

(IgG Westernblot with 5 Strains)

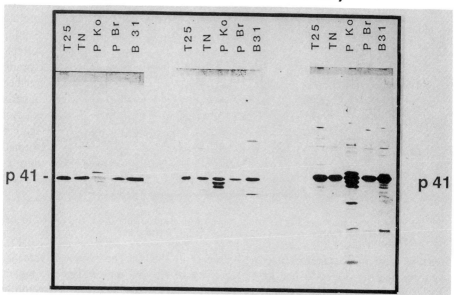

(a) Early immune response (stage II)

Figure 4.6 Westernblot analysis of the humoral immune response in Lyme borreliosis using different *B. burgdorferi* strains as antigen; 3 sera were tested with 5 different strains (T25-B31) in IgM and IgG Westernblot respectively

ACRODERMATITIS (n = 3)

(IgG Westernblot with 5 Strains)

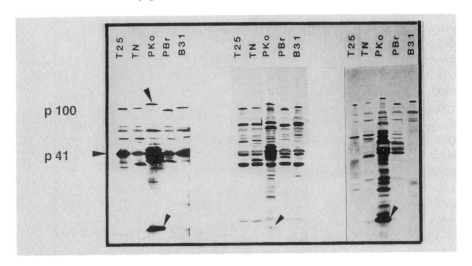

LYME ARTHRITIS (n = 3)

(IgG Westernblot with 5 Strains)

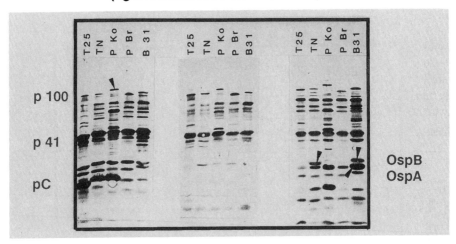

(b) Late immune response (stage III); sera from patients with acrodermatitis (n = 3) and Lyme arthritis (n = 3) were tested with 5 different strains (T25-B31) in the IgG Westernblot

reactive with pC compared to p41 (Wilske et al 1989a). The reverse is true for neuroborreliosis stage II. The lower reactivity of the pC may reflect the higher antigenic diversity of CSF isolates compared to skin isolates. IgM antibodies to the pC have also been demonstrated in patients from whom pC negative isolates were cultured (Wilske et al 1986a, 1988a). This may indicate expression of pC in vivo, but not in vitro.

In principle, IgG antibody-positive sera (by ultrasonicate ELISA or IFA) do have IgG antibodies reactive with p41 in the Westernblot. However, as shown in Fig. 4.6, striking differences in the degree of the reactivity are observed in the 40 kDa region. This may reflect antigenic diversity of the flagellum as also shown by Mab L41 1D3 (Fig 4.4). In late disease (arthritis or acrodermatitis) a broad spectrum of antibodies is usually detected by the Westernblot (Wilske et al 1988b). Many of them are also detected with immune sera against unrelated bacteria. IGg antibodies to p100 are present in most sera from patients with late manifestations (Table 4.2). No obvious strain-dependent differences (except for tick isolate TN) were observed with various p100 components, indicating that sera from patients usually recognize common epitopes of this component. Part of the gene encoding the p100 has been cloned in *E. coli* and a polypeptide reactive with Mab L100 1D4 was expressed by the clone (Fuchs et al unpublished results). A recombinant p100 may provide a highly specific antigen in the future. Sera from patients with acrodermatitis are predominantly reactive with the serotype 2 strain (PKo). Part of the better reactivity is due to reaction with p17. A comparable antigenic component is only rarely observed with other strains. The combination of p100 and p17 provided positive results in all 17 cases of late LB tested.

Antibodies to OspA and OspB are only rarely observed in European patients in all stages of the disease. This may be explained in different ways: (i) low immunogenicity or antigenic mimicry, (ii) degradation of OspA and OspB in the tissue, (iii) antigenic heterogeneity, (iv) antigenic variation in the host.

In diagnosis of HIV infection the Westernblot is widely used as a confirmatory test of high specificity. For diagnosis of LB, however, the Westernblot is less specific, since interpretation of the blot is impaired by cross-reacting proteins if whole cell lysates of *B. burgdorferi* are used as antigen. Another critical point is that the use of different serotypes as antigen may result in very different reactivity patterns.

At present we use the Westernblot, especially for demonstration of intrathecal antibody production in neuro-Lyme-borreliosis. By parallel testing of CSF and serum diluted to the same immunoglobin content in the Westernblot it can be shown whether intrathecal antibody production is present and against which proteins the

Table 4.2 Late manifestations (n = 17). (Reactivity with major immunodominant proteins in the IgG Western blot using different strains as antigen)

	T25 type 7	TN type 6	PKo type 0	PBr type 3	B31 type 1	at least 1 strain reactive
Arthritis (n = 10)						
p100	10	10	10	10	10	10
p41	10	10	10	10	9	10
OspB	—	—	—	—	1	1
OspA	—	1	—	—	1	1
pC	2	3	3	2	3	3
p17	1	—	4	—	—	5
Acrodermatitis (n = 7)						
p100	3	5	5	5	5	
p41	5	5	5	5	5	5
OspB	—	—	—	—	—	—
OspA	—	—	—	—	—	—
pC	—	—	—	—	—	—
p17	—	—	7	—	—	7
All cases (n = 17)						
p100 or p17	15	13	17	15	15	17

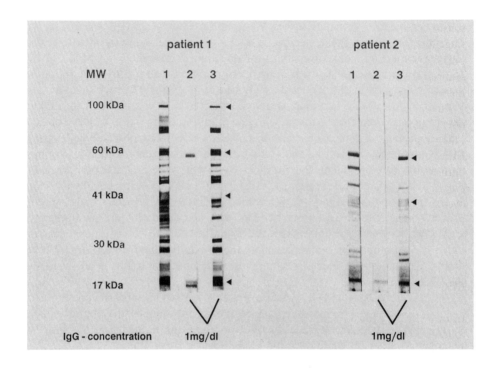

patient 1   patient 2

MW   1 2 3   1 2 3

1:          serum diluted to 1 : 100

2 and 3:   serum (2) and CSF (3) diluted to equal IgG concentrations

Figure 4.7 Westernblot for detection of intrathecal antibodies against *B. burgdorferi* in neuro-Lyme borreliosis, stage III

Note stronger reactivity of CSF compared to serum! CSF and serium were diluted to the same IgG content.

antibodies are directed (Wilske et al 1986b). This technique is especially useful in diagnosis of neuro-Lyme borreliosis stage III (chronic progressive encephalomyelitis) (Fig 4.7).

Previously, a higher specificity of the Westernblot was obtained by using sarcosyl-extracted borrelia cells as antigen. By this procedure p100 and pC components are enriched and cross-reacting antigens, especially the 60-70 kDa range proteins, are mostly eliminated (Wilske et al unpublished results). Possibly the best standardization may be achieved by using certain recombinant proteins (i.e. p100, p41 and pC).

SEROLOGICAL TESTS

The most frequently used techniques to detect antibodies to *B. burgdorferi* are indirect immunofluorescence (IFA) and ELISA, though specificity of both the IgG IFA and the IgG ultrasonicate ELISA is impaired by cross-reactions. Specificity may be increased by pre-absorption of sera with *T. phagedenis* (which is especially helpful for elimination of crossreaction with *T. pallidum*) (Wilske et al 1984). Increases in sensitivity and specificity were described by Coleman & Benach (1987), who used flagellum-enriched antigen preparations and by Hansen et al (1988b) who used purified flagellae instead of crude ultrasonicate antigen for the ELISA. According to Hansen the gain in specificity was due to elimination of cross-reaction antigens, i.e. the 60 kDa common antigen.

Purified p41 may also be obtained by affinity chromatography (using a Mab for p41) (Fuchs et al 1990) or purified pC by anion exchange chromatography. IgG and IgM positive sera from patients with early LB were tested with the pC and the p41 ELISA. With few exceptions the sera were reactive with p41 and pC, indicating that both are suitable antigens. However, in all these techniques cultivation of *B. burgdorferi* in considerable amounts is needed. The use of recombinant proteins may overcome this problem.

RECOMBINANT *B. burgdorferi* ANTIGENS

In order to obtain recombinant antigens for standardized ELISA techniques, the following recombinant polypeptides derived from skin isolate PKo were produced in *E. coli*: p41, OspA and pC.

p41 (Flagellum Associated Protein)
Oligonucleotides were synthesized according to a previously published sequence of the flagellum protein p41 (Gassmann et al 1989), of the American strain B31 and used as primers for amplification of the flagellum encoding gene of the European skin isolate PKo. The gene was cloned in *E.coli*. The p41 component was efficiently expressed and obtained in purified form by anion exchange chromatography. The recombinant protein was immunologically reactive.

OspA (Outer Surface Protein)
OspA was cloned from a *B. burgdorferi* genomic library obtained from the skin isolate PKo. An OspA-producing clone was detected by the OspA specific Mab L32 2E7 previously produced in our laboratory. The recombinant protein was purified by cation exchange chromatography. The purified OspA was sequenced (Zumstein et al unpublished results) and differs from the OspA encoding gene of the American strain B31 (Bergström et al 1989).

pC (Membrane Associated Protein)
Oligonucleotides were synthesized according to amino acid sequences obtained from tryptic cleavage products of the pC-component. Using PCR the gene encoding pC was amplified from strain PKo DNA. The pC encoding gene was cloned, expressed in *E. Coli* and recombiant pC-protein obtained in purified form by anion exchange chromatography (Fuchs et al unpublished results). Immune reactivity of the recombinant pC is shown in Fig. 4.8. The pC encoding gene was sequenced by Jauris (unpublished results) and was shown to differ from the OspA encoding gene of strain PKo.

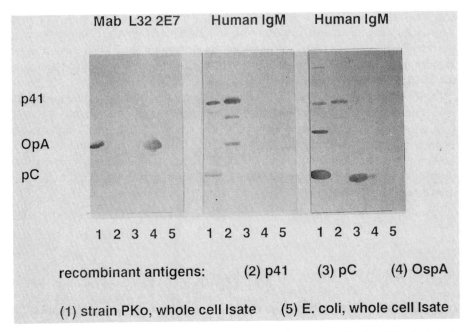

Figure 4.8 Immune reactivity of recombinant *B. burgdorferi* polypeptides (p41, pC and OspA) derived from strain PKo

Recombinant antigens (p41, pC and OspA) and whole cell lysates from strain PKo and *E. coli* were tested by Westernblot using Mab L32 2E7 for detection of OspA and two human IgM positive sera for detection of p41 and pC respectively.

ELISA TESTS

The suitability of the three recombinant antigens was tested in comparison to the ultrasonicate ELISA (Wilske et al 1989b) and the flagellum ELISA (Hansen et al 1988a). The recombinant ELISAs were performed as described for the ultrasonicate ELISA. In order to compare the different ELISA techniques we used a panel of clinically defined sera from 74 patients with erythema migrans, which were not pre-selected by serology. Blood donor sera (n = 100) from the Munich area served as controls; sera from patients and controls were tested in the same assay.

In both IgM and IgG ELISA, the use of single antigens enabled the sensitivity of the antibody detection to be increased when compared to the ultrasonicate ELISA. The best single antigen test was the flagellum ELISA, followed by the recombinant pC ELISA and the recombinant p41 ELISA (Table 4.3). As expected the OspA ELISA was highly insensitive. However, the highest detection rate was provided by combining recombinant pC ELISA and recombinant p41 ELISA. Decreased sensitivity of the recombinant p41 ELISA compared to the native flagellum ELISA may be due to the use of a denatured antigen. Another possibility is that exposure of cross-reactive epitopes in the denatured antigen account for a higher background reactivity and therefore for lower sensitivity. Possibly, the future use of recombinants not bearing the cross-reactive epitopes, as also discussed by Wallich et al (1990), may overcome this problem.

Table 4.3 Detection of IgM- and IgG antibodies in patients with erythema migrans (n = 74) using different antigens for the ELISA

ELISA antigen	erythema migrans (n = 74)				controls (n = 100)	
	IgM			IgG	IgM	IgG
ultrasonicate	20	27.0%	17	22.9%	5	5
flagellum	29	39.1%	30	40.5%	5	5
p41 (recomb.)	22	29.7%	23	31.1%	5	5
OspA (recomb.)	7	9.4%	6	8.1%	5	5
pC (recomb.)	26	35.1%	27	36.5%	5	5
p41 and/or pC (recomb.)	34	45.9%	34	45.9%	5	5

The cut off for the positive test was determined as an OD value above the 95% percentile of the OD values of 100 blood donor sera from the Munich area. To evaluate whether combining two recombinant antigen ELISAs may increase the sensitivity of antibody detection the cut off levels for the p41 and the pC ELISA were increased in order to retain the 95% percentile cut off of the blood donor panel.

Our study has shown that recombinant proteins as pC and p41 may be used as effective antigens for early antibody detection. However, further studies are needed concerning patients suffering from LB stage II and stage III. Additionally, and especially in later stages of LB, the use of alternative recombinant proteins such as p100 or p17 should be considered.

SUMMARY AND CONCLUSIONS

1. SDS-PAGE analysis of whole cell lysates of *B. burgdorferi* shows two major proteins with constant molecular weight—p41 (flagellin) and p60 (broadly cross-reacting antigen). These proteins are common to all *B. burgdorferi* isolates so far tested. Three further major proteins, OspA, OspB and pC, are proteins with variable molecular weights of about 30 and 20 kDa. *B. burgdorferi* strains have at least an OspA or a pC component.

2. Species-specific epitopes of *B. burgdorferi* are recognized by monoclonal antibodies against OspA and pC components. The OspA specific antibody was reactive with OspA-positive strains (> 50), the pC specific antibody with about 50% of OspA-positive and all OspA negative strains (four strains available).

3. A 100 kDa range protein (minor protein in SDS-PAGE) has common species-specific epitopes reactive with a monoclonal antibody.

4. These antibodies may provide—in combination (Mab against OspA, pC) or alone (Mab against p100)—effective reagents for identification of the species *B. burgdorferi*. They may also improve antigen detection in infected tissues or body fluids.

5. Antigenic heterogeneity of major *B. burgdorferi* proteins (p41, OspA and pC) was demonstrated by differences in the reactivity with monoclonal antibodies. A serotyping system was based on the reactivity with OspA specific monoclonal antibodies and confirmed the previous description of seven OspA-Types. Antigenic heterogeneity has to be considered with respect to serodiagnosis or development of a vaccine.

6. Immunodominant proteins for the early immune response in patients with Lyme borreliosis are p41 and pC. In late disease, p41, p100 and p17 are predominantly recognized.

7. For antibody detection in early LB purified p41- and pC-components are comparably sensitive antigens for the ELISA as whole cell ultrasonicate.

8. Genes encoding p41, pC and OspA components of a European strain (PKo) have been cloned in *E. coli*.

9. The respective clones do produce immune reactive polypeptides. Use of recombinant pC and p41 as ELISA antigen improved sensitivity of antibody detection compared to the conventional ultrasonicate ELISA in patients with early LB.

10. Recombinant polypeptides may also be used for development of a vaccine or research on the pathogenesis of the disease.

REFERENCES

Anderson J F, Magnarelli L A, McAninich J B 1988 New *Borrelia burgdorferi* antigenic variant isolated from *Ixodes dammini* from upstate New York. Journal of Clinical Microbiology 26: 2209-2212

Anderson J F, Magnarelli L A, LeFebvre R B et al 1989 Antigenically variable *Borrelia burgdorferi* isolated from cottontail rabbits and *Ixodes dentatus* in rural and urban areas. Journal of Clinical Microbiology 27: 13-20

Barbour A G, Schrumpf M E 1986 Polymorphisms of major surface proteins of *Borrelia burgdorferi*. Zentralblatt fur Bakteriologie, Mikrobiologie und Hygiene A 263: 83-91

Barbour A G, Tessier S L, Todd W J 1983 Lyme disease spirochetes and ixodid tick spirochetes share a common surface antigenic determinant defined by a monodonal antibody. Infection and Immunity 41: 795-804

Barbour A G, Tessier S L, Hayes S F 1984 Variation in a major surface protein of Lyme disease spirochetes. Infection and Immunity 45: 94-100

Barbour A G, Hayes S F, Heiland R A, Schrumpf M E, Tessier S L 1986 A Borrelia-specific monoclonal antibody binds to a flagellar epitope 52: 549-554

Benach J L, Bosler E M, Hanrahan J P et al 1983 Spirochetes isolated from the blood of two patients with Lyme disease. New England Journal of Medicine 308: 740-742

Bergström S, Bundoc V G, Barbour A G 1989 Molecular analysis of linear plasmid-encoded major surface proteins, OspA and OspB, of the Lyme disease spirochaete *Borrelia burgdorferi*. Molecular Microbiology 3: 479-486

Bissett M L, Hill W 1987 Characterization of *Borrelia burgdorferi* strains isolated from *Ixodes pacificus* ticks in California. Journal of Clinical Microbiology 25: 2296-2301

Bundoc V G, Barbour A 1989 Clonal polymorphisms of outer membrane protein OspB of *Borrelia burgdorferi*. Infection and Immunity 57: 2733-2741

Burgdorfer W, Barbour A G, Hayes S F, Benach J L, Grunwald E, Davis J P 1982 Lyme disease—a tick-borne spirochetosis? Science 216: 1317-1319

Cluss R G, Boothby J T 1990 Thermoregulation of protein synthesis in *Borrelia burgdorferi*. Infection and Immunity 58: 1038-1042

Coleman J L, Benach J L 1987 Isolation of antigenic components from the Lyme disease spirochete: Their role in early diagnosis. Journal of Infectious Diseases 155: 756-765

Duray P H, Kusnitz A, Ryan J 1985 Demonstration of the Lyme disease spirochete by a modified Dieterle stain method. Laboratory Medicine 16: 685-687

Fuchs R, Wilske B, Preac-Mursic V, Schierz G in press Purification of *B. burgdorferi* flagellum by use of a monoclonal antibody. Molecular and Cellular Probes

Gassmann G S, Kramer M, Göbel U B, Wallich R 1989 Nucleotide sequence of a gene encoding the *B. burgdorferi* flagellin. Nucleic Acids Research 17: 3590

Hansen K, Bangsborg J M, Fjordvang H, Pederson N S, Hindersson P 1988a Immunochemical characterization and isolation of the gene for a *Borrelia burgdorgeri* immunodominant 60-kilodalton antigen common to a wide range of bacteria. Infection and Immunity 56: 2047-2053

Hansen K, Hindersson P, Pedersen N S 1988b Measurement of antibodies to the *Borrelia burgdorferi* flagellum improves serodiagnosis in Lyme disease. Journal of Clinical Microbiology 26: 338-346

Johnson R C, Schmidt G P, Hyde F W, Steigerwald A G, Brenner D J 1984 *Borrelia burgdorferi* sp. nv.: Etiologic agent of Lyme disease. International Journal of Systemic Bacteriology 34: 436-497

Karlsson M, Hovind-Hougen K, Svenungsson B, Stiernstedt G 1990 Cultivation and characterization of spirochetes from cerebrospinal fluid of patients with Lyme borreliosis Journal of Clinical Microbiology 28: 473-479

Karlsson M, Möllegard I, Stiernstedt G 1988 Characterization of antibody response in patients with Borrelia meningitis. Serodiagnostics and Immunotherapy 2: 375-386

Malloy D C, Nauman R K, Paxton H 1990 Detection of *Borrelia burgdorferi* using the polymerase chain reaction. Journal of Clinical Microbiology 28: 1089-1093

Preac-Mursic V, Wilske B, Schierz G 1986 European *Borrelia burgdorferi* isolated from humans and ticks: Culture conditions and antibiotic susceptibility. Zentralblatt fur Bakteriologie, Mikrobiologie und Hygiene A 263: 112-118

Rosa P A, Schwan T G 1989 A specific and sensitive assay for the Lyme disease spirochete *Borrelia burgdorferi* using the polymerase chain reaction. Journal of Infectious Diseases 160: 1018-1029

Steere A C, Grodzicki R L, Kornblatt A N et al 1983 The spirochetal etiology of Lyme disease. New England Journal of Medicine 308: 733-740

Wallich R, Moter S E, Simon M M, Ebnet K, Heiberger A, Kramer M D 1990 The *Borrelia burgdorferi* flagellum-associated 41-kilodalton antigen (flagellin): molecular cloning, expression, and amplication of the gene. Infection and Immunity 58: 1711-1719

Wilske B, Schierz G, Preac-Mursic V, Weber K, Pfitster H-W, Einhäupl K 1984 Serological diagnosis of erythema migrans disease and related disorders. Infection 5: 331-337

Wilske B, Preac-Mursic V, Schierz G, von Busch K 1986a Immunochemical and immunological analysis of European *Borrelia burgdorferi* strains. Zentralblatt fur Bakteriologie, Mikrobiologie und Hygiene A 63: 92-102

Wilske B, Schierz G, Preac-Mursic V, Weber K, Pfitster H-W, Einhäupl K 1984 Serological diagnosis of erythema migrans disease and related disorders. Infection 5: 331-337 lymphocytic meningoradiculitis (Bannwarth's syndrome). Journal of Infectious Diseases 153: 304-314

Wilske B, Preac-Mursic V, Schierz G, Gueye W, Herzer P, Weker K 1988a Immunochemische Analyse der Immunantwort bei Spätmanifestationen der Lyme borreliose. Zentralblatt für Bakteriologie, Mikrobiologie und Hygiene A 267: 549-558

Wilske B, Preac-Mursic V, Schierz G, Kühbeck R, Barbour A G, Kramer M 1988b Antigenic variability of *Borrelia burgdorgeri*. Annals of the New York Academy of Science 539: 126-143

Wilske B, Preac-Mursic V, Schierz G, Liegl G, Gueye W 1989a Detection of IgM and IgG antibodies to *Borrelia burgdorferi* using different strains as antigen. Proceedings of the Lyme borreliosis update Europe. Baden 2-4 Juni 1987. Zentralblatt fur Bakteriologie (Suppl) 18: 299-309

Wilske B, Schierz G, Preac-Mursic V, Pfister H W, Weber K, von Busch K, Baruschke A 1989b IgM- and IgG immune response to *Borrelia burgdorferi* in erythema migrans and neuroborreliosis. Proceedings of the Lymeborreliosis update Europe. Baden 2-4 Juni 1987. Zentralblatt fur Bakteriologie (Suppl) 18: 290-298

Discussion of paper presented by B. Wilske

Discussed by E. Guy
Reported by P. K. Peterson

Those people who are perhaps not involved in the front line of Lyme disease may have the impression that the problems of serodiagnosis are great—they are! Serodiagnosis is one area which is holding back our understanding of the disease. In terms of epidemiology it is difficult to do seroprevalence studies with a test that is not 100% trustworthy, and there are also problems for clinicians both in diagnosis and in trying to define the spectrum of the disease.

A recent letter in the Lancet reported a case of Raynaud's syndrome with a positive Lyme serology. The link between that disease and Lyme disease was based on one test from one commercial kit. False positives are often a problem where a number of clinical symptoms supposedly associated with Lyme disease are implicated on the basis of tests that may not be 100%.

I shall try to summarize some of the problems. Diagnosis is one—the problem being to try to develop better tests. In early Lyme disease we often see low levels of antibody. Johnson showed some Westernblots with poor antibody response in the disease and, indeed, picking out the low-level specific antibodies is a problem where relatively high levels of antibody binding are seen in the sera of healthy adults.

It has been mentioned that the flagellin protein cross-reacts heavily on Western blot. A number of heat-stress proteins in Lyme disease also can cause problems. We have analyzed Western blots of Forestry Commission workers in an endemic area in the UK. In those people chronically exposed, we see a very characteristic pattern of antibody binding to the flagellin and to Wilske's pC protein. (A Swedish strain of the organism was used in the Western blot.) The problem with serodiagnosis is that none of these people was ever ill with any symptoms of Lyme disease. This underlines one of the particular problems in diagnosing disease in endemic areas—people may come in who will have specific antibodies, well-developed immune responses to Lyme disease, but their symptoms may be due to another aetiology, e.g., as in facial palsy. We have had patients with facial palsies not due to Lyme disease but who had positive serologies due to previous *B. burgdorferi* infection.

We do have a problem with the pC protein. If our sample had been sent in with symptoms consistent with early Lyme disease we would have a serious problem in trying to ascertain whether it was a true case of Lyme disease. Also, we have a number of proteins in the range 60-85KDa—the stress proteins—which can also cause problems in the tests.

Looking at clinical cases of Lyme disease, we have studied sera from five patients, four of whom remembered having a tick bite. All five had erythema migrans; all developed flu-like symptoms and all developed facial palsy, three left-sided, one right-sided and one bilateral. All responded to treatment with antibiotics. So, as best as we can tell these are good clinical cases of Lyme disease.

The samples were all taken at between 3 and 5 months after onset of symptoms and in at least two of the cases it was very easy to diagnose Lyme disease, bearing in mind that patients living in endemic areas may have antibodies in any event. To overcome that problem we have to consider IgM antibodies as well, and in this sample at least two of the patients have only antibodies to flagellin and to 60KDa protein, which some would claim is highly cross-reactive. Whether that is the common antigen protein I am not convinced.

Five other sera tested were from syphilis patients. Syphilis sera cross-react heavily in the Lyme test. This is not a major problem in diagnosis but it illustrates clearly the potentially large number of *B. burgdorferi* proteins that can be detected by non-specific sera.

A number of the new strategies for diagnosing Lyme disease concentrate more on how the antigen is presented in the test. Current popular methods of immunofluorescence and ELISA tend to use wholesale sonicated or unsonicated antigen. The new generation tests, including that described by Wilske, use flagellin ELISA, which is apparently better when compared with its cross-reactivity on Western blot. The apparent superiority of flagellin ELISA is due to the antigen being non-denatured, or essentially non- denatured. On Western blot we look at sequential or continuous epitopes, whereas with the flagellin ELISA we look at discontinuous epitopes, which are apparently more *B. burgdorferi* specific. We have investigated the sera from well defined Lyme cases and the syphilis sera in an immunoprecipitation assay. Viable cells of *B. burgdorferi* were surface labelled with ^{125}I and the proteins disaggregated under mild detergent conditions (to conserve as much of the native conformation as possible). These were then reacted with the patients' sera, immunoprecipitated, the immunoprecipitated proteins run out on GL followed by autoradiography. The resulting bands were the surface exposed or surface associated proteins of *B. burgdorferi* that are detected by the sera.

The results were fairly clear-cut. Sera from all Lyme disease patients reacted to some extent with some of the surface exposed proteins of *B. burgdorferi* under the conditions of the assay. The syphilis sera did not react at all, suggesting that most of the cross-reacting epitopes with which the syphilis sera reacts are occluded when the antigen is presented in this form. This may explain why some tests—the Dako flagellin ELISA test and the Sigma enriched flagellin ELISA test—may be improving matters by conserving *B. burgdorferi* specific epitopes, but are also cutting down on a number of accessible cross-reacting epitopes.

One point of caution. If we look at the Lyme sera no one protein reacts well with all of the sera. A Sigma representative would say that his kit is better than the Dako kit because it includes several antigens, whereas the Dako kit includes only one. I am told that in the USA, cases have been seen where Lyme disease patients have no detectable antibody to the flagellin protein—a point which must be borne in mind if we are to develop new tests.

Until now it has been generally accepted where tests are available that looking at different strains does not have too much effect on the results, particularly on ELISA. On Western blot the proteins have different molecular weights and some proteins will be detected and others not. However, it appears that if we are to begin developing more specific tests, we may also need tests that are more strain specific. Hence the work that Wilske is carrying out is so important—that we do characterize and understand these epitopes, immunodominant epitopes, in different strains of the organism.

In closing, we are discussing new technologies and it would be wrong not to include PCR. This may be a very useful technique, particularly in animal model studies for evaluating tissue infiltration by the organism, and perhaps in incidence studies in animal reservoirs and in tick vectors. I suspect too that many people are now looking urgently at clinical samples to try to determine whether there is a good clinical use for PCR in diagnosis. The PCR primers that I have designed were based on the American strain B31, the sequence from the OspA protein. I tried to choose sequences that I thought would be conserved between different strains. Studies to date suggest that the PCR primers, if chosen carefully, can detect different strains of the organism.

Section II:
Vaccines

Chairman: K. P. W. J. McAdam

5. Polysaccharide vaccines: vaccines needed for the 1990s

A. A. Lindberg

INTRODUCTION

Carbohydrates are found in the cell envelope of bacteria either as pure carbohydrates in the form of a capsule, or covalently linked to lipid forming a glycoconjugate named lipopolysaccharide (LPS). Carbohydrates are ideal as carriers of individuality. Whereas three amino acids can be combined into six peptides, three hexoses can combine into 1056 different oligosaccharides. This is due to the ability of hexoses to form covalent linkages with any of five carbon atoms in the hexose ring, and to do it in either the α- or β-configuration. This inherent variability is recognized in the great number of polysaccharide structures, with different antigenic epitopes, which are formed in different bacteria.

The polysaccharides are bacterial virulence factors and are used as such by the bacteria to evade host defences. The evasion mechanism can either be to resist phagocytosis by mononuclear host cells, as for pneumococci and meningococci, or to be able to multiply intracellularly and spread to adjacent tissues, as for salmonellae. The rationale for attempting to develop vaccines against these and other bacteria is the observation that repeated exposure to a particular bacterium results in a diminished host susceptibility caused by an acquired immunity as a result of the exposure.

The potential of using polysaccharides as vaccines was demonstrated in 1945 when MacLeod et al showed that immunization with pneumococcal polysaccharides was followed by type-specific protection against the acquisition of pneumococcal infection. This landmark observation coincided, however, with the advent of antimicrobial agents, and halted polysaccharide vaccine development for several decades. However, in time the medical community became aware of some of the shortcomings of antibiotic treatment: the emergence of bacterial strains which were resistant to used antimicrobial agents, and that sometimes the treatment of a disease caused by a sensitive strain either left the patient with serious sequelae like deafness and mental retardation after a bacterial meningitis, or even worse, was fatal. In this paper current strategies for vaccine development, the nature of the immune response against polysaccharides, and prospects for development of more efficacious vaccines are described.

POLYSACCHARIDE VIRULENCE DETERMINANTS IN BACTERIAL PATHOGENS

Both *Streptococcus pneumoniae* and *Haemophilus influenzae* are encapsulated bacteria which are recognized as major pathogens in acute respiratory tract infections, meningitis, otitis media, etc. World-wide such infections are most common in the very young and the very old. Our knowledge of the actual disease burden caused by these organisms is incomplete, and particularly so in developing countries. A recent attempt to estimate the size of the problem was made by the Institute of Medicine's Committee on Issues and Priorities for New Vaccine Development, and their findings were published in 1986 (New Vaccine Development 1986) A summary of the number of deaths for four pathogens is given in Table 5.1 and discussed below.

S. pneumoniae is by a wide margin the bacterial pathogen where most infections may have a fatal outcome. More than one-third of these occur in children below the age of 5 years. The estimated number of fatalities caused by *H. influenzae* with the serotype b capsule is considerably smaller. But here 90% of the infections terminating in death are seen in children under 5 years. It should be noted that the figures are estimates of death in all types of infections caused by these bacteria.

Neisseria meningitidis causes almost exclusively bacterial meningitis and accounts for about one-third of all cases of bacterial meningitis world-wide. It is a very severe disease which untreated has a mortality approaching 100%. Meningococcal disease appears as endemic (caused by capsular polysaccharide types A, B, C, Y and W135) all over the world. The greatest frequency is seen in infants and very young children. In epidemics, which occur sporadically but where the incidence may be as high as 500 per 100 000 population, one epidemic strain is spread and then older children and young adults are also taken ill.

Typhoid fever caused by *Salmonella typhi* is an enteric fever more than a diarrhoeal disease. *S. typhi* is unique among more than 2000 serotypes of the genus *Salmonella* in being a strict human pathogen, and in having the Vi capsular antigen which is a homopolymer of *O*- and *N*-acetylated β1, 4-linked *N*-acetylgalactosaminuronic acid (Heyns et al 1959). Typhoid fever, although occurring in all age groups, has its greatest mortality in school-children and adults (Table 5.1). The prospects for vaccination against typoid fever are treated separately in Chapter 6.

Table 5.1 Estimated number of deaths (from New Vaccine Development, 1986) resulting from bacterial pathogens with polysaccharide virulence determinants and with prospects for vaccine development

Pathogen	No. of deaths in thousands per age group (years)			
	< 5	5-14	15-59	≥ 60
Streptococcus pneumoniae	3687	1858	1949	3115
Haemophilus influenzae type b	131	5	7	2
Neisseria meningitidis	9	10	14	2
Salmonella typhi	35	215	319	12
Total	3862	2088	2289	3131

MECHANISMS IN ANTICARBOHYDRATE IMMUNITY

Humoral antibody defences

The mechanisms of host defence against encapsulated and/or lipopolysaccharide-containing organisms are multiple and complex. Polysaccharides are immunogenic and induce type-specific immunity when given to adults. This holds true for polyvalent pneumococcal vaccine (Austrian et al 1976, Bolan et al 1986), the polyribosylribitol phosphate capsule of *H. influenzae* type b (Peltola et al 1984) and meningococcal types A and C polysaccharides (Gotschlich et al 1969a). However, when given to children under 2 years the immune response is low and inconsistent (Gotschlich et al 1969a, Austrian et al 1976, Cowan et al 1978, Peltola et al 1984, Bolan et al 1986). The insufficient ability of young children to mount an efficient antibody response coincides with their great susceptibility to infections with these organisms. Acquisition by age of resistance based on immune mechanisms can thus be considered as a developmental process. The factors and mechanisms behind this process are complex, and have only recently started to become understood.

The two main families of immunocompetent cells which are stimulated to proliferation and differentiation when recognizing non-self antigens via their cell surface receptors are the B and T lymphocytes. The B cells are responsible for the humoral immunity, whereas the T cells are responsible for cell-mediated immunity plus the regulation of the humoral immunoresponse via T-helper and T-suppressor cells. Bacterial polysaccharide and lipopolysaccharide antigens appear not to require T lymphocytes for antibody induction (which most protein antigens or hapten-protein conjugates do). They instead trigger B cell activation directly without participation of T cells and are classified as T-independent antigens. Salient characteristics of T-independent and T-dependent antigens are listed in Table 5.2.

Polysaccharide antigens

The characteristics of T-independent antigens have largely been worked out using the murine model (Mosier & Subbarao 1982). The studies have demonstrated that there are two separate classes of T-independent antigens: class I, of which lipopolysaccharides are an example; and class II, represented by pure polysaccharide antigens (Mosier & Subbarao 1982, Subbarao & Mosier 1982). By the early 1970s it was

Table 5.2 Characteristics of T-independent and T-dependent antigens

Type of antigen	T-independent Type I lipopolysaccharide	T-independent Type II Polysaccharide	T-dependent Protein or saccharide-protein complex
T lymphocytes required for antibody induction	−	−	+
IgG subclass distribution	IgG3/IgG2b	IgG3	IgG1/IgG2a
IgM to IgG switch	−	−	+
Booster/anamnestic effect	−	−	+
Response in athymic nude mice	+	+	−
Response in CBA/N mice	+	−	+
Response in infants	+	−	+
Requirement of Lyb5+ mature B cell subset	−	+	−

recognized that CBA/N mice are unresponsive to polysaccharide antigens (Scher 1982). The mechanism behind the unresponsiveness was the apparent lack of a subset of mature B cells which have the Lyb5 cell surface marker. This B cell subset appears to be essential for a response to polysaccharide antigens. Normal neonatal mice also respond poorly to polysaccharide antigens. This is, however, caused by immaturity and at the age of 8-10 weeks normal antibody levels are achieved.

However, there is a constant presence of specific B-cell precursors throughout development as studied with a dextran preparation (Lundqvist et al 1986). The addition to the immaturity of a diminished amplifier B cell activity and an excessive T-suppressor activity to pneumococcal type 3 polysaccharide has been observed in neonatal mice (Baker et al 1977).

Lipopolysaccharide antigens
In contrast to pure polysaccharides the lipopolysaccharide antigens elicit a T-independent type I response (Table 5.2). This is recognized as an ability to elicit an antibody production in athymic as well as CBA/N mice. Otherwise both type I and II responses are characterized by IgG3 antibody responses, with type I responses also seen in the IgG2b subclass. Downregulation of the amount of antibody produced by suppressor T cells and clonal expansion by amplifier T cells has been observed both for *Escherichia coli* and *Pseudomonas aeruginosa* lipopolysaccharide (Type I) and pneumococcal and meningococcal polysaccharides (Type II) antigens (Elkins et al 1987, Muller & Apicella 1988, Taylor & Bright 1989). The strict classification of the polysaccharide responses as either T1 or T2 has been challenged by Nossal & Pike (1984) who argued that the antigens form a spectrum rather than two sharp nodal groups.

Saccharide-protein conjugates
The observation that protein or hapten-protein complexes are T-dependent antigens which stimulate a response in CBA/N mice, do not require the Lyb5 + B cell subset and display a memory function, has stimulated the conversion of polysaccharides to saccharide-protein conjugates and hereby from T independence to T dependence (Table 5.2) (Braley-Mullen 1980). The first study done with pneumococcal polysaccharide conjugates (Braley-Mullen 1980) was soon followed by meningococcal group C ( ) and *H. influenzae* type b saccharide-protein conjugates (Beuvery et al 1982). The conjugate antigens elicit an increased total antipolysaccharide antibody response, an enhanced response to booster injection, an antibody response in young individuals and an increased IgG/IgM ratio in induced antibodies (Table 5.2).

Glycoconjugate antigens
Polysaccharides used as vaccines have been isolated as the large macromolecular complexes in which they are found on the bacterial cell envelope, or in the cell culture supernatant. For the production of glycoconjugates a number of questions are relevant: (i) what saccharide size is optimal? (ii) which immunogenic carrier protein should be chosen? (iii) what coupling method is optimal and acceptable? (iv) what saccharide/protein ratio is optimal? (v) are adjuvants needed? (vi) what is the optimal dose? The optimization of all these parameters in humans, and in particular

Table 5.3 Structures of some *Streptococcus pneumoniae* capsular polysaccharides (for references see Jennings 1990)

Serotype	Structure
3	→4)βD-Glc*p*(1→3)βD-Glc*p*A(1→

6A
$$\rightarrow 2)\alpha\text{D-Gal}p(1\rightarrow3)\alpha\text{D-Gle}p(1\rightarrow3)\alpha\text{L-Rha}p(1\rightarrow3)\text{Ribitol(5-P-O-}$$
with
$$\overset{\text{O}}{\underset{\overset{\|}{\text{O}}}{|}}$$

6(B)
$$\rightarrow 2)\alpha\text{D-Gal}p(1\rightarrow3)\alpha\text{D-Glc}p(1\rightarrow3)\alpha\text{L-Rha}p(1\rightarrow4)\text{Ribitol(5-P-O-}$$
with
$$\overset{\text{O}}{\underset{\overset{\|}{\text{O}}}{|}}$$

7F
→6)αDGal*p*(1→3)βL-Rha*p*(1→4)βD-Glc*p*(1→3)βD-Gal*p*NAc(1→

```
      2             2                    4
      ↑             |                    ↑
      1            AcO                   1
   βD-Galp              αD-GlcpNAc(1→2)αL-Rhap
```

| 8 | →4)βD-GlepAc(1→4)βD-Glc*p*(1→4)αD-Glc*p*(1→4)αD-Gal*p*(1→ |

19F
$$\rightarrow 4)\beta\text{D-Man}p\text{NAc}(1\rightarrow4)\alpha\text{D-Glc}p(1\rightarrow2)\alpha\text{L-Rha}p(1\text{-P-O-}$$
with
$$\overset{\text{O}}{\underset{\overset{\|}{\text{O}}}{|}}$$

23F
```
             αL-Rhap
               1
               ↓
               2
→4)βDGlcp(1→4)βD-Galp(1→4)βL-Rhap(→
               3
               |
               O
               |
           O=P-O-2-Glycerol
               |
               O
```

in infants, is limited by ethical constraints since we are obliged to study only such candidates as have good prospects of inducing immunity. Hence, data on structure-immunogenicity relationships have to be obtained either from animal studies, or by the difficult comparison of different conjugates (which differ in several variables) used in human trials.

It is possible that characteristics of the conjugate are the underlying cause of observations such as that the conjugate elicits an Ig subclass response typical of a T-independent rather than T-dependent type (Mäkelä et al 1987). Probably the most difficult variable to control is that of the saccharide component. The saccharides are almost exclusively derived through chemical degradations of the isolated macromolecular complex. Our ability to degrade is then a consequence of whether there are linkages that can be cleaved (by acid hydrolysis or endoenzymes) or not, whether this procedure does destroy other structures (like sialic acid residues) or not, etc. Can we by such procedures manufacture equal size-equal structure saccharides? Unfortunately so far synthetic chemistry cannot provide saccharides larger than three to four sugars at a reasonable price. The fact that the biosynthetic process of saccharides requires synthesis of nucleotide sugars, glycosyl transferases and often repeating unit polymerases and that the genes for these products are scattered over the bacterial chromosome has delayed the use of recombinant-DNA and cloning techniques.

The functional classification of the conjugates as T-dependent antigens fails to define the cellular mechanisms that are involved. An understanding of the mechanisms whereby saccharide-specific B cells are activated by saccharide-protein conjugates will be critical both for evaluation of immune responses and for minimizing generation of saccharide-specific suppressor cells.

In a systematic attempt to study the antibody response with respect to (i) size of the saccharide moiety, (ii) the saccharide/protein ratio, and (iii) the coupling method, Seppälä & Mäkelä (1989) studied the immunogenicity of 13 α1, 6-dextran-chicken serum albumin conjugates in mice. The strongest responses were seen with conjugates with small dextran molecules (mol. wt 1000-4000) coupled to the protein via the reducing end, and with carbohydrate/protein ratios in the range 0.17-0.49. The molecular background for the 10-fold better antigenicity of the small dextran is unknown. A possible explanation is that the small dextran does not interfere with the cell collaboration which probably is necessary for a good antibody response (Lanzavecchia 1985, Buus et al 1987). A comparative study along the same lines was done using various *H. influenzae* polyribosylribitol-phosphate conjugates in infants and will be discussed next (Anderson at al 1989).

Mucosal immune defence

Humoral antibodies form the main host defence by promotion of phagocytosis, aided by the complement system, of invading encapsulated bacteria like pneumococci, meningococci and *H. influenzae*. However, the host defence mechanisms which protect against disease caused by non-encapsulated bacteria which are intracellular pathogens like salmonellae and shigellae are less well understood. The host-defence mechanism which is primarily mobilized is the local secretory response with IgA and IgM antibodies (Brandtzaeg et al 1987). The secretory IgA plays the most important role in this defence, and since it does not activate complement (or only very little), it acts as a non-inflammatory antibody. The fact that there are 10^{10} immunoglobulin-producing cells per metre of intestine as compared to altogether 2.5×10^{10} such cells in the bone marrow, spleen and lymph nodes points to the importance of this host defence mechanism. Approximately 40 mg of secretory IgA is secreted into the gut per kg body weight per day compared with a total daily production of 30 mg IgG per kg. It is evident that IgA (secretory plus monomeric IgA in the circulation and intestinal tissues) is the dominating antibody class.

Immunoglobulin-producing plasma cells in mucosal membranes and exocrinic glands are developed from circulating B lymphocytes. They are found in lymphoepithelial structures in the intestine—aggregates of which are called Peyer's patches—and collectively known as gut-associated lymphoid tissues (GALT). In the respiratory tract they are known as bronchus-associated lymphoid tissues (BALT). Both GALT and BALT do contain MHC class II-positive antigen-presenting cells plus T-helper and T-suppressor cells. Therefore all components required for an immune response are present in the mucosal tissues. There are also cells involved in the switch of B-lymphocytes from IgM to IgA synthesis. Antigen-stimulated cells migrate from the mucosa via lymph nodes to the circulation before reaching the lamina propria of the intestine and other glandular tissues (Mestecky 1987). There they mature to plasma cells which secrete IgA for less than a week. This migration of antigen-stimulated B cells, in particular from GALT, to the respiratory tract, the mammary and other exocrine glands, is actually an active dissemination of secretory immunity to all mucosal surfaces.

However, bacteria which overcome the local sIgA (IgM) host defence invade the epithelial cells. In the non-immune host intracellular multiplication, and subsequent dissemination to adjacent cells, the lymphatics and circulation eventually lead to cell death and bacteraemia. In immune individuals the multiplication and subsequent dissemination is controlled. The mechanism(s) behind this intracellular control are not understood. Antibody-dependent cytotoxicity has been proposed as one possible mechanism. Should the bacteria manage to penetrate into the circulation, antibodies plus complement form a final barrier acting with bactericidal and/or opsonizing mechanisms.

PNEUMOCOCCAL VACCINES

The revival of the capsular polysaccharide vaccine against *Streptococcus pneumoniae* can be attributed to Austrian (1988). Among the 83 capsular serotypes of pneumococci first 14, and subsequently 23, were incorporated in the vaccine which contains 50 μg of each polysaccharide. The absence of antigenic competition among the T-independent antigens makes it possible to subject the immune system to such a heavy load. The protective efficacy against the serotypes represented in the vaccine has been investigated intensively and adequately demonstrated for adults (Austrian et al 1976, Bolan et al 1986). In children the protective efficacy is not sufficiently high, as was amply demonstrated in a study in Australian children (Douglas & Miles 1984). Another study in a community in the developing world by Riley et al (1986) showed that the 14-valent vaccine caused a 37% reduction in pneumonia and an 87% reduction in mortality. Likewise, in a study in Finland on the protective efficacy against otitis media, a partial protection (against certain pneumococcal serotypes) was observed (Mäkelä et al 1981).

The inadequate protective effect of either the 14- or the 23-valent vaccine correlates with the inability of the young child to elicit an humoral antibody response. In this respect the lack of the immune system in the infant to respond is similar to that of neonatal mice: a child under 2 years is similar to a mouse <10 weeks old. However, the immaturity is not seen with all polysaccharides since young children (and mice) respond at the age of 2-6 months (and 2-4 weeks) to the type 3 polysaccharide (Douglas et al 1983, Barrett et al 1984). Intermediate responses were seen against the type 23 polysaccharide, whereas no response in either IgG or IgM was seen against the polysaccharides of types 6 (6A or 6B), 18 and 19. The response to the type 6 (A or B) polysaccharides may in fact be delayed until the child has reached school age (Kaplan et al 1982). The structure of the saccharides (Table 5.3) has so far failed to reveal a structure-immunogenicity relationship. This differential responsiveness against the various pneumococcal polysaccharides suggests that different factors control the immune response. The differences most likely must be sought in the structural (and conformational) features of the polysaccharides. Available evidence indicates that the ontogeny of human immune responses against polysaccharide antigens may parallel the T-independent type I system of the mouse.

Protection against pneumococcal infection correlates with the appearance of appropriate antibody titres in serum. Both IgM and IgG antibodies are formed, and among the IgG isotypes the IgG2 antibody (which is equivalent to IgG3 in the mouse) has been found to dominate (Barrett & Ayoub 1986). The preimmunization titres against IgG2 were up to fourfold higher than the IgG1, IgG3 and IgG4 titres. Post-immunization a significant fourfold rise was seen in IgG2 titre, whereas the titres of the other subclasses were unchanged. This IgG2 dominance was noted against types 3, 6, 18, 19 and 23 polysaccharides.

Recent studies where adult volunteers were given the 23-valent vaccine showed that systemic immunization also induces serum and secretory IgA responses predominantly of the IgA2 isotype (Heilmann et al 1988, Lue et al 1988). The observed responses were most likely dependent on previous exposure to and priming with pneumococci which are known colonizers of the airways of most individuals, particularly in childhood when up to 100% may be carriers (Austrian 1988). The antibody-secreting cells have the ability to 'home' to mucosal tissues for eventual secretion of sIgA. Here the antibodies may be effective in controlling colonization of the mucosal surface. Such an affect of sIgA is likely a more effective host defence mechanism than phagocytosis as a result of a binding of IgA to the cell envelope since IgA is known as a poor opsonizing antibody.

The persistence of elicited antipneumococcal antibody titres was studied in 21 subjects one decade after a single dose of a polyvalent vaccine (Mufson et al 1987). Only titres against types 7F and 8 were significantly higher ($P < 0.01$) than preimmunization titres, whereas titres against types 1, 3, 4, 12F 14 and 19F had declined. However, the individual variations were obvious. These data confirm earlier observations about the persistence of antipolysaccharide antibody titres, but indicate that variations both in individuals and in titres against particular serotypes can be expected. The question of whether reimmunization shall be recommended for the pneumococcal vaccine, and when, cannot yet be answered.

The poor immunogenicity of most pneumococcal polysaccharides stimulated the idea of making glycoconjugate vaccines composed of pneumococcal saccharides linked to an immunogenic carrier thereby creating a T-dependent vaccine (Table 5.2). To achieve this a smaller portion of the polysaccharide—6 to 25 monosaccharides—obtained through cleavage of the macromolecule should be made reactogenic to be covalently linked to the carrier molecule. Although a hexasaccharide (equivalent to three repeating units) of the type 3 polysaccharide was coupled to bovine serum albumin almost 10 years ago and found immunogenic and eliciting protection in a mouse model (Snippe et al 1983), the development has been slow. This is most likely so for the following reasons: (i) a series of conjugates would have to be produced, (ii) several pneumococcal polysaccharides are not easily degraded to smaller fragments (iii) synthetic alternatives to degraded saccharides are not available.

Besides the type 3 saccharide only saccharides of the type 6A and 6B capsular polysaccharides (Table 5.3), and generated by acid hydrolysis, have been converted into glycoconjugates and tested (Porro et al 1985, Sarnaik et al 1990). Children with sickle cell anaemia, and with defective or absent splenic function, do not elicit a significant antibody response to the group 6 (6A or 6B) polysaccharide up to the age of 6 years. The 6B conjugate elicited antibodies after the first injection and booster responses were stimulated (Sarnaik et al 1990). It appears that conjugates may confer protective immunity both to normal individuals and to patients with partial immunodeficiencies not responding to the polysaccharide vaccine.

In view of the disease and death burden of pneumococcal infections (Table 5.1) there is no doubt that the development of a pneumococcal vaccine containing glycoconjugates representing at least the 'infant types' 6A, 6B, 14, 18C, 19A, 19F and 23F has the highest priority. It holds the prospect of being a powerful asset in reducing morbidity and mortality in pneumococcal disease.

Haemophilus influenzae TYPE B VACCINES

The total mortality in invasive *H. influenzae* infection, almost exclusively caused by type b bacteria, is not as overwhelming as that of pneumococcal infection (Table 5.1). However, the fact that up to one-third of those surviving their meningitis, in spite of adequate antibiotic treatment, have permanent neurological sequelae has made development of an effective *H. influenzae* type b capsular polysaccharide vaccine important. Intense efforts during the last decade have been successful and today effective and extremely safe vaccines are available.

The capsule polysaccharide of type b is a relatively simple structure, being a D-ribofuranosyl-D-ribitol phosphate polymer (PRP) (Table 5.4). Endgroup phosphoric esters detected in the capsule may have functioned as the original linkage to the outer membrane (Egan et al 1982).

The use of an isolated purified PRP polysaccharide as a vaccine proved its efficacy in children over 2 years and adults (Peltola et al 1984). However, the poor immunogenicity in infants and the appearance of 'vaccine failures' in adequately

Table 5.4 Structures of some *Haemophilus influenzae* and *Neisseria meningitidis* capsular polysaccharides (for references see Jennings 1990)

Serotype	Structure
H. influenzae b	$\begin{array}{c} O \\ | \\ \rightarrow 3)\beta\text{D}\text{Rib}f(1 \rightarrow 1)\text{D-Ribitol}(5\text{-P-O-} \\ || \\ O \end{array}$
N. meningitidis A	$\begin{array}{c} \text{OAc} \\ | \qquad O \\ 3 \qquad | \\ \rightarrow 6\alpha\text{D-Man}p\text{Ac}(1\text{-P-O-} \\ || \\ O \end{array}$
N. meningitidis B	$\rightarrow 8)\alpha\text{D-Neu}p\text{NAc}(2\rightarrow$
N. meningitidis C	$\begin{array}{c} \text{OAc} \\ | \\ 7/8 \\ \rightarrow 9)\alpha\text{D-Neu}p\text{NAc}(2\rightarrow \end{array}$

vaccinated older children propelled the development of conjugate vaccine candidates (Schneerson et al 1980). This development was much facilitated by the fact that there is only one structure to be recognized and chemically it is relatively simple. Today there are at least four different conjugates under evaluation (Eskola et al 1987, Anderson et al 1989, Smith et al 1989, Tudor-Williams et al 1989, Madore et al 1990, Vella et al 1990). They differ in their composition with respect to the protein carrier, the size of the hapten saccharide, the type of linkage between the hapten and carrier, and the ratio of saccharide to protein (see Smith et al 1989, Table 1). Although all information is not yet in, it appears as if a key factor is that the saccharide should be oligomeric (not T-independent) and coupled with a high hapten load onto the carrier (Anderson et al 1989). Such conjugates (i) have a greater immunogenicity than the PRP in adults, (ii) are immunogenic in young infants as early as 2 months of age, (iii) elicits an IgG1 response which is both bactericidal and promotes opsonization and is protective, (iv) elicit an antibody response which is long-lived and can be boostered, (v) elicit antibody responses also in children with impaired antibody responses, i.e. 'vaccine failures' either for unidentified reasons or individuals who lack the Km (1) allotype (Weinberg & Granoff 1990). The protective efficacy in Finland appears to be complete (P H Mäkelä, personal communication).

The molecular basis for the effectiveness of using the mutant diptheria toxin (CRM197) as a carrier is just beginning to be understood. A peptide region encompassing 14 amino acids (CRM370-383) was found to contain a T cell epitope of the CRM protein (Bixter et al 1989). This means that a synthetic 13 amino acid long peptide representing a defined T cell epitope of CRM197 can be used as carrier. Hereby a glycoconjugate vaccine defined by physicochemical parameters can be produced.

Another leading candidate vaccine utilizes a *Neisseria meningitidis* serogroup B outer membrane protein complex (proteins P1.2, P2a and P4) (Vella et al 1990). Besides being a good T cell-dependent immunogen, immunization with the conjugate has the potential to elicit protective immunity against *N. meningitidis* serogroup B against whose capsular polysaccharide (Table 5.4) humans of all ages fail to respond (see later).

With commonly used vaccination schemes it is reasonable to assume that children will not have developed antibody titres which can be considered protective (a titre of >1.0 μg/ml is widely accepted as correlating with protection) until they are 3-4 months old. Up to then maternal antibodies may confer protection.

The conclusions which can be reached are that there are commercially available *H. influenzae* type b glycoconjugate vaccines which appear to be ready for public health use. As such they are well suited to be included in the routine immunization schemes used for young children (equivalent to the Expanded Programme on Immunization, EPI).

Neisseria meningitidis GROUPS A, B AND C VACCINES

The development of the vaccines against groups A and C meningococcal capsular polysaccharides was a successful achievement during the 1960s. The polysaccharides can be obtained in high-molecular-weight immunogenic form by precipitation from the culture medium, and this property is critical to their effectiveness as vaccines (Kabat & Bezer 1958, Gotschlich et al 1969b). The large size is due to the presence of lipid substituents on these chains which causes micelle formation of individual polysaccharide chains (Gotschlich et al 1981). A bivalent vaccine containing groups A and C polysaccharides was prepared and successfully used in prevention of meningitis (Gotschlich et al 1969a, Artenstein et al 1970).

It was recognized early that, although the groups A and C meningococcal polysaccharides are efficacious in older children and adults, their effectiveness in infants is only marginal (Goldschneider et al 1973). As discussed earlier for pneumococcal and *H. influenzae* type b polysaccharides, this is most likely so because of an immaturity of the infant immune system. The solution to this problem will probably reside in the development of glycoconjugate vaccines.

The relatively simple structures of the groups A and C polysaccharides (Table 5.4) have facilitated their covalent linkage to carrier proteins (Jennings & Lugowski 1981). After controlled periodate oxidation of the group A polysaccharide, the terminal 2-acetamido-2-deoxy-D-mannose residue of each saccharide was coupled to tetanus toxoid by reductive amination. This method minimizes the possibility of polysaccharide modification, which is important in conjugate production, and also eliminates the risk for cross-linking. The meningococcal A and C conjugates when used for immunization of mice elicited polysaccharide-specific IgG responses suggesting that they had been converted to T-dependent antigens (Jennings & Lugowski 1981). It is likely that the conjugates should be equally immunogenic in young infants.

The group B meningococcal polysaccharide, an α 2,8-linked sialic acid homopolymer (Table 5.4), was found to be poorly immunogenic in man (Wyle et al 1982). The most likely explanation for this is that the structure, which is also found in a brain glycoprotein involved in neural cell adhesion (Edelman 1983, Finne et al 1983) is recognized as 'self' by the human immune system and, as a consequence, antibody production against the homopolymer is suppressed. The fact that conversion of the group B polymer from a T-independent polysaccharide to a T-dependent antigen by conjugation to tetanus toxoid through its terminal non-reducing sialic acid failed to enhance its immunogenicity (Jennings & Lugowski 1981) is in strong support for the 'self' hypothesis.

Because of the incidence of group B meningococcal meningitis, attempts have been made to modify the structure so that it is not recognized as 'self' but still elicits an antibody response which would recognize the native B polysaccharide (Jennings et al 1986). The common epitope on the group B polysaccharide is only contained in a saccharide of at least 10 sialic acid residues, which suggests that it is conformationally controlled (Finne & Mäkelä 1985, Jennings et al 1985). The

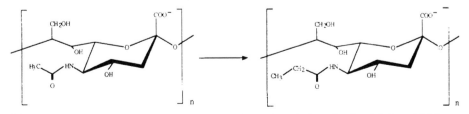

Figure 5.1 *Neisseria meningitidis* group B polysaccharide (left) and *N*-propionylated derivate (right).

antigenicity of the B saccharide was found to be dependent on the retention of both carboxylate and N-carbonyl groups (Fig. 5.1, Jennings et al 1986). Removal of the N-acetyl groups of the sialic acid residues by strong base followed by replacement with N-propionyl groups and subsequent coupling to tetanus toxoid gave a neoglycoconjugate. Mice immunized with the N-propionylated conjugate responded with much higher titres of B polysaccharide-specific antibodies than the native B polysaccharide conjugate (Jennings et al 1985). A pronounced booster effect was noticeable after three injections. The antibodies elicited in mice were found to be bactericidal for group B meningococci (Jennings et al 1987).

The sialic acid homopolymer is also found in the capsular polysaccharide of *Escherichia coli* K1 bacteria which cause neonatal meningitis. A N-propionylated B saccharide conjugate vaccine would therefore be expected to be able to elicit an immune response protective against both meningococcal group B and *E. coli* K1 meningitis. Concerns about the risk that immunization could break tolerance against the fetal brain glycopeptide have caused hesitation against a possible use of this prototype vaccine.

STREPTOCOCCUS GROUP B

Infections caused by group B streptococci are, together with *E. coli* K1 infections, a leading cause of neonatal sepsis and meningitis, and are associated with a significant morbidity and mortality (Baker & Edwards 1983). Since the infection is neonatal the infant is not the target for vaccination. The observation that infants born to mothers with high titres of antipolysaccharide antibodies are less likely to fall ill in group B infection (Kasper & Jennings 1982) has stimulated attempts to develop a vaccine. The target group for a group B streptococcal vaccine is pregnant women or young women before pregnancy.

The group B streptococci have capsular polysaccharides which distinguish them as types Ia, Ib, II, III, and IV. The structures of these polysaccharides have been determined, with the exception of type IV (Jennings 1990). Streptococci with serotypes I to III are all considered as invasive, but type III strains are most commonly isolated from infants. In particular, in infants with meningitis, type III strains account for almost 90% of all isolates (Baker & Kasper 1985). The structure of the type III polysaccharide is as follows:

$\rightarrow$4)βD-Glc$p$(1$\rightarrow$6)βD-Glc$p$NAc(1$\rightarrow$3)βD-Gal$p$(1$\rightarrow$

$\qquad$ 4

$\qquad$ $\uparrow$

$\qquad$ 1

aD-Neu$p$NAc(2$\rightarrow$3)βD-Gal$p$

The branch disaccharide with a sialyl residue in the terminal non-reducing end in the type III polysaccharide (and also in types Ia and Ib saccharides) is the same as the endgroup oligosaccharide in human blood group M and N glycoproteins (Sadler et al 1979). The acquisition of this disaccharide in the group B streptococcal polysaccharides, as of an α2, 8 sialic acid homopolymer in group B meningococci (see earlier), is most likely a potent virulence factor. Through molecular mimicry the bacterium masquerades as 'self', thereby evading the host's immune defence mechanisms.

The asialo-trisaccharide repeating unit of the type III polysaccharide is identical to that of pneumococcal type 14 capsular polysaccharide (Fisher et al 1978). However, only antibodies directed against the native type III polysaccharide showed a high correlation with protection in human sera (Kasper et al 1979). This does not imply that the immunity is directed against the 'self' sialylated disaccharide, but indicates that the disaccharide is a conformational element controlling the entire polysaccharide and thereby its epitopes (Jennings et al 1984).

So far no group B streptococcal vaccine is commercially available. It would be preferable to have a conjugate vaccine but the development of the saccharide portion is faced with the problems of retaining the extremely acid-labile sialyl residue.

CONCLUSIONS AND PROSPECTS FOR THE FUTURE

Development, particularly during the 1980s, has demonstrated that production of glycoconjugate vaccines which consist of a relatively small saccharide (6 to 25 monosaccharides) covalently linked to immunogenic carrier proteins has considerably improved prophylactic immunization. Compared with the native macromolecular polysaccharide vaccines, which are T-independent, the glyco-conjugate vaccines, which are T-dependent, are immunogenic in infants and elicit high boosterable antibody titres in them and also in older children and adults who are poor responders (vaccine failures) using polysaccharide vaccines (Table 5.5).

Today, efficacious vaccines which hold the prospect of being effective and extremely safe in prophylaxis of *H. influenzae* type b infections are ready for the market. For an improved pneumococcal vaccine, where glycoconjugates should be developed for certain of the 'poorly immunogenic' capsular types, the technology is available. Such a vaccine would globally probably have the largest public health impact on morbidity and mortality of all bacterial infections. Meningococcal group A and C glycoconjugate vaccines are also being developed. A prototype vaccine against group B meningococci has been developed and awaits further testing, depending on immunological considerations concerning the risk of a possible break of tolerance. A vaccine against streptococcal group B infections requires more developmental work.

Despite the progress we should be aware that the mechanisms behind the T

Table 5.5 Characteristics of human antibody responses against pure polysaccharides and saccharide-protein conjugates

Polysaccharides	Saccharide-protein conjugates
Poor response in children < 2 years	Good responses in infants and young children
Elicit moderate antibody responses of restricted isotype	Elicit high antibody responses
No induction of memory function	Induction of memory function with enhanced secondary responses
Poor responses in children with immunodeficiency diseases (lacking G2m(n) or Km(l) allotypes)	Good responses in individuals lacking Km(l) and G2m(n) allotypes

dependence are not yet understood. Such knowledge may be of importance for conjugate strategies aimed at maximizing the antibody production and minimizing the risk of eliciting suppressor mechanisms. The development of potent adjuvants will also be followed with great interest.

More polysaccharides in bacterial cell envelopes, as capsules or lipopolysaccharides, are being subject to conversion into conjugates from organisms like *Staphylococcus aureus, Klebsiella, E. coli, S. typhi, Shigella* and others.

The immunization with polysaccharides and glycoconjugates is directed towards elicitation of bactericidal and opsonizing antibodies. These vaccines have little potential for utilization of the possibility to elicit immune defence mechanisms operating at mucosal surfaces. Hereby the possibility of fending off invasive microorganisms at their port of entry is not utilized. Present attempts to deliver antigens via the oral route, in live attenuated bacteria or viruses, stimulating GALT and BALT, should be followed with interest. An effective mucosal immune system would benefit the mother, perhaps preventing her from being colonized in the genital tract with group B streptococci or *E. coli* K1 bacteria, as well as the infant influencing colonization patterns in early childhood.

ACKNOWLEDGEMENTS

This work has been supported by the Swedish Medical Research Council (grant no. 16X-656). The skilled secretarial assistance of Rose-Marie Hellberg is gratefully appreciated.

REFERENCES

Anderson P W, Pichichero M E, Stein E C et al 1989 Effect of oligosaccharide chain length, exposed terminal group, and hapten loading on the antibody response of human adults and infants to vaccines consisting of *Haemophilus influenza* type b capsular antigen uniterminallly coupled to the diphteria protein CRM 197, Journal of Immunology 142:2464-2468
Artenstein M S, Gold R, Zimmerly J G, Wyle F A, Schneider H, Harkins C 1970 Prevention of meningococcal disease by group C polysaccharide vaccine. New England Journal of Medicine 282:417-420
Austrian R 1988 Life with the pneumococcus. University of Pennsylvania Press, Philadelphia
Austrian R, Douglas R M, Schiffman G et al 1976 Prevention of pneumococcal penumonia by vaccination. Transactions of the Association of American Physicians 89:184-192
Baker C H, Edwards M S 1983 Group B streptococcal infections. In: Remington J S, Klein J O (eds) Infectious diseases of the fetus and newborn infant, 2nd edn. Saunders, Philadelphia, USA, pp 820-881
Baker C J, Kasper D L 1985 Group B streptococcal vaccines. Reviews of Infectious Diseases 7:458-467
Baker P J, Morse H C III, Cross S S, Stashak P W, Trescott B 1977 Maturation of regulatory factors influencing magnitude of antibody response to capsular polysaccharide of type III *Streptococcus penumoniae*. Journal of Infectious Diseases 136:220-224
Barrett D J, Ayoub E M 1986 IgG2 subclass restriction of antibody to pneumococcal polysaccharides. Clinical and Experimental Immunology 63:127-134
Barrett D J, Lee C G, Amman A A, Ayoub E M 1984 IgG and IgM pneumococcal polysaccharide antibody repsonses in infants. Pediatric Research 18:1067-1071
Beuvery E C, van Rossum F, Nagel J 1982 Comparison of the induction of immunoglobulin M and G antibodies in mice with purified pneumococcal type III and meningococcal group C polysaccharides and their protein conjugates. Infection and Immunity 37:15-22
Bixler G S Jr, Eby R, Dermody K M 1989 Synthetic peptide representing a T cell epitope of CRM197 substitutes as carrier molecule in a *Haemophilus influenzae* type B (HIB) conjugate vaccine. Advances in Experimental Medical Biology 251:175-180

Bolan G, Broome C V, Facklam R, Plikaytis M S, Fraser D W, Schlech W F III 1986 Pneumococcal vaccine efficacy in selected populations in the United States. Annals of Internal Medicine 104:1-6

Braley-Mullen H 1980 Antigen requirements for priming of IgG producing B memory cells specific for type III pneumococcal polysaccharide. Immunology 40:521-527

Brandtzaeg P, Baklien K, Bjerke K, Rognum T O, Scott H, Valnes K 1987 Nature and properties of the human gastrointestinal immune system. In: Miller K, Nicklin S (eds) Immunology of the gastrointestinal tract. CRC Press, Boca Raton pp 1-85

Buus S, Sette A, Colon S M, Miles C, Grey M H 1987 The relation between major histocompatibility complex (MHC) restriction and the capacity of Ia to bind immunogenic peptides. Science 235:1353-1358

Cowan M J, Amman A J, Wara D W et al 1978 Pneumococcal polysaccharide immunization in infants and children. Pediatrics 62:721-727

Douglas R M, Miles H B 1984 Vaccination against Streptococcus pneumoniae in childhood: lack of demonstrable benefit in young Australian children. Journal of Infectious Diseases 149:861-869

Douglas R M, Paton J C, Duncan S J, Hausman D J 1983 Antibody response to pneumococcal vaccination in children younger than five years of age. Journal of Infectious Diseases 148:131-137

Edelman G 1983 Cell adhesion molecules. Science 219:450-457

Egan W, Schneerson R, Werner K E, Zon G 1982 Structural studies and chemistry of bacterial capsular polysaccharides. Investigations of phosphodiester-linked capsular polysaccharides. Journal of the American Chemistry Society 104:2898-2910

Elkins K L, Stashak P W, Baker P J 1987 Mechanisms of specific immunological unresponsiveness to bacterial lipopolysaccharides. Infection and Immunity 55:3093-3102

Eskola J, Peltola H, Takala A K et al 1987 Efficacy of Haemophilus influenzae type b polysaccharide-diphtheria toxoid conjugate vaccine in infancy. New England Journal of Medicine 317:717-722

Finne J, Mäkelä P H 1985 Cleavage of the polysialosyl units of brain glycoproteins by a bacteriophage endosialidase. Journal of Biological Chemistry 260:1265-1270

Finne J, Leinohen M, Mäkelä P H 1983 Antigenic similarity between brain components and bacteria causing meningitis. Lancet ii:355-357

Fisher G W, Lowell G M, Cumrine M H, Bars J W 1978 Demonstration of opsonic activity and in vivo protection against group B streptococci type III by Streptococcus pneumoniae type 14 antisera. Journal of Experimental Medicine 148:776-786

Goldschneider I, Lepow M L, Gotschlich E C, Mauck F T, Bachl F, Randolph M 1973 Immunogenicity of the group A and group C meningococcal polysaccharides in human infants. Journal of Infectious Diseases 128:769-776

Gotschlich E C, Goldscheider I, Artenstein M C 1969a Human immunity to the meningococcus. IV. Immunogenicity of group A and C meningococcal polysaccharides in human volunteers. Journal of Experimental Medicine 129:1367-1384

Gotschlich E C, Liu T-Y, Artenstein M S 1969b Human immunity to meningococcus. III. Preparation and immunochemical properties of the group A, group B and group C meningococcal polysaccharides. Journal of Experimental Medicine 129:1349-1365

Gotschlich E C, Fraser B A, Nishimura O, Robbins J B, Liu T-Y 1981 Lipid on capsular polysaccharides of gram-negative bacteria. Journal of Biological Chemistry 256:8915-8921

Heilmann C, Barington T, Sigsgaard T 1988 Subclass of individual IgA-secreting human lymphocytes. Investigation of in vivo pneumococcal polysaccharide-induced and in vitro mitogen-induced blood B cells by monolayer plaque-forming cell assays. Journal of Immunology 140:1496-1499

Heyns K, Kielling G, Lindenberg W, Paulsen H, Webster M E 1959 D-Galaktosaminuronsäure (2-amino-2-desoxy-D-galakturonsäure) als Baustein des Vi-antigens. Chemische Berichte 92:2435-2437

Jennings H J 1990 Capsular polysaccharides as vaccine candidates. Current Topics in Microbiology and Immunology 150:97-127

Jennings H J, Lugowski C 1981 Immunochemistry of group A, B and C meningococcal polysaccharide-tetanus toxoid conjugates. Journal of Immunology 127:1011-1018

Jennings H J, Katzenellenbogen E, Lugowski C, Michon F, Roy R, Kasper D L 1984 Structure, conformation and immunology of sialic acid containing polysaccharides of human pathogenic bacteria. Pure and Applied Chemistry 56:893-905

Jennings H J, Roy R, Michon F 1985 Determinant specificities of the groups B and C polysaccharides of Neisseria meningitidis. Journal of Immunology 134:2651-2657

Jennings H J, Roy R, Gamian A 1986 Induction of meningococcal group B polysaccharide-specific IgG antibodies in mice by using an N-propionylated B polysaccharide-tetanus toxoid conjugate vaccine. Journal of Immunology 137:1708-1713

Jennings H J, Gamian A, Aston FE 1987 N-propionylated group B meningococcal polysaccharide mimics a unique epitope on group B Neisseria meningitidis. Journal of Experimental Medicine 165:1207-1211

Kabat E A, Bezer A E 1958 The effect of variation in molecular weight on the antigenicity of dextran in man. Archives of Biochemistry and Biophysics 78:306-318

Kaplan J, Frost H, Sarnaik S, Schiffman G 1982 Type-specific antibodies in children with sickle cell anemia given polyvalent pneumococcal vaccine. Journal of Pediatrics 100:404-406

Kasper D L, Jennings H J 1982 Immunological, immunochemical and structural studies of the type III and group B streptococcal polysaccharides. In: Easmon CSF, Jeljaszewig J (eds) Medical Microbiology, vol. 1. Academic Press, New York, pp 183-216

Kasper D L, Baker C J, Baltimore R S, Crabb J H, Schiffman G, Jennings H J 1979 Immunodeterminant specificity of human immunity to type III group B *Streptococcus*. Journal of Experimental Medicine 149:327-339

Lanzavecchia B 1985 Antigen-specific interaction between T and B cells. Nature 314:537-539

Lue C, Tarkowski A, Mestecky J 1988 Systemic immunization with pneumococcal polysaccharide vaccine induces a predominant IgA2 response of peripheral blood lymphocytes and increases of both serum and secretory anti-pneumococcal antibodies. Journal of Immunology 140:3793-3800

Lundqvist I, Holmberg D, Ivars F, Coutinho A 1986 The immune response to bacterial dextrans. III. Ontogenic development and strain distribution of specific clonal precursors. European Journal of Immunology 16:957-962

MacLeod C M, Hodges R G, Heidelberger M, Bernhard W G 1945 Prevention of pneumococcal pneumonia by immunization with specific capsular polysaccharides. Journal of Experimental Medicine 82:445-465

Madore D V, Johnson C L, Phipps D C, Pennridge pediatric associates, Popejoy L A, Eby R, Smith D H 1990 Safety and immunologic response to *Haemophilus influenzae* type b oligosaccharide CRM 197 conjugate vaccine in 1-to-6-month old infants. Pediatrics 85:331-337

Mäkelä P H, Leinonen M, Pukander J, Karma P 1981 A study of pneumococcal vaccine in prevention of clinically acute attacks of recurrent otitis media. Reviews of Infectious Diseases 3:S124-130

Makela O, Mattila P, Rautonen N, Seppälä J, Eskola J, Käyhty H 1987 Isotype concentrations of human antibodies to *Haemophilus influenzae* type b polysaccharide (Hib) in young adults immunized with the polysaccharide as such or conjugated to a protein (diphtheria toxoid). Journal of Immunology 139:1999-2004

Mestecky J 1987 The common mucosal immune system and current strategies for induction of immune responses in external secretions. Journal of Immunology 7:265-276

Mosier D E, Subbarao B 1982 Thymus-independent antigens: complexity of β-lymphocyte activation revealed. Immunology Today 3:217-222

Mufson M A, Krause H E, Schiffman G, Hughey D F 1987 Pneumococcal antibody levels one decade after immunization of healthy adults. American Journal of the Medical Sciences 293:279-289

Muller E, Apicella M 1988 T-cell modulation of the murine antibody resopnse to *Neisseria meningitidis* group A capsular polysaccharide. Infection and Immunity 56:259-266

New vaccine development establishing priorities. Vol.II. Diseases of importance in developing countries 1986. National Academy Press, Washington DC, pp 1-432

Nossal G J V, Pike B 1984 A re-appraisal of 'T-independent' antigens. II. Studies on single hapten-specific B cells from neonatal CBA/N mice fail to support classification into TI-1 and TI-2 categories. Journal of Immunology 132:1696-1701

Peltola H, Käyty H, Virtanen M, Mäkelä P H 1984 Prevention of *Haemophilus influenzae* type b bacteremic infections with the capsular polysaccharide vaccine. New England Journal of Medicine 310:1561-1566

Porro M, Constantino P, Viti S, Vannozzi F, Naggi A, Torri G 1985 Specific antibodies to diphtheria toxin and type 6A pneumococcal capsular polysaccharide induced by a model of semi-synthetic glycoconjugate antigen. Molecular Immunology 22:907-919

Riley I D, Alpers M P, Gratten H, Lehmann D, Marshall T F, Smith D 1986 Pneumococcal vaccine prevents death from acute lower-respiratory-tract infections in Papua New Guinean chidren. Lancet ii:877-881

Sadler J E, Paulsen J C, Hill R L 1979 The role of sialic acid in the expression of human MN blood group antigens. Journal of Biological Chemistry 254:2112-2119

Sarnaik S, Kaplan J, Schiffman G, Bryla D, Robbins J B, Schnerson R 1990 Studies on pneumococcus vaccine alone or mixed with DTP and on pneumococcus type 6B and *Haemophilus influenzae* type b capsular polysaccharide-tetanus toxoid conjugate in 2-to-5-year-old children with sickle cell anemia. Pediatric Infectious Disease Journal 9:181-186

Scher I 1982 The CBA/N mouse strain: an experimental model illustrating the influence of the X-chromosome on immunity. Advances in Immunology 33:1-71

Schneerson R, Barrera O, Sutton A, Robbins J B 1980 Preparation, characterization, and immunogenicity of *Haemophilus influenzae* type b polysaccharide-protein conjugates. Journal of Experimental Medicine 152:361-376

Seppälä I, Mäkelä O 1989 Antigenicity of dextran-protein conjugates in mice. Effect of molecular weight of carbohydrate and comparison of two modes of coupling. Journal of Immunology 143:1259-1264

Smith D H, Madore D V, Eby R, Anderson P W, Insel R A, Johnson C L 1989 Haemophilus b oligosaccharide-CRM 197 and other Haemophilus b conjugate vaccines: a status report. In: Atassi MZ (ed) International symposium on the immunobiology of proteins and peptides: vaccines-mechanisms, designs, and applications. Alberta. Advances in Experimental Medical Biology 251:65-82

Snippe H, van Houte A-J, van Dam J E G, de Reuver M J, Jansze M, Willers J M N 1983 Immunogenic properties in mice of hexasaccharide from the capsular polysaccharide of *Streptococcus pneumoniae* type 3. Infection and Immunity 40:856-861

Subbarao B, Mosier D E 1982 Lyb antigens and their role in B lymphocyte activation. Immunological Reviews 69:81-97

Taylor C E, Bright R 1989 T-cell modulation of the antibody response to bacterial polysaccharide antigens. Infection and Immunity 57:180-185

Tudor-Williams G, Frankland J, Isaacs D et al 1989 *Haemophilus influenzae* type b conjugate vaccine trial in Oxford: implications for the United Kingdom. Archives of Disease in Childhood 64:520-524

Vella P P, Staub-J M, Armstrong J et al 1990 Immunogenicity of a new *Haemophilus influenzae* b conjugate vaccine (meningococcal protein conjugate). (Pedvax HIB ™). Pediatrics 85:668-675

Weinberg G A, Granoff D M 1990 Immunogenicity of *Haemophilus influenzae* type b polysaccharide-protein conjugate vaccines in children with conditions associated with impaired antibody responses to type b polysaccharide vaccine. Pediatrics 85:654-661

Wyle F A, Artenstein M S, Brandt B L et al 1982 Immunologic response of man to group B meningococcal polysaccharide vaccines. Journal of Infectious Diseases 126:514-521

D

Discussion of paper presented by A. A. Lindberg

Discussed by E. R. Moxon
Reported by K. P. W. J. McAdam

In reviewing Lindberg's presentation, Moxon picked out a few issues requiring emphasis and further discussion. Considered in global terms, most existing polysaccharide vaccines are marginal in their immunogenicity, but the application of the hapten-carrier approach of Avery and Goebels to produce conjugate vaccines provides an approach of huge potential importance with respect to two important diseases: meningitis and pneumonia. The prospect of safe and effective vaccines is a tremendous step forward, although issues of cost and implementation present substantial problems.

Moxon indicated the considerable achievement of the successful conjugate *H. influenzae* b (Hib) vaccine. Protective immunity to invasive *H. influenzae* disease is type-specific, since serotype b strains cause the majority of infections (e.g. meningitis). However, young infants who contract invasive disease often do not develop protective immunity and are susceptible to further episodes of invasive Hib infections, although these are rare. Thus, to protect young infants against Hib infections by immunization requires the vaccine to be more efficient as an immunogen than the effect of systemic infection with naturally acquired Hib organisms. In fact, conjugate vaccines have been shown to achieve a superior result to immunization with a whole organism. This is impressive and it should be emphasized that conjugate vaccines are extremely safe, arguably the safest proposed for routine use.

Much is still unknown about the basic immunology and the immunogenicity of conjugate vaccines. Compared to what is known about peptides, the interaction of carbohydrate antigens—whether pure or conjugated—is a relatively neglected area. Bacterial capsular polysaccharides are comparatively simple polymers comprising one or two repetitive sugar units and behave as T-independent antigens. However, the manner is which these polysaccharides interact with cells is not well understood. They are not efficient immunogens, do not induce memory and the ability to produce antibody matures slowly in infants. As a result, when maternally-acquired immunity wanes, there is a period of heightened susceptibly to infection with encapsulated bacteria. Covalent linkage of the polysaccharide or oligosaccharide to a protein converts the hapten into a T-dependent antigen, but the mechanisms involved are not understood. The choice of protein, the linkage, the size of the carbohydrate antigen and other variables each affect immunogenicity. Moxon emphasized that both T-dependent and T-independent mechanisms are likely to be involved in the immune response to conjugates. Indeed, in developing countries the primary response to the first immunization with conjugate vaccine reflecting T-independent mechanisms may be crucial, since early protection is needed and the opportunities for carrying out immunization are limited. Substantial differences in the timing and magnitude of immune responses in infants immunized with conjugate Hib vaccines have become apparent and understanding of these differences is vital in order to design optimal vaccines.

A further issue discussed was the need to induce mucosal as well as serum antibodies. This is especially important when considering protection against pneumococcal disease such as otitis media. A possible approach might involve the choice of the carrier protein capable of inducing antibodies acting at the mucosal level. Serum antibodies may diffuse into mucosal secretions, especially if there is inflammation, a possibility that may circumvent the difficulties of inducing secretory IgA or IgM immunoglobulins. Moxon also raised the practical issues of quality control for conjugate vaccines, since the relationship between the formulation, immunogenicity and protective efficacy is poorly defined. He considered conjugates as biological, rather than pharmaceutical products. Moreover, the integration of the increasing numbers of the conjugate vaccines with the WHO recommended immunization schedules is an important issue for further discussion.

Lindberg elaborated further on immunogenicity of glycoconjugates and the mechanisms behind T- and B-cell cooperation. The saccharide portion is not processed by macrophages, but has a variable conformation which may be linear or helical, extended or condensed, consequently occupying more or less space. It is therefore difficult to predict the optimal size of a glycoconjugate vaccine, and this may have to be determined individually for each saccharide and conjugate. As a consequence some vaccines will have to be well defined in physicochemical terms and considered as pharmaceutical, rather than biological products, he suggested. In terms of cost the vaccine market is small, as is the profit margin. The producers have to consider the risk of litigation because of vaccine side-effects and glycoconjugate vaccines are not and will not, in the forseeable future, be inexpensive. However, they are very safe and the benefits of such vaccines may make the costs acceptable to Public Health Authorities worldwide. Lindberg forecast plans to launch the concept of a child's vaccine containing immunogens against more than ten childhood infectious diseases during the 'Child Summit' in New York in September 1990.

Makela then presented the results of a randomized prospective trial in Finland in which about 55 000 children participated in each of the control and vaccine groups. The vaccine group received primary series of immunizations at 3, 4 and 6 months of age (the same result has been obtained by giving the vaccine at 4 and 6 months, though at least two doses are required). In the fully vaccinated children, there were 4 cases of invasive *H. influenzae* type b disease and 37 cases among the controls, translating into a 90% efficacy following the basic immunization before the age of 7 months. A booster dose given 1 year later provided even more solid immunity, so that there were no cases in the vaccinated children and 29 cases in the controls. This is a convincing demonstration that this conjugate vaccine could do what a polysaccharide vaccine had not done, that is, to protect children between the ages of

6 and 18 months. The conjugate vaccine (PRP-D) was composed of *Haemophilus influenzae* polysaccaride conjugated to diphtheria toxoid prepared by Connaught.

This vaccine trial had influenced the disease, demonstrating efficacy in a field trial and in the public health setting. During the period 1987-1988, half of the children less than 5 years old in Finland had received this vaccine. During the period that followed, i.e. in 1989, 90% of the children aged less than 5 years old had received the vaccine. *H. influenzae* bacteraemia in children of this age had been continuously high until the vaccination programme started, at which point numbers began to fall, from 180 cases before vaccination to only 29 cases during the following year. However, despite this decrease in the under-5s, bacteraemic *H. influenzae* disease continued in older children and in adults who had not been vaccinated, at a rate of about 30 cases each year. The current practice in Finland is to immunize all infants at 4 and 6 months, with a booster at 18 months. Makela went on to discuss nasopharyngeal carriage rates of *H. influenzae* which occur at about 5% in the general population and is common in children in close contact with cases. When the carriage rate was compared, between 1976 and 1986 in 3-year-old children, *H. influenzae* were found in about 5% in each case, although no carriers were found in those children who had been fully immunized. In contrast, carriage rates of non-encapsulated *H. influenzae* and *Pneumococcus* at the same times was not influenced by the *H. influenzae* vaccination, which only reduced the Hib type-specific carriage rate. Makela assumed that this resulted from antibodies reaching the mucosa and preventing colonization. Lagrange pointed out that mucosal antibodies are also produced with glycoconjugate vaccines and the sub-type of IgA mucosal antibody is important, with IgA 1 predominating. It is unclear whether IgA 1 or IgA 2 is more effective at preventing colonization.

The question of revaccination against pneumococcus using a multivalent vaccine was also discussed. A few capsular polysaccharide titres had remained high, even after ten years, but serological responses to other capsular polysaccharides dropped to pre-immunization levels. Since there is no anamnestic response to polysaccharides, each vaccination has to be considered as a primary vaccination. The ultimate solution to this problem is to manufacture glycoconjugate vaccines. After splenectomy, antibody titres drop more quickly, with 3 to 5 years given as a rough guide. Responses to type 6 and 19 are almost always inadequate.

Immunization of pregnant women with transfer of antibodies to the foetus, will protect the child for no longer than the first few months after birth. It is in this window that the child should be vaccinated with glycoconjugate vaccines against pneumococcal, meningococcal and *Haemophilus influenza* type b infections.

6. Salmonella vaccines

M. M. Levine   D. Hone   C. O. Tacket   C. Ferreccio
S. Cryz and G. Losonsky

INTRODUCTION

Salmonella infections, depending on serotype, cause three clinico-epidemiological syndromes in humans: acute gastroenteritis, enteric fever and septicaemic/metastatic foci. Acute *Salmonella* gastroenteritis, of which *S. typhimurium* is a major causative serotype, is prevalent in industrialized as well as less-developed countries; in the healthy host above 3 months of age the illness is usually self-limited. In young infants (below 3 months of age) (Rice et al 1976) and in immunocompromised hosts, including patients with acquired immunodeficiency syndrome (Glaser et al 1985), non-typhoidal *Salmonella* serotypes such as *S. typhimurium* and *S. cholerasuis* can cause septicaemic disease leading to metastatic foci of infection (e.g. empyema and osteomyelitis) (Rhame et al 1973). However, worldwide, the major public health burden of *Salmonella* infection is due to the enteric (typhoid and paratyphoid) fevers. *S. typhi*, the agent of acute typhoid fever, is by far the major culprit.

TYPHOID FEVER DISEASE BURDEN

Human beings are the only reservoir and host for typhoid fever. Three groups at particular risk of typhoid fever constitute the reference populations targeted for eventual use of new typhoid vaccines. These include school-age children in less-developed countries, persons from industrialized countries who travel to developing areas of the world (Rice et al 1977, Taylor et al 1983), and clinical microbiology technicians worldwide (Blaser et al 1980).

It has been estimated that 33 million cases and more than half a million deaths due to typhoid fever occur throughout the developing world annually, mainly in school-age children (Institute of Medicine 1986). Recent epidemiological data show that clinically overt typhoid infection is much more common than previously thought. For example, in some recent field trials, culture-confirmed annual incidence rates of 700-1000 per 100 000 population were recorded among school-age children and young adults (Acharya et al 1987, Klugman et al 1987).

Case reporting in typhoid-endemic locales usually reveals little typhoid in children less than 24 months of age. However, a recent epidemiological study in Chile involving the systematic collection of a single blood culture from all children < 24 months of age who presented to health centres with fever, irrespective of their clinical symptoms, showed that 3.5% of the febrile infants and toddlers had 'benign' bacteraemic infections due to *S. typhi* or *S. paratyphi* (Ferreccio et al 1984). In none was enteric fever suspected on clinical grounds; rather, 'viral syndrome' was the typical diagnosis.

Because of increased travel to less-developed countries, typhoid fever is increasingly recognized as a risk for travellers from industrialized countries. It is also known that clinical microbiology technicians are at increased risk of acquiring *S. typhi* infection (Blaser et al 1980). The World Health Organization (WHO) has targeted as a high priority the development of improved vaccines to prevent typhoid fever.

Shortcomings of the parenteral killed whole cell vaccines
As recently reviewed (Levine et al 1989a), the parenteral killed whole cell vaccines, containing heat-phenolized or acetone-treated *Salmonella typhi*, significantly protected (51-88% vaccine efficacy) against typhoid fever in randomized, controlled field trials sponsored by the WHO in the 1960s and early 1970s. While protective, these vaccines are unpopular public health tools for the routine immunization of children and travellers because they elicit adverse reactions at high frequency, including fever and malaise in approximately 20-25% and local reactions in about 40-50% of vaccinees.

NEW GENERATIONS OF TYPHOID VACCINES

During the past 15 years there has been a resurgence of research in typhoid vaccine development with two distinct approaches having each achieved success (Levine et al 1989b): (i) the use of purified Vi polysaccharide as a parenteral vaccine, (ii) the use of attenuated strains of *S. typhi* as live oral vaccines. How prototype vaccines of these two generic varieties have served a pathfinder function, stimulating the development of a whole generation of exciting new vaccine candidates is discussed here.

Vi capsular polysaccharide as a parenteral vaccine

Properties of the Vi antigen
The Vi polysaccharide α-1,4, 2-deoxy-2-*N*-acetyl galacturonic acid, found as a capsule on clinical isolates of *S. typhi*, is a virulence property (Felix & Pitt 1951, Robbins & Robbins 1984). However, until recently its role as a protective antigen was the subject of debate, because of conflicting observations. In the early 1950s, Landy (Landy et al 1954, 1961) suggested that to assess the role of Vi as a protective antigen it should be purified and employed as a parenteral vaccine. Webster et al (1952) purified Vi by chemical procedures that unwittingly denatured the antigen, resulting in loss of *O*-acetyl and *N*-acetyl moieties. Their Vi vaccine elicited Vi antibodies in man but failed to protect chimpanzees or volunteers from experimental challenge (Gaines et al 1961, Hornick et al 1970).

In the 1970s it became possible to purify Vi without denaturation, yielding

Table 6.1 Culture-confirmed typhoid fever in persons immunized with *Salmonella typhi* Vi polysaccharide or control (pneumococcal or meningococcal) polysaccharide parenteral vaccine in two randomized, controlled field trials

Vaccine group	No. vaccinated	Cases of typhoid	Incidence per 10^3	Vaccine efficacy	Period of surveillance
*Nepal trial**					
Vi	3457	9	2.6	72%	17 months
		$p = 0.004$		(CI, 42.1-86.4%)[+]	
pneumococcal	3450	32	9.3	–	
*South Africa trial***					
Vi	5692	16	2.8	64%	21 months
		$p < 0.001$		(CI, 35.9-79.3%)	
meningococcal	5692	44	7.7		

*Participants were randomized to receive a 0.5 ml intramuscular inoculation containing either 25 μg of purified Vi or 23-valent pneumococcal polysaccharide. This study in Nepal utilized active surveillance methods in which health workers visited the households of participants every two days (except · Sundays) to detect cases of typhoid fever (Acharya et al 1987).
**Participants were randomized to receive a single 25 μg intramuscular dose of Vi or a 50 μg dose of meningococcal polysaccharide vaccine. This trial used a combination of active and passive surveillance methods (Klugman et al 1987).
+95% confidence interval (CI).

products for clinical trials (Wong et al 1974, Robbins & Robbins 1984). Tacket et al (1986) reported the immunogenicity of two non-denatured Vi lots prepared at the National Institutes of Health, Bethesda, Maryland and at l'Institut Merieux, Lyon, France. The former was 95% and the latter 99.8% free of contaminating LPS. Both lots elicited high titres of Vi antibody in about 90% of recipients. However, the less pure lot also stimulated O antibody in >80% of vaccinees, some of whom manifested systemic adverse reactions attributed to the contaminating LPS. In contrast, the 99.8% pure preparation was well tolerated and stimulated O antibody in <20% of vaccinees. Tacket et al (1989) showed that the Vi antibodies generated by the vaccine persisted for at least three years. Vi antibody of the levels elicited by the parenteral purified Vi vaccine are seen in nature only in chronic typhoid carriers; curiously, only about one-fourth of patients convalescent from acute typhoid fever develop elevated titres of Vi antibody (Losonsky et al 1987).

Field trials with purified Vi vaccine
Two randomized, controlled field trials document the safety and efficacy of Vi vaccine produced at l'Institut Merieux; in both trials the vaccine was well tolerated (Acharya et al 1987, Klugman et al 1987.) As summarized in Table 6.1, in Nepal, a single 25 μg intramuscular dose of Vi vaccine provided 72% protection for at least 17 months against culture-confirmed typhoid fever in a study involving both children and adults. Similar results were obtained in a field trial in South Africa, where a single 25 μg intramuscular dose of Vi polysaccharide conferred 64% protection against culture-confirmed typhoid fever in schoolchildren for at least 21 months.

Vi polysaccharide-protein conjugate vaccines
Szu et al (1987, 1989) are attempting to increase the immunogenicity of Vi as a parenteral antigen by conjugating it to carrier proteins such as tetanus toxoid, diphtheria toxoid and cholera toxin, thereby conferring T-dependent properties on the polysaccharide. In tests in two animal species, weanling mice and juvenile rhesus

monkeys, conjugate vaccines elicited higher levels of antibodies than purified Vi alone. Immunized animals responded to booster inoculations with the conjugate vaccines by exhibiting further increases in Vi antibody titre; in contrast, booster doses of the purified Vi polysaccharide alone failed to increase the level of Vi antibody. Clinical studies in humans with such conjugates are in progress.

TY21a, a pioneer live oral typhoid vaccine

Characteristics of the vaccine strain

In 1975, Germanier and Furer described a mutant *S. typhi* strain, Ty2la, harbouring a mutation in the *galE* gene, and proposed that it might serve as a live oral vaccine. Derived by chemical mutagenesis, Ty2la is entirely deficient in activity of the enzyme UDP-glucose-4-epimerase, the *galE* gene product involved in the reversible isomerization of UDP-galactose to UDP-glucose. As a consequence of the non-specific action of nitrosoguanidine, the chemical mutagen used, Ty2la has many other mutations, in addition to that in the *galE* gene; Ty2la also lacks the Vi polysaccharide.

In preliminary safety and immunogenicity studies in adult North Americans (Gilman et al 1977) Ty2la grown in the presence of low concentrations of galactose was well tolerated, even with oral doses as high as 10^{11} organisms; and it was immunogenic. The uptake of galactose leads to production of smooth lipopolysaccharide (LPS), making the strain immunogenic; however, it also results in an intrabacterial accumulation of gal-1-phosphate and UDP-galactose, which culminates in bacteriolysis; this is believed to explain the failure to recover vaccine organisms in coprocultures of persons who ingest the typical dose of 1-5 x 10^9 organisms. It was previously assumed that the safety of Ty2la was due to the combination of the of the *galE* mutation and the lack of Vi. However, this appears not to be so. Hone et al (1987) found that typhoid fever occurred in two of four volunteers who ingested an analogous Vi− *galE* deletion mutant of *S. typhi* prepared by recombinant techniques; thus, these mutations by themselves cannot account for the safety of Ty2la.

Field trials with Ty2la

Field trials with Ty2la have clearly shown that the level of efficacy that can be achieved is markedly influenced by the formulation of vaccine, the number of doses administered and the immunization schedule. The first field trial of efficacy of Ty2la (Wahdan et al 1982) was carried out in Alexandria, Egypt, where approximately 32 000 schoolchildren 6-7 years of age were randomized to receive three 10^9 organism doses of vaccine or placebo administered every other day. Each dose of lyophilized vaccine or placebo *in vacuo* in glass vials was reconstituted in the field with a diluent to create a liquid suspension that was imbibed by the child one minute after chewing a 1.0 g tablet of $NaHCO_3$ (to neutralize gastric acid and enhance survival of vaccine organisms transiting the stomach into the small intestine). No significant adverse reactions attributable to vaccine were noted. During three years of surveillance, a vaccine efficacy of 96% against culture-confirmed typhoid fever was recorded (Table 6.2).

Regrettably, the formulation of vaccine used in the Alexandria trial was not

Table 6.2 The efficacy of three doses of Ty2la oral typhoid vaccine in a liquid formulation or in enteric-coated capsules given within one week in field trials in Alexandria, Egypt, and Area Occidente, Santiago, Chile

	Vaccine	Placebo	p value
*Alexandria, Egypt, trial**			
n	*16* 486	15 902	
Cases	1	22	< 0.001
Incidence/10^5	6.1	138.3	
Efficacy	95.6%	—	
95% confidence interval	77.1-99.2		
*Santiago, Chile trial***			
n	22 170	21 906	
Cases	49	130	< 0.0000001
Incidence/10^5	221.0	522.8	
Efficacy	62.8%	—	
95% confidence interval	49.8-76.6		

* 36 months of surveillance, Wahdan et al 1982.
** 80 months of surveillance, Levine et al 1987a and authors unpublished data.
All cases noted above were bacteriologically confirmed.

amenable to large-scale manufacture. Consequently, the Swiss Serum and Vaccine Institute prepared two other formulations of Ty2la. One consisted of gelatin capsules containing a dose of lyophilized vaccine accompanied by two additional gelatin capsules each containing 0.4 g of $NaHCO_3$. The second new formulation, which requires no accompanying buffer, consists of enteric-coated capsules containing lyophilized vaccine organisms.

The efficacy of Ty2la in the gelatin capsule/$NaHCO_3$ and enteric-coated capsule formulations was directly compared in a randomized, placebo-controlled, large-scale field trial in Area Occidente (Western administrative area) of Santiago, Chile (Levine et al 1987a). After three years of surveillance, the enteric-coated capsule formulation (three doses within one week) showed an efficacy of 67% against bacteriologically confirmed typhoid fever; this was significantly higher than the gelatin capsule formulation (19% efficacy). As shown in Table 6.2, after 80 months of surveillance, comprising seven typhoid seasons, three doses of Ty2la in enteric-coated capsules given within one week in Area Occidente still show a cumulative level of protection of 63% vaccine efficacy; this is an impressive demonstration of long-lived protection.

Another field trial in Santiago, involving more than 212 000 schoolchildren, compared the relative efficacy of two, three or four doses of Ty2la in enteric-coated capsules given within a period of 8 days (Ferreccio et al 1989). Four doses were significantly more protective than three or two doses. This trial documented the practicality of large-scale, school-based immunization with Ty2la as a public health tool. In the USA the Food and Drug Administration recently licensed the enteric-coated capsule formulation of Ty2la with a recommended immunization schedule of four doses given every other day.

A comparison of data from the two field trials summarized in Table 6.2 suggested that administration of Ty2la in a liquid suspension might be an important factor responsible for the increased protection observed in the Egyptian trial. Accordingly, another field trial was conducted in Santiago to address the question of formulation: schoolchildren were randomized to receive three doses of Ty2la within one week in enteric-coated capsules or in a liquid formulation (Levine et al unpublished data).

Table 6.3 Comparison of the efficacy of three doses of Ty21a live oral typhoid vaccine given in enteric-coated capsule or liquid formulations. 24 months of surveillance of a randonized, controlled, double-blind trial in Area Sur Oriente and Area Norte, Santiago, Chile

	Liquid	Enteric capsules	Placebo*
No. children	36 623	34 696	10 302
Cases	13	39	20
Incidence/10^5	35.5[a]	112.4[b]	194.1[c]
Efficacy	81.7%	42.1%	–
95% confidence interval	(64–91)	(1–66)	

* Combined liquid and enteric-coated placebo groups.
a vs c, $p < 0.0000001$; b vs c, $p = 0.032$ by Chi square with Yates correction, single-tail test.
a vs b, $p = 0.00025$, Chi square with Yates correction, two-tail test.
Levine et al unpublished data.

Results of two years of surveillance in this field trial are summarized in Table 6.3; the liquid formulation was significantly more protective. It is expected that a liquid formulation of Ty21a similar to that used in the Chilean trial will become available in the near future.

A laboratory correlate of protection
The seroconversion rate of IgG-ELISA *S. typhi* O antibody in young adult Chileans increases with each additional dose (from one to four) of Ty21a ingested within a period of 8 days and the seroconversion rate roughly correlates with the level of protection encountered in field trials in Chile (Levine et al 1989a). This antibody is not believed to mediate protection *per se*; nevertheless, it serves as a useful correlate to compare dosage regimens.

Drawbacks of Ty21a
While safe and protective, Ty21a suffers from several drawbacks. Multiple doses are required to achieve a satisfactory level of protection; the yield of viable organisms is low when it is fermented and lyophilized in large-scale manufacture; the basis of its attenuation is not known. Finally, with respect to its possible use as a carrier strain for the expression of foreign antigens, it is cumbersome in genetic manipulations: it grows slowly, is difficult to transform and exhibits a low recombination frequency.

The pathogenesis of *S. typhi* infection
Understanding the pathogenesis of *S. typhi* infection allows a rational approach to the development of new generations of attenuated vaccine strains. Our reconstruction of events in the pathogenesis of *S. typhi* infection is derived from four main sources: clinico-pathological studies (Mallory 1898, Salas et al 1960), experimental infection of chimpanzees (Gaines et al 1968), a volunteer model of experimental typhoid fever (Hornick et al 1970), and studies of the 'mouse typhoid' model employing *S. typhimurium* or *S. enteriditis* (Collins 1972, Carter & Collins 1974).

Following ingestion by a susceptible host, typhoid bacilli must successfully transit the stomach where gastric acid and proteolytic enzymes comprise a potent non-specific defence barrier. Upon arrival in the small intestine, *S. typhi* translocate from the lumen to reach the lamina propria and the mesenteric lymph nodes by two mechanisms. *S. typhi* readily associate with M-cells that overlie the Peyer's patches and other organized lymphoid tissue in the small intestine (Kohbata et al 1986). They invade and destroy the M-cells and enter the lymphoid tissue below, many being ingested by macrophages. Other *S. typhi* invade enterocytes of the small intestine and become engulfed by pinocytotic vesicles (Takeuchi 1971). These vesicles migrate from the luminal surface of the cell to its basal surface to discharge the bacteria into the lamina propria, without death of the enterocyte. The presence of *S. typhi* in the lamina propria causes an infiltration of macrophages to the site of the bacteria whereupon most of the bacilli are ingested. These macrophages drain into mesenteric lymph nodes. Both within macrophages and perhaps as free bacteria, typhoid bacilli enter the lymph circulation, pass into the thoracic duct and from there enter the bloodstream in a clinically silent primary bacteraemia. Typhoid bacilli are removed from the blood by fixed macrophages of the reticuloendothelial system in the liver, spleen, bone marrow, and lymph nodes. Intramacrophagic residence shields typhoid bacilli from the effects of antibody and complement. Within the macrophages the *Salmonella* are contained within phagolysosomes (Fields et al 1989). Pathogenic *Salmonella* possess virulence properties that allow them to evade the microbicidal properties of these professional phagocytes and to survive and grow for many days. After approximately 8-14 days, corresponding to the incubation of typhoid fever, a secondary bacteraemia occurs accompanied by the clinical symptoms of typhoid fever including increasing fever, headache, malaise and abdominal discomfort.

Attenuated *Salmonella* strains that function as successful vaccines mimic all of the above steps, including intracellular survival, except for the occurrence of clinical illness and secondary bacteraemia. While there are many notable similarities between the behaviour of *S. typhimurium* in mice and *S. typhi* in humans, there also exist important differences. Consequently, mutations that adequately attenuate virulent *S. typhimurium* for mice do not necessarily predict that analogous mutations will also successfully attenuate *S. typhi* for humans (Hone et al 1988a).

NEW ATTENUATED *S. typhi* STRAINS AS VACCINE CANDIDATES AND EXPECTATIONS FOR SUCH STRAINS

Investigators are trying various strategies to attenuate *S. typhi* both for use as a live vaccine to prevent typhoid fever and to serve as live carrier vaccines for the expression of foreign antigens. The usual approach is to make mutations analogous to those that have been shown to attenuate reliably *S. typhimurium* for mice (or other natural hosts of that serotype) in the hope that those mutations may similarly attenuate *S. typhi* for humans. Several new attenuated *S. typhi* vaccine strains will be entering clinical trials within the next few years. Ideally, we would expect an optimal vaccine strain to have the following characteristics:

1. To confer protective immunity after ingestion of a single oral dose. If used as a carrier vaccine, protection should not only be against typhoid fever but also against the unrelated pathogen whose antigens are expressed in the *S. typhi* carrier strain.
2. The vaccine should be well tolerated and cause no serious adverse reactions.

3. The strain should have two separate mutations that independently attenuate. These should be located in genes sufficiently far apart on the chromosome such that a single recombinational event (an extremely unlikely event under any circumstances) could not restore pathogenicity.

4. The attenuating mutations must be well characterized and preferably should represent deletions.

5. The strain should be readily amenable to genetic manipulations (such as transformation, recombination and electroporation).

6. The strain should allow good expression of foreign antigens following integration of foreign DNA into the chromosome or stabilization of plasmids coding genes for the foreign antigen.

7. The strain should harbour no clinically relevant antibiotic resistances nor should there be Hfr in the chromosome.

8. A high yield should be obtainable following fermentation and lyophilization of the vaccine strain at the industrial scale.

With these expectations in mind, it is relevant to describe some of the new constructs and proposed attenuating mutations that are under investigation.

Vi+ Ty21a

Cryz et al (1989) hoped to improve upon the immunogenicity and efficacy of Ty21a, while not sacrificing safety, by genetically restoring the ability of Ty21a to make Vi polysaccharide. This Vi+ variant of Ty21a was evaluated for safety and immunogenicity in clinical trials; preliminary data are shown in Table 6.4. The vaccine candidate was well tolerated except for two of 15 vaccinees who developed mild diarrhoea at a dose of 10^9 organisms. No rises were detected in serum Vi antibody. However, the rate of seroconversion of serum IgG O antibody in recipients of three doses (67%) was somewhat greater than in Maryland adults who received three doses of Vi- Ty21a (25%) ($p = 0.08$) (Table 6.4).

cya, crp mutants

Curtiss & Kelly (1987) have prepared a *cya, crp* mutant of *S. typhi* analogous to the

Table 6.4 The clinical and serological response of healthy US adult volunteers following immunization with live oral typhoid vaccine candidate Vi+ Ty21a and with well-established parent vaccine strain Vi- Ty21a

Vaccine	Dose no. organisms	No. doses	No. subjects	Fever	Diarrhoea	No. with significant rises in serum IgG O antibody
Vi+ Ty21a	10^9	3[a]	9	0	1	6 (67%)
	10^9	1	6	0	1	1 (17%)
	10^{5-7}	1	6	0	0	2 (17%)
Vi- Ty21a	10^9	4[b]	27	0	0	15 (56%)
	10^9	3[c]	16	0	0	4 (25%)
	10^9	2[c]	30	0	0	2 (7%)
	10^9	1[c]	30	0	0	5 (14%)

[a] Data from Tacket et al (in preparation).
[b] Authors unpublished data.
[c] Black et al (1983).

S. typhimurium strains that they have shown to be safe, immunogenic and protective in mice and chickens (Curtiss et al 1988). This attenuation is based on the fact that the expression of numerous genes of *Salmonella* is dependent on the availability of cyclic AMP and the cyclic AMP receptor protein (CRP). CRP functions as a positive activator of transcription for many genes including those for carbohydrate and amino acid transport, glycogen synthesis and the synthesis of fimbriae, flagella and certain outer membrane proteins that play a role in the pathogenicity of the organism. Phase 1 safety/immunogenicity studies in healthy adults with a *aro, cya,* mutant of *S. typhi* strain Ty2 (the pathogenic parent of Ty2la) will commence in 1990.

phoP mutants

Fields et al (1989) identified *phoP* as a chromosomal locus that controls the resistance of *S. typhimurium* to microbicidal proteins (defensins) present in the phagosomes in which the bacteria are located following their ingestion by macrophages. Fields et al (1989) and others (Galan & Curtiss 1989; Miller et al 1989b) have shown that *phoP* are attenuated in mice and sometimes provide at least partial protection against challenge with virulent *S. typhimurium*. Miller et al (1989b) have shown evidence that a two-component gene regulatory system, *phoP/phoQ,* regulates the expression of several genes involved in the pathogenicity of *S. typhimurium*, including its ability to survive intracellularly within macrophages. Mutants of *S. typhi* harbouring deletions in *phoP* are being constructed for clinical studies to ascertain whether they are attenuated and immunogenic for humans. If so, strains harbouring deletions in *phoP* along with a second independent attenuation mutation may make attractive candidates for clinical studies in humans.

ompR mutants

The *ompR* and *envZ* genes are believed to form a two-gene regulatory system where *envZ* gene may sense the the osmolarity of the environment and transmit a signal to *ompR* which then regulates transcription of various genes (Dorman et al 1989). Among the *ompR*-dependent genes are several coding for major outer membrane porin proteins, including *ompC* and *ompF*. The expression of these porins is inversely regulated by the osmolarity of the culture medium in a manner that is dependent on *ompR*. In environments of high osmolarity the level of *ompC* is elevated while *ompF* is diminished. In contrast, in an ambience of low osmolarity *ompC* expression is repressed and *ompF* is increased. It has been hypothesized that through such regulation *S. typhimurium* adapt to transition from a free-living (low osmolarity) environment to that of the intestine (high osmolarity). *S. typhimurium* strains mutated in *ompR* lack this osmotic regulatory capability and are markedly avirulent when fed orally to mice; in the hands of some investigators such mutants successfully protect immunized mice against oral challenge with virulent *S. typhimurium* (Dorman et al 1989). If further studies of *ompR* mutants in outbred mice and other animal models document the attenuating effect of this mutation, deletion mutants of *S. typhi* should be evaluated in humans.

aro mutants, pur mutants and aro, pur mutants

Other investigators are pursuing the development of Aro− *S. typhi* strains because of the exceptional safety and immunogenicity of Aro- *S. typhimurium* and *S. dublin* strains (Hoiseth & Stocker 1981, Robertson et al 1983, Eisenstein et al 1984, Killar & Eisenstein 1985, Dougan et al 1987, 1988) which have been attenuated by inactivation of *aro* genes that control the synthesis of aromatic amino acids. Interruption of this synthetic pathway renders the *Salmonella* auxotrophic for 2, 3-dihydroxybenzoate (DHB) and *para* -aminobenzoic acid (PABA), substrates not available to the bacteria in mammalian tissues. As a consequence of this auxotrophy, the bacteria cannot sustain proliferation within mammalian cells. Yet they reside and grow intracellularly long enough to stimulate protective immune responses.

Strains of *S. typhimurium* mutated in *aroA* , when used as live oral vaccines, are safe in mice and calves, stimulate both antibody and cell-mediated immune responses, and protect these animals against otherwise lethal challenges with virulent *S. typhimurium* (Hoiseth & Stocker 1981, Robertson et al 1983, Eisenstein et al 1984, Killar & Eisenstein 1985, Dougan et al 1988).

Based on the success of the *aro* mutants of *S. typhimurium* in animals, Edwards & Stocker (1988) prepared an *aroA* deletion mutant of *S. typhi* . The deletions in *aro* that they made involved insertion of transposon Tn*10* in *aroA*, spontaneous illegitimate excision of the transposon leading to a small deletion in *aroA*, transfer of the *aro* mutation (using closely linked *ser* C::Tn*10* for selection) from *S. typhimurium* to *S. typhi* by means of a transducing phage P22, and finally, selection of a *ser* C$^+$ tetracycline-sensitive strain designated 523Ty. They transduced in a deletion on *purA*, to provide a second independent attenuating lesion in their candidate vaccine to guard against the possible restoration of pathogenicity by a random DNA transfer event; for example, with wild-type *Salmonella* (that might in theory be ingested by and colonize the intestine of a vaccinee shortly after vaccination). The deletion in *purA* created a requirement for the purine adenine (or an assimilable adenine compound such as adenosine) which is not sufficiently supplemented *in vivo* . The *aro*, *pur* mutants of *S. typhi* were fed to volunteers as both Vi+ (strain 54lTY) and Vi- (strain 543Ty) variants (Levine et al 1987b). Unfortunately, in humans the *aro*, *pur* vaccine was hyperattenuated; it was well tolerated and elicited specific cell-mediated immune responses to *S. typhi* (detected by lymphocyte stimulation assays) but the serological responses were meagre, if they occurred at all (Levine et al 1987b). Subsequently, O'Callaghan et al (1988) demonstrated in mice that *pur* or *pur*, *aro* mutants of *S. typhimurium* are poorly protective, while in contrast, *aro* mutants are highly protective. The selection of *purA* as a second attenuating mutation, therefore, was unfortunate because such mutants of *Salmonella* are hyperattenuated, poorly immunogenic and not protective.

Double mutants with inactivation of two aro genes
The aromatic amino acid biosynthesis pathway can be equally well inactivated at several loci (Dougan et al 1988, Miller et al 1989a). Since these genes are widely separated on the chromosome, deletions in two carefully selected *aro* genes of *S. typhi* should yield vaccine candidates that are attenuated by means of two independent mutations.

SALMONELLA AS A LIVE CARRIER FOR EXPRESSION OF FOREIGN ANTIGENS

Attenuated *S. typhi* are particularly attractive as carrier strains to express foreign antigens and deliver them to the human immune system for the following reasons: (i) They are administered orally. (ii) They stimulate a broad immune response that includes serum antibody (Black et al 1983, Sarosombath et al 1987, Levine et al 1989a), SIgA intestinal antibody (Sarosombath et al 1987, Forrest, 1988), cell-mediated immunity (Levine et al 1987b, Murphy et al 1987) and antibody-dependent cytotoxicity (ADCC) (Tagliabue et al 1986, Levine et al 1987b). (iii) There is a large clinical experience attesting to the safety, immunogenicity and efficacy of attenuated *S. typhi* vaccine strains. (iv) Much is known about methods to manipulate genetically *Salmonella*: plasmid vectors developed for use with *Escherichia coli* are generally suitable for use with *Salmonella*; methods to stabilize plasmids exist (Nakayama et al 1988); techniques are available to integrate foreign DNA into the chromosome (Hone et al 1988b). (v) Considerable experience from immunization of mice with attenuated *S. typhimurium* expressing foreign antigens provides ample precedent and a base of knowledge for analogous studies with attenuated *S. typhi* in humans (Clements & El-Morshidy 1984, Brown et al 1987, Dougan et al 1987, Maskell et al 1987, Curtiss et al 1988).

SITE OF EXPRESSION OF THE FOREIGN ANTIGENS

Systems have been designed that allow foreign antigens to be expressed so that they are exposed on the surface of the attenuated *Salmonella* carrier strain. These include inclusion of the foreign antigen in subunits of fimbriae (DeGraaf 1988, Thiry et al 1989), in subunits of flagella (Newton et al 1989), or as part of the LamB outer membrane protein (Charbit et al 1987). It is also possible to utilize fusion proteins to assure that foreign antigens are at least transported to the periplasmic space (Schodel & Will 1989). The importance of such manipulations has not been established with respect to increasing a particular type of immune response, e.g. SIgA intestinal antibodies, ADCC, cell-mediated immunity.

SALMONELLA HYBRID VACCINES EXPRESSING FOREIGN ANTIGENS

Attenuated *S. typhimurium* constructs expressing foreign antigens have been used to immunize mice and stimulate serum and intestinal antibody and cell-mediated immune responses to the foreign antigen (Clements & El-Morshidy 1984, Brown et al 1987, Maskell et al 1987, Curtiss et al 1988, 1989). Sadoff et al (1988) immunized mice with attenuated *S. typhimurium* harbouring the cloned gene for the circumsporozoite protein of *Plasmodium berghei*. When challenged with infective sporozoites of *P. berghei*, the immunized mice were significantly protected. Since protection occurred in the absence of humoral antibody responses, this fact indirectly suggests that the hybrid vaccine successfully stimulated protective cell-mediated responses against the expressed foreign plasmodial antigen (Sadoff et al 1988). It has since been shown that such constructs indeed elicit MHC I-restricted CD8$^+$ cytotoxic lymphocyte responses to the plasmodial antigen.

The only two constructs tested so far in humans have utilized attenuated *S. typhi* strain Ty2la to express foreign O antigens. The first such construct was developed by Formal et al (1981) who introduced the 120 Md plasmid of *Shigella sonnei* into Ty2la and achieved plasmid stability and expression of the *S. sonnei* O antigen. In this *Shigella* species, genes responsible for expression of the O polysaccharide are located on the plasmid. The hybrid vaccine was well tolerated, moderately immunogenic and protective in experimental challenge studies in volunteers (Black et al 1987). However, variability occurred from lot-to-lot in the protective efficacy of the vaccine (Herrington et al in press). For this reason, field trials of efficacy were not undertaken. A drawback to this construct is that the *S. sonnei* O antigen is not expressed as a complete lipopolysaccharide anchored in the bacterial outer membrane (Seid et al 1984); rather it is expressed as an O polysaccharide that is intermeshed with the lipopolysaccharide O antigen of *S. typhi* (Seid et al 1984). Nevertheless, this vaccine clearly demonstrated the potential of *Salmonella* to serve as a carrier of foreign antigens. Investigators in Adelaide, Australia, modified strain Ty2la to express the lipopolysaccharide O antigen of *Vibrio cholerae* O1 serotype Inaba (Forrest et al 1989). In this construct the *rfa* locus of the Ty2la chromosome was replaced with the homologous region from *E. coli* K-12. A plasmid containing the genes encoding the O antigen of *V. cholerae* O1 serotype Inaba and a *thyA*$^+$ gene was stabilized in Ty2la that was *thyA* deficient. This hybrid vaccine was well tolerated and stimulated modest antivibrio antibody titres when volunteers ingested three 10^{10} organism doses given every other day (Forrest et al 1989, Tacket et al in press). One month after vaccination, a group of vaccinees and 13 unimmunized controls were challenged with 10^6 organisms of pathogenic strain El Tor Inaba N16961 (Tacket et al in press). Diarrhoea occurred in all 13 controls and in 6 of 8 vaccinees (25% vaccine efficacy). However, the severity of diarrhoea (measured as the mean diarrhoeal stool volume) and the excretion of the pathogen (determined as the mean number of *V. cholerae* per gram of stool) were significantly diminished ($p < 0.05$) in the vaccinees compared with the controls. Although the level of protection was not marked, there was clearly a biological effect stimulated by this hybrid vaccine. This is more notable when one considers that only a single antigen of *V. cholerae* was expressed in the carrier vaccine.

While neither of the two attenuated *S. typhi* hybrid vaccines tested so far in clinical studies in humans involved the expression of foreign protein antigens, studies with multiple such constructs are expected to be initiated in the near future using attenuated *S. typhi* carriers other than Ty2la.

SUMMARY

In recent years there has been a resurgence of research to develop new and improved vaccines against typhoid fever. Two distinct approaches have both proved successful: parenteral vaccines based on stimulating serum antibodies against the Vi capsular polysaccharide; and attenuated strains used as oral vaccines to elicit serum antibody, intestinal SIgA antibody and cell-mediated immune responses. The attenuated strains also offer great promise as live carrier vaccines to express foreign antigens and deliver them to the immune system.

REFERENCES

Acharya V L, Lowe, C U, Thapa R et al 1987 Prevention of typhoid fever in Nepal with the Vi capsular polysaccharide of *Salmonella typhi*. A preliminary report. New England Journal of Medicine 317: 1101-1104

Black R E, Levine M M, Young C et al (Chilean Typhoid Committee) 1983 Immunogenicity of Ty21a attenuated *Salmonelli typhi* given with sodium bicarbonate or in enteric-coated capsules. Developments in Biological Standardization 53: 9-14

Black R E, Levine M M, Clements M L et al 1987 Prevention of shigellosis by a *Salmonella typhi-Shigella sonnei* bivalent vaccine. Journal of Infectious Diseases 155: 1260-1265

Blaser M, Hickman F W, Farmer J J, Brenner D J, Balows A, Feldman R A 1980 *Salmonella typhi* : the laboratory as a reservoir of infection. Journal of Infectious Diseases 142: 934-938

Brown A, Hormaeche C E, Demarco De Hormaeche et al 1987 An attenuated *aroA Salmonella typhimurium* vaccine elicits humoral and cellular immunity to cloned beta-galactosidase in mice. Journal of Infectious Diseases 155: 86-92

Carter P B, Collins R M 1974 The route of enteric infection in normal mice. Journal of Experimental Medicine 139: 1189-1203

Charbit A, Sobczak E, Michel M-L, Molla A, Tiollas P, Hofnung M 1987 Presentation of two epitopes of the preS2 region hepatitis B on live recombinant bacteria. Journal of Immunology 139: 1658-1664

Clements J D, El-Morshidy S 1984 Construction of a potential live oral bivalent vaccine for typhoid fever and cholera-*Escherichia coli*-related diarrheas. Infection and Immunity 46: 564-569

Collins F M 1972 Salmonellosis in orally infected specific pathogen-free C57Bl mice. Infection and Immunity 5: 191-198

Cryz S J Jr, Furer E, Baron L S, Noon K F, Rubin F A, Kopecko D J 1989 Construction and characterization of a Vi-positive variant of the *Salmonella typhi* live oral vaccine strain Ty21a. Infection and Immunity 57: 3863-3878

Curtiss R III, Kelly S M 1987 *Salmonella typhimurium* deletion mutants lacking adenylate cyclase and cyclic AMP receptor protein are avirulent and immunogenic. Infection and Immunity 55: 3035-3043

Curtiss R III, Goldschmidt R M, Fletchall N B, Kelly S M 1988 Avirulent *Salmonella typhimurum* delta cya delta crp oral vaccine strains expressing a streptococcal colonization and virulence antigen. Vaccine 6: 155-160

Curtiss R III, Kelly S M, Gulig P A, Nakayama K 1989 Selective delivery of antigens by recombinant bacteria. Current Topics in Microbiology and Immunology 146: 35-49

DeGraaf F K 1988 Fimbrial structures of enterotoxigenic *E. coli*. Antonie von Leeuwenhoek 54: 395-404

Dorman C J, Chatfield S, Higgins C F, Hayward C, Dougan G 1989 Characterization of porin and *ompR* mutants of a virulent strain of *Salmonella typhimurium*: *ompR* mutants are attenuated in vivo. Infection and Immunity 57: 2136-2140

Dougan G, Hormaeche C E, Maskell D J 1987 Live oral Salmonella vaccines: potential use of attenuated strains as carriers of heterologous antigens to the immune system. Parasite Immunology 9: 151-160

Dougan G, Chatfield S, Pickard D, Bester J, O'Callaghan D, Maskell D 1988 Construction and characterization of vaccine strains of *Salmonella* harbouring mutations in two different aro genes. Journal of Infectious Diseases 158: 1329-1335

Edwards M F, Stocker B A D 1988 Construction of del aroA his del pur strains of *Salmonella typhi*. Journal of Bacteriology 170: 3991-3995

Eisenstein T K, Killar L M Stocker B A D, Sultzer B M 1984 Cellular immunity induced by avirulent *Salmonella* in LPS-defective C3H/HeJ mice. Journal of Immunology 133: 958-961

Felix A, Pitt R M 1951 The pathogenic and immunogenic activities of *Salmonella typhi* in relation to its antigenic constituents. Journal of Hygiene (Camb) 49: 92-109

Ferreccio C, Levine M M, Manterola A et al 1984 Benign bacteremia caused by *Salmonella typhi* and *paratyphi* in children younger than 2 years. Journal of Pediatrics 104: 899-901

Ferreccio C, Levine M M, Rodriguez H, Contreras R, (Chilean Typhoid Committee) 1989 Comparative efficacy of two, three of four doses of Ty21a live oral typhoid vaccine in enteric-coated capsules. A field trial in an endemic area. Journal of Infectious Diseases 159: 766-769

Fields P I, Groisman E A, Heffron F 1989 A Salmonella locus that controls resistance to microbicidal proteins from phagocytic cells. Science 243: 1059-1062

Formal S B, Baron L S, Kopecko D J, Washington O, Powell C, Life C A 1981 Construction of a potential bivalent vaccine strain: introduction of *Shigella sonnei* form I antigen genes into the *galE Salmonella typhi* Ty21a typhoid vaccine strain. Infection and Immunity 34: 746-750

Forrest B 1988 The identification of an intestinal immune response using peripheral blood lymphocytes. Lancet i: 81-83

101

Forrest B, LaBrooy J T, Attridge S R et al 1989 A candidate live oral typhoid/cholera hybrid vaccine is immunogenic in man. Journal of Infectious Diseases 159: 145-146

Gaines S, Landy M, Edsall G, Mandel A D, Trapani R J, Benenson A S 1961 Studies on infection and immunity in experimental typhoid fever. III. Effect of prophylactic immunization. Journal of Experimental Medicine 114: 327-342

Gaines S, Sprinz H, Tully J G, Tiggertt W D 1968 Studies on infection and immunity in experimental typhoid fever. VII. The distribution of *Salmonella typhi* in chimpanzee tissue following oral challenge and the relationship between the numbers of bacilli and morphologic lesions. Journal of Infectious Diseases 118: 293-306

Galan J, Curtiss R III 1989 Virulence and vaccine potential of phoP mutants of *Salmonella typhimurium*. Microbial Pathogenesis 6: 433-443

Germanier R, Furer E 1975 Isolation and characterization of gal E mutant Ty21a of *Salmonella typhi*: a candidate strain for a live oral typhoid vaccine. Journal of Infectious Diseases 141: 553-558

Gilman R H, Hornick R B, Woodward W E et al 1977 Immunity in typhoid fever: evaluation of Ty21a—an epimeraseless mutant of *S. typhi* as a live oral vaccine. Journal of Infectious Diseases 136: 717-723

Glaser J B, Morton-Kute L, Berger S et al 1985 Recurrent *Salmonella typhimurium* bacteremia associated with the acquired immunodeficiency syndrome. Annals of Internal Medicine 102: 189-193

Herrington D, Van De Verg L, Formal S B et al in press Studies in volunteers to evaluate candidate *Shigella* vaccines: Further experience with a bivalent *Salmonella typhi-Shigella sonnei* vaccine and protection conferred by previous *Shigella sonnei* disease. Vaccine

Hoiseth S, Stocker B A D 1981 Aromatic-dependent *Salmonella typhimurium* are non-virulent and effective as live vaccines. Nature (London) 292: 238-239

Hone D, Attridge S R, Forrest B et al 1988a A *galE via* (Vi-negative) mutant of *Salmonella typhi* Ty2 retains virulence in man. Infection and Immunity 56: 1326-1333

Hone D, Attridge S, Van den Bosch L, Hackett J 1988b A chromosomal integration system for stabilization of heterologous genes in *Salmonella* based vaccine strains. Microbial Pathogenesis 5: 407-418

Hornick R B, Greisman S E, Woodward T E, DuPont H L, Dawkins A T, Snyder M J 1970 Typhoid fever; pathogenesis and control. New England Journal of Medicine 283: 686-691

Institute of Medicine 1986 New vaccine development: establishing priorities. Vol II. Diseases of important in developing countries. National Academy Press, Washington, DC. Appendix D-14, Prospects for immunizing against *Salmonella typhi*, pp 1-10

Killar L M, Eisenstein T K 1985 Immunity to *Salmonella typhimurium* infection in C3H/HeJ and C3H/HeNCr1BR mice: Studies with an aromatic-dependent live *S. typhimurium* strain as a vaccine. Infection and Immunity 47: 605-612

Klugman K, Gilbertson I T, Koornhof H J et al (Vaccination Advisory Committee) 1987 Protective activity of Vi capsular polysaccharide vaccine against typhoid fever. Lancet ii: 1165-1169

Kohbata S, Yokoma, Yabuchi E 1986 Cytopathogenic effect of *Salmonella typhi* GIFU 10007 on M cells of murine ileal Peyer's patches in ligated ileal loops: an ultrastructural study. Microbiology and Immunology 30: 125-1237

Landy M 1954 Studies on Vi antigen. VI. Immunization of human beings with purified Vi antigen. American Journal of Hygiene 60; 52-62

Landy M, Gaines S, Seal J P, Whiteside J E 1954 Antibody responses of man to three types of antityphoid immunizing agents. American Journal of Public Health 44: 1572-1579

Landy M, Johnson A G, Webster M E 1961 Studies on Vi antigen. VIII. Role of acetyl in antigenic activity. American Journal of Hygiene 73: 55-65

Levine M M, Ferreccio C, Black R E, Germanier R, (Chilean Typhoid Committee) 1987a Large-scale field trial of Ty21a live oral typhoid vaccine in enteric-coated capsule formulation. Lancet i: 1049-1052

Levine M M, Herrington D, Murphy J R et al 1987b Safety, infectivity, immunogenicity, and in vivo stability of two attenuated auxotrophic mutant strains of *Salmonella typhi*, 541Ty and 543Ty, as live oral vaccines in man. Journal of Clinical Investigation 79: 888-902

Levine M M, Ferreccio C, Black R E, Tacket C O, Germanier R (Chilean Typhoid Commission) 1989a Progress in vaccines against typhoid fever. Reviews of Infectious Diseases 11 (suppl. 3): S552-S567

Levine M M, Taylor D N, Ferreccio C 1989b Typhoid vaccines come of age. Pediatric Infections Disease Journal 8: 374-381

Levine M M, Ferreccio C, Cryz S, Ortiz E A randomized, controlled field trial comparing three doses of Ty21a live oral typhoid vaccine administered in enteric-coated capsule or liquid formulations (submitted)

Losonsky G, Kaintuck S, Kotloff K L, Kainruk S, Robbins J B, Levine M M 1987 Evaluation of an enzyme-linked immunosorbent assay for detection of chronic typhoid carriers. Journal of Clinical Microbiology 25: 2266-2269

Mallory F B 1898 A histological study of typhoid fever. Journal of Experimental Medicine 3: 611-638

Maskell D, Sweeney K J, O'Callaghan D, Hormaeche C, Liew F Y, Dougan 1987 *Salmonella typhimurium aroA* mutants as carriers of the *Escherichia coli* heat-labile enterotoxin B subunit to the murine secretory and systemic immune systems. Microbial Pathogenesis 2: 211-221

Miller I A, Chatfield S, Dougan G, Desilva L, Joysey H S, Hormaeche C 1989a Bacteriophage P22 as a vehicle for transducing cosmid gene banks between smooth strains of Salmonella typhimurium: use in identifying a role for aroD in attenuating virulent Salmonella strains. Molecular and General Genetics 215: 312-316

Miller S I, Kurral A M, Mekalanos J J 1989b A two-component regulatory system *(phoP phoQ)* controls *Salmonella typhimurium* virulence. Proceedings of the National Academy of Sciences (USA) 86: 5054-5058

Murphy J R, Baqar S, Munoz C, et al 1987 Characteristics of humoral and cellular immunity to *Salmonella typhi* in residents of typhoid-endemic and typhoid-free regions. Journal of Infectious Diseases 156: 1005-1009

Nakayama K, Kelly S M, Curtiss R III 1988 Construction of an ASd$^+$ expression-cloning vector: stable maintenance and high level expression of cloned genes in a Salmonella vaccine strain. Biotechnology 6: 693-697

Newton S M, Jacob C O, Stocker B A D 1989 Immune response to cholera toxin epitope inserted in *Salmonella* flagellin. Science 244: 70-72

O'Callaghan D, Maskell D, Liew F Y, Easmon CSF, Dougan G 1988 Characterization of aromatic- and purine-dependent *Salmonella typhimurium*: attenuation, persistence, and ability to induce protective immunity in BALB/c mice. Infection and Immunity 56: 419-423

Rhame F S, Root R K, Maclowry J D, Dadisman T, Bennett J V 1973 Salmonella cholerasuis septicemia outbreak caused by platelet transfusions from a hematogenous carrier. Annals of Internal Medicine 78:633-641

Rice P A, Craven P C, Wells J G 1976 *Salmonella heidelberg* enteritis and bacteremia. American Journal of Medicine 60: 509-516

Rice P A, Baine W B, Gangarosa E J 1977 *Salmonella typhi* infections in the United States. 1967-1972: increasing importance of international travellers. American Journal of Epidemiology 106: 160-166

Robertson J A, Lindberg A A, Hoiseth S, Stocker B A D 1983 *Salmonella typhimurium* infection in calves: Protection and survival of virulent challenge bacteria after immunization with live or inactivated vaccines. Infection and Immunity 41: 742-750

Robbins J D, Robbins J B 1984 Reexamination of the protective role of the capsular polysaccharide Vi antigen of *Salmonella typhi*. Journal of Infectious Diseases 150: 436-449

Sadoff J, Ballou W R, Baron L et al 1988 Oral *Salmonella typhimurium* vaccine expressing circumsporozoite protein protects against malaria. Science 240: 336-338

Salas M, Angulo O, Villegus J 1960 Patologia de la fiebre tifoidea en los ninos. Boletin Medico del Hospital Infantil de Mexico 17: 63-98

Sarosombath S, Banchuin N, Tassannee S, Vanaduringhan S, Rungpitarangsi B, Dumhavibhat B 1987 Systemic and intestinal immunities after different typhoid vaccinations. Asian Pacific Journal of Allergy and Immunology 5: 53-61

Schodel F, Will H 1989 Construction of a plasmid for expression of foreign epitopes as fusion proteins with subunit B of *Escherichia coli* heat-labile toxin. Infection and Immunity 57: 1347-1350

Seid R, Kopecko D J, Sadoff J C, Schneider L, Baron L S, Formal S B 1984 Unusual lipopolysaccharide antigens of a *Salmonella typhi* oral vaccine strain expressing the *Shigella sonnei* form I antigen. Journal of Biological Chemistry 259: 9028-9034

Szu S C, Stone A L, Robbins J D, Schneerson R, Robbins J B 1987 Preparation and characterization of conjugates of the Vi capsular polysaccharide and carrier proteins. Journal of Experimental Medicine 166: 1510-1524

Szu S C, Li X, Schneerson R, Vickers J H, Bryla D, Robbins J B 1989 Comparative immunogenticities of Vi polysaccharide-protein conjugates composed of cholera toxin or its b subunit as a carrier bound to high- or lower-molecular-weight Vi. Infection and Immunity 57: 3823-3827

Tacket C O, Ferreccio C, Robbins J B et al 1986 Safety and characterization of the immune response to two *Salmonella typhi* Vi capsular polysaccharide vaccine candidates. Journal of Infectious Diseases 154: 342-345

Tacket C O, Levine M M, Robbins J B 1989 Persistence of Vi antibody titres three years after vaccination with Vi polysaccharide against typhoid fever. Vaccine 6: 307-308

Tacket C O, Forrest B, Morona et al in press Safety, immunogenicity and efficacy against cholera challenge in man of a bivalent typhoid-cholera hybrid vaccine derived from Ty2la. Infection and Immunity

Tacket C O, Losonsky G, Taylor D N et al Lack of immune response to the Vi component of a Vi-positive variant of the *Salmonella typhi* live oral vaccine strain Ty2la in volunteer studies. In preparation

Tagliabue A, Villa L, De Magistris M T et al 1986 IgA-driven T cell-mediated anti-bacterial immunity in man after live oral Ty2la vaccine. Journal of Immunology 137: 1504-1510

Takeuchi A 1971 Penetration of the intestinal epithelium by various microorganisms. Current Topics in Pathology 54: 1-27

Taylor D N, Pollard R A, Blake P A 1983 Typhoid in the United States and the risk to the international traveller. Journal of Infectious Diseases 148: 599-602

Thiry G, Clippe A, Scaecez T, Petro J 1989 Cloning of DNA sequences encoding foreign peptides and their expression in the K88 pili. Applied and Environmental Microbiology 55: 984-993

Wahdan M H, Serie C, Cerisier Y, Sallam S, Germanier R 1982 A controlled field trial of live *Salmonella typhi* strain Ty2la oral vaccine against typhoid; three year results. Journal of Infectious Diseases 145: 292-296

Webster M E, Landy M, Freeman M E 1952 Studies on Vi antigen. II. Purification of Vi antigen from *Escherichia coli* 5396/38. Journal of Immunology 69: 135-142

Wong K H, Feeley J C, Northrup R S, Forlines M E 1974 Vi antigen from *Salmonella typhosa* and immunity against typhoid fever. I. Isolation and immunologic properties in animals. Infection and Immunity 9: 348-353

Discussion of paper presented by M. M. Levine

Discussed by H. Makela
Reported by K. P. W. J. McAdam

During her discussion, Makela noted that 65% to 70% efficacy of typhoid vaccines was not ideal and considered rational ways in which they may be improved. She pointed out that *S. typhimurium* in mice has many similarities to typhoid fever in man, and also addressed the issue of immunizing against salmonella-caused enteritis, rather than systemic typhoid fever. Finally, she discussed the use of salmonella vaccines as carriers of foreign antigens.

Salmonella infection is a multi-stage disease. An ideal vaccine would attack the organism at each of the different stages. In the first stage the bacteria are in the intestines where they need to adhere to the surface. At stage two, they traverse the Peyer's patches, enter the tissue space, the local lymph nodes and the blood. By the third stage, they become phagocytosed in the Kupffer cells of the liver and the macrophages of the spleen, where they undergo the multiplication that is the critical part of the infection and is important for the creation of immunity when live vaccines are used. The evidence for these multiple stages of infection is derived from the mouse model and has not been studied in man. It seems clear, however, that a vaccine strain is needed that will be able to survive for long enough at the proliferative phase in the liver and spleen, perhaps for several days. Vaccine strains that are more rapidly eliminated will not cause the long-lasting immunity required to eliminate the salmonellae.

Vaccine strategies should aim to interrupt all three phases of the disease, different mechanisms of immunity operating at each stage. In the first and second phases protection is antibody-mediated. The specificity of the antibody is mainly anti-O and by analogy it is believed to be anti- Vi in typhoid fever. The Vi antigen does not occur in the strains causing infection in the mouse in which the corresponding function is mediated by the capsular-like, smooth O-antigen. In the third phase of the disease, cell-mediated immunity is required. This is not O-antigen specific, but is directed at protein antigens, as yet undefined.

Mouse studies show that passive antibodies can provide a 100-fold protection, increasing the LD_{50} by a factor of 100. However, if the challenge dose is higher, antibody-mediated immunity is overwhelmed so that the infection proceeds to the third stage. This might be similar to the case where Vi antigen vaccine may protect against light infection, but in developing countries where the infectious dose can be very high, antibody-mediated immunity is overwhelmed in some children.

Cell-mediated immunity in the mouse is also capable of increasing the LD_{50} by about 100-fold and in this case the immune mechanism cannot be overwhelmed by a higher infective dose. If both antibody- and cell-mediated immunity are stimulated, they act synergistically. Presumably, antibody reduces the infective dose considerably and cellular responses deal with the rest. If immunization mechanisms induce antibody in the intestine and blood and also cell-mediated immunity in the liver and spleen, it is likely that even heavy infectious doses will be effectively controlled.

Current oral live vaccines produce fairly high local antibody responses, but lower antibody responses in the serum and a good cell-mediated immunity, provided the vaccine strain is not attenuated too much. With the parenteral killed vaccine, such as the Vi vaccine, there are high antibody levels in the serum and some of the antibody is likely to seep through the mucosal surfaces to act in the gut. However, there is no cell-mediated immunity generated by these killed vaccines. A rational strategy would involve utilizing both types of mechanisms to give the body the best chance of killing the invading organisms.

Preventing salmonella enteritis would require antibody at the mucosal surface and also enough antibody in the serum to mop up any organisms that penetrate the gut. Cellular immunity would not be necessary, since the enteritis-causing salmonellae do not multiply in macrophages causing systemic disease. While oral immunization may be sufficient to produce antibody dependent immunity, this needs to be serotype-specific, requiring many antigens to be included in the vaccine. Using live carrier vaccines requires that the vaccine strain survives sufficiently long in the body to stimulate effective cellular immunity. Since live vaccine strains do cause cell-mediated immunity, it may be possible to immunize only once with a live strain against, for example, salmonellosis, cholera and hepatitis B carried by the vaccine strain. But then the recipient would be immune to salmonella, irrespective of which new antigens it carries and this might prevent the second use of a salmonella vaccine carrying other antigens. It is unclear whether oral vaccine strains generate serotype-specific immunity which will again require multiple different O-antigenic types to be effective against all salmonellae.

Blaser raised the issue of herd immunity and cross-immunity with other group D salmonellae. Levine commented that there were few bacteraemic infections other than *paratyphi*, indicating few group D salmonella infections in that age group. He commented that in Chile a major environmental cause of endemic typhoid is the sewage system. About 80% of the houses of typhoid cases are connected to the municipal open sewage system which has no subsequent sewage treatment. In the dry summers all water is recycled to cultivate vegetables. It is little wonder that salmonella infection is endemic. He hypothesized that when hundreds of thousands of individuals are immunized the total load of *Salmonella typhi* that goes into the sewage system is diminished. Herd immunity is not caused by transmission of the vaccine strain, since the strain is not excreted but self-destructs when grown in the presence of galactose. Other live strains may be shed in the stool for a couple of days and it is unclear whether they are picked up by farm animals, because *S. typhi* is so host specific. Some vaccine strains fed to calves can be found for 6 to 8 weeks in manure. Survival of *aroA, aroC* or *aroD* is about the same as the wild type strain since the mutations or deletions do not impair their survival.

Levine provided evidence of cross-protection between *S. paratyphi B* and *S. typhi* in Chile during the seven years' surveillance following oral vaccination. The 35% protection against *S. paratyphi B* is attributed to the sharing of O-antigens with partial cross-protection.

Makela commented that cellular immunity correlated with reaction to the protein coded by the virulence plasmid in *S. typhimurium*, but not to flagellin in the mouse model. Levine pointed out that in *S. typhi* there is no virulence plasmid but cellular immune responses had been detected specific for terminal O-polysaccharides. Dogma suggests that T-cells do not respond to polysaccharide and the question of contaminating peptides was raised.

Section III:
Mucosal surface infections

Chairman: S. R. Norrby

7. The role of bacterial adherence in urinary tract infections

G. K. Schoolnik

INTRODUCTION

The purpose of this chapter is to discuss newer aspects of bacterial adherence as these pertain to the pathogenesis of urinary tract infections. However, in order to provide detailed information at the molecular level, the scope of the chapter will, of necessity, be narrow. For example, only studies with *Escherichia coli* will be discussed. Although *E. coli* is responsible for 85-95% of all urinary tract infections in normal individuals, it causes only about one-half of urinary tract infections occurring in hospitalized patients, patients with structural or neurological abnormalities of the urinary tract and patients with a recurrent pattern of infections. However, far more is known about *E. coli* pathogenicity than the pathogenicity of other urinary tract pathogens. In addition, only infections occurring in patients with normal urinary tracts will be considered and by-and-large, only infections of the upper urinary tract, i.e. pyelonephritis. These limitations on the scope of this discussion are regrettable, but necessary. It is regrettable because infections of the lower urinary tract, particularly bladder infections (cystitis) are far more common, albeit less severe, clinical problems than pyelonephritis. Moreover, pyelonephritis in patients with abnormalities of the urinary tract including ureteral reflux, obstruction, and calculi is far more likely to cause loss of renal function than pyelonephritis occurring in patients without these abnormalities. However, thus far most animal urinary tract infection models have simulated upper tract infections in normal women, and as discussed later, the use of these models has helped to establish the pathogenic significance of bacterial adherence. Unfortunately, well-characterized animal models have not been established for cystitis or for infections in the structurally or neurologically abnormal urinary tract. Finally, although pathogenicity is now viewed as a series of events including adherence, invasion, cell-death and the subversion of host defences, we shall only consider the first of these. This is a little like being asked to describe a symphony by reference to the notes played by the trumpet section of the orchestra. However, at present, we have little understanding of how the other *E. coli* virulence determinants harmonize or indeed, how many may exist and what their roles might be. Adherence is nonetheless the linchpin of *E. coli* pathogenesis and as such is an appropriate focus for new therapeutic and preventive strategies.

THE ADHERENCE MODEL OF UROPATHOGENICITY

Studies from many laboratories during the last decade have shown that the adherence of *E. coli* to host cell surfaces is a virulence factor in urinary tract infection. Characterization of this process at the molecular level has led to a model that specifies the existence of two components which together mediate the adherence process. These are surface proteins of the bacterium, termed 'adhesins' and their corresponding epithelial cell 'receptor' molecules. In addition, soluble analogues of these receptor compounds may be present in urine or in mucus; there, they may bind bacterial adhesins and thus act as competitive antagonists of the adherence process. In this way, adherence can be viewed as a function of the specificity, concentration and affinities of bacterial adhesins and the presence and density of the corresponding adhesin receptors both on the epithelial surface and as soluble, fluid-phase compounds in urine or mucus. In previously infected or vaccinated hosts, anti-adhesin antibodies might also influence the adherence process. The attractiveness of this model is that it reduces a complex process to the interaction of identifiable molecules; characterizes adherence in thermodynamic terms; provides a rational basis for the development of new anti-infectives; and offers an explanation for well-established clinical and pathological observations. Among these are the tissue-tropism exhibited by uropathogenic *E. coli* for the mucous membranes of the human urinary tract and the apparent susceptibility of a small fraction of otherwise healthy women for highly recurrent urinary tract infections. In spite of the simplicity of this model, complexity arises from the fact that individual bacterial strains produce several adhesins with different receptor specificities whose regulation of expression may be controlled by chemical or physical cues found in different microenvironments of the host. This capability, together with subtle differences in the receptor specificity of closely related adhesin molecules seems to have evolved to allow these bacteria to adapt to the receptor repertoire of different hosts and tissues.

THE ADHESINS OF UROPATHOGENIC *E. coli*

E. coli adhesins can be classified by their ultrastructural appearance and receptor specificities. Ultrastructurally, they may exist either as filaments termed pili or fimbriae that project from the bacterial surface or as a non-pilus, proteinaceous, surface-exposed component of the organism's outer membrane. A more informative classification system is based on receptor specificity, where this has been determined. As discussed later, most *E. coli* isolated from the urine of patients with pyelonephritis can simultaneously express type 1 pili, which bind host glycoproteins containing α-mannose residues, and P pili which bind globoseries glycolipids containing galabiose which has the structure α-Gal-(1,4)-β-Gal (Leffler & Svanborg-Eden 1980, Kallenius et al 1980). More recently, additional adhesin specificities of uropathogenic *E. coli* have been identified, including S pili, which bind glycoproteins with a terminal α-NeuNAc-(2,3)-β-Gal structure (Korhonen et al 1984), and M pili which bind glycophorin A molecules that specify the human blood group antigen M (Vaisanen et al 1982), where the pilus binding site of this receptor glycoconjugate is comprised of galactose, *N*-acetylgalactosamine, sialic acid and serine residues. For each of these pilus types it is apparent that *E. coli* adhesins are proteins that bind carbohydrates and thus they are functionally analogous to lectins.

Epidemiological studies of the receptor specificities of *E. coli* adhesins have been conducted by many groups using strains isolated from the urine of patients with pyelonephritis, cystitis or asymptomatic infections of the urinary tract as well as strains obtained from the faeces of healthy control subjects. All such strains, if grown under optimal conditions, can express type 1 pili; thus, this pilus type is not uniquely associated with any particular clinical syndrome. In contrast, a representative study of this kind showed that P pili are expressed by most pyelonephritis strains, by about 65% of cystitis strains, but by only one-fifth of strains isolated from patients with asymptomatic bacteriuria (Leffler 1980, O'Hanley et al 1985a). Thirty per cent of normal fecal *E. coli* were also found to express P pili. This and many other studies of both adults and children have documented the statistical association of P piliated *E. coli* with infections of the upper urinary tract. Nearly a decade ago these observations led to the proposal by workers in Sweden that this association was due to the presence of globoseries glycolipids in the human kidney, especially in the collecting ducts and the epithelia of the renal medulla (Hanssen et al 1980, Leffler & Svanborg-Eden 1980, Breimer 1985). An important caveat of all such studies is that this correlation only exists for patients with normal urinary tracts; in the presence of ureteral reflux for example, infections of the upper urinary tract can be established by *E. coli* lacking P pili (Lomberg et al 1989). Moreover, relatively little is known about the in situ expression of these pilus types, although antibodies to P pili have been found in the sera of patients with pyelonephritis, indicating that in vivo expression of P pili probably occurs (De Ree & Van Den Bosch 1987). The epidemiological significance of S- and M-piliated *E. coli* strains have not been as thoroughly studied. Accordingly, only the type 1 and P pili adhesins will be discussed here.

PATHOGENIC SIGNIFICANCE OF *E. coli* TYPE 1 AND P PILI

The probable significance of P pili for the virulence of uropathogenic *E. coli* is implied by their association with pyelonephritis, as discussed earlier. Direct experimental proof of this has come from studies with isogenic *E. coli* strains expressing either the P pilus or type 1 pilus types using the BALB/c murine model of pyelonephritis (O'Hanley et al 1985b). The gene clusters encoding either P pili or type 1 pili expression were isolated from a fully virulent human pyelonephritis strain and cloned into an avirulent, non-piliated *E. coli* recipient strain. Functional, biochemical and ultrastructural studies showed that each of the two resulting recombinant strains expressed either P pili or type 1 pili, but lacked other virulence determinants of the parent pyelonephritis strain including haemolysin production and resistance to the bactericidal action of normal serum. Each of the strains was then assessed for infectivity and virulence by instillation of a graded inocula into the bladders of BALB/c mice.

This model was designed to simulate an ascending mode of infection, similar to that which occurs in humans with anatomically normal urinary tracts. Moreover, as discussed below, receptors for type 1 and P pili were shown to be present in the epithelia of the bladder, ureters, renal medulla and collecting ducts of this murine species in a distribution that resembled their distribution in the human urinary tract. Finally, the urine of BALB/c mice, like human urine, was shown to contain type 1 pilus-binding glycoconjugates. The results of this study are as follows. The original pyelonephritis strain infected bladder urine, renal epithelia and caused haemorrhage and micro-abscess formation within the medulla of the kidney, indicative of the strain's invasive capacity. The same inoculum of the P pili expressing recombinant strain caused infection of the bladder urine and renal epithelia, but did not result in parenchymatous invasion. In contrast, the same inoculum of the type 1 piliated recombinant strain infected only the bladder urine. Only when the type 1 piliated strain was administered in concentrations 100-fold greater than the original challenge inoculum was infection of the renal epithelia evident in about one-half of the animals; however, invasion of the renal parenchyma did not occur. These studies led to the following conclusions. First, P pili confer infectivity of bladder urine and renal epithelial surfaces. In contrast, type 1 pili confer infectivity of the renal epithelium, but only when the challenge inoculum is large. The difference in the efficiency of infectivity between the P and type 1 piliated recombinants can be ascribed to the effect of soluble type 1 pilus receptor analogues in urine; these mannose-containing glycoconjugates appear to reduce the capacity of type 1 pili to bind epithelial cell surface receptor compounds. Second, infectivity can be dissociated experimentally from invasiveness. In these studies, infectivity was conferred by P pili whereas invasiveness, which was only evident in the fully virulent pyelonephritis strain, was conferred by virulence determinants other than pili. The significance of this observation for the immunoprophylaxis of pyelonephritis is described later.

Additional proof for the pathogenic role of the P versus the type 1 pilus types was sought through the study of vaccines containing pili purified from each of the two recombinant strains described above. Only the P pili vaccine prevented infection of the bladder urine and the renal epithelia by the fully virulent pyelonephritis strain. Of greater importance, the P pili vaccine also prevented bacterial invasion of renal parenchyma (O'Hanley et al 1985b). Similar findings have also been reported using a primate model of pyelonephritis (Roberts et al 1984). Taken together, these studies not only provide additional evidence for the pathogenic significance of P pili, but also demonstrate that a vaccine that prevents infectivity—presumably by blocking the attachment of bacteria to host epithelial cells—also can prevent invasion of tissue. This, in turn suggests that the colonization of epithelial surfaces by bacteria both precedes and is a necessary prerequisite for, bacterial invasion. In a more general sense, by providing evidence for the efficacy of anticolonization vaccines, these results also are pertinent for the protection of mucosal surfaces elsewhere, including respiratory, gastrointestinal and genital tissues. Pyelonephritis vaccines will be discussed in greater detail in a following section.

STRUCTURE, BIOGENESIS AND ANTIGENIC ANALYSIS OF P PILI

Elegant work by Normark and colleagues has shown that each P pili filament is in fact a macromolecular assembly comprised of several different polypeptides, each specified by a gene within the P pili operon; in turn, this operon functions as a single transcriptional unit (Hultgren et al 1989) within the *E. coli* chromosome. Studies with type 1 and S pili indicate that they have a similar genetic and structural arrangement.

The Pap A subunit of P pili is present in about 1000 copies per pilus filament; it thus constitutes the major structural polypeptide of the pilus polymer. Each Pap A subunit is comprised of approximately 170 amino acids and contains an intra-molecular disulphide loop in the first one-third of the molecule. When the primary structures of Pap A subunits from different strains are compared, the N- and C-terminal regions are found to be conserved, but structural diversity is evident in the middle section of the molecule. This structural diversity, the associated antigenic diversity and the fact that most of the mass and surface area of a P pilus filament is comprised of polymerized Pap A subunits causes Pap A to be the immuno-dominant polypeptide of the filament. As a result, at least 16 P pilus serotypes have been defined using monoclonal antibodies. The significance of this antigenic diversity for vaccine development will be discussed in a later section.

The Pap G protein of P pili is located at the distal tip of the pilus filament, is present in one to a few copies per filament and constitutes the galabiose-binding subunit of the pilus. Thus, Pap A subunits form a linear polymer that serves to present the functionally important Pap G subunit to the host epithelial cell receptor. Structure-function analysis of the Pap G subunit indicates that it is a 35 000 dalton protein with two domains (Hultgren et al 1989). The galabiose-binding domain appears to be located within the N-terminal 155 amino acids of the subunit. The C-terminal region of the molecule interacts with the Pap D protein; this protein exists in the periplasm where it serves to stabilize several of the pilus subunits before they are incorporated into the pilus filament. Structural and serological analysis of the Pap G protein from three P pilus serotypes reveals only 45% homology between the PapG protein of the F13 serotype and the Pap G proteins from the F11 and F7 serotypes. In contrast, the Pap G proteins of the F11 and F7 serotypes differed by only five amino acids out of a total of 316 amino acids (Lund et al 1988a). The Pap G protein is far less immunogenic than the Pap A protein. However, antisera to whole pilus filaments contain antibodies to the Pap G protein and these bind the tip of the filament. The Pap G protein (Hoschutzky et al 1989) and a Pap G-Pap D complex (Lund et al 1988a) have now been isolated. The use of the former as a pyelonephritis vaccine will be considered below.

The Pap E protein is also present in a few copies per filament, is located at the tip of the pilus, serves to link Pap G to the filament and exhibits both structural and antigenic diversity. The role of the Pap F protein is less defined. However, its presence is required for the normal receptor binding function of Pap G, it also is located at the pilus tip and unlike the Pap A, Pap G and Pap E proteins, it is structurally and antigenically conserved between P pilus serotypes. The Pap H protein is located at the base of the pilus filament where it anchors the filament to the outer membrane of the bacterium. As noted above, the Pap D protein is an 'accessory' protein, necessary for the biogenesis of the filament. Similarly, Pap C appears to function as a channel in the outer membrane through which other polypeptides are conducted for assembly on the bacterial surface.

Vaccine efficacy studies have been conducted with murine and primate models designed to simulate infection of the anatomically normal, upper urinary tract. As noted above, vaccines comprised of purified P pili conferred homologous protection, i.e. prevented infection by virulent pyelonephritis *E. coli* strains expressing serologically identical P pili (Roberts et al 1984, O'Hanley et al 1985b). Purified P pili can also confer heterologous protection providing the challenge strains express P pili that contain serologically cross-reacting antigenic determinants (Pecha et al 1989). However, as expected, no protection is conferred for strains expressing serologically unrelated P pili. When these vaccine studies are taken together the following conclusions are evident. First, systemic immunization with purified P pili prevents renal colonization and invasion by uropathogenic *E. coli* carrying serologically identical or closely related P pili. However, neither the duration of the protective effect nor the mechanism of protection is known. It seems clear that antibodies are elicited by these vaccines; that these antibodies are directed primarily to the Pap A subunit of the pilus filament; that they are present in serum and urine; and that they are principally of the IgG class. When the function of these antibodies is examined in vitro, they do not appear to block the galabiose-binding function of the pilus. Rather, they appear to bind quite densely along the longitudinal axis of the pilus filament in a location that might cause the agglutination of these filaments and P piliated bacteria. Thus, the protective efficacy of P pili vaccines seems to be unrelated to the adhesive role of P pili per se. Instead, with regard to protective immunity, efficacy seems to be due to the fact that P pili are a surface-exposed antigen of the bacteria that can be readily bound by specific antibody. In turn, it seems likely that the bound antibodies perturb the bacterial surface in some important way that is critical for pathogenesis.

Because the Pap A subunit is the immunodominant polypeptide of P pili and carries protective epitopes, antigenic analysis of it has been performed using synthetic peptides corresponding to regions of the Pap A sequence from one P pilus serotype (Schmidt et al 1985, 1988). Peptides corresponding to residues 5 to 12 and 65 to 75 bound intact pili, indicating that these regions of the Pap A sequence are surface-exposed and encode linear antigenic determinants. Antisera to peptide 5-12 bound seven of eight heterologous P pili (including representatives of four different P pili serotypes), indicating that this N-terminal region contains a P pili cross-reacting epitope. In contrast, antisera to peptide 65-75 bound only the homologous pilus filament, indicating that this region contains a type-specific epitope. Both peptides conferred homologous protection in the previously described murine model of pyelonephritis. Because peptide 5-12 contains a cross-reacting protective epitope and corresponds to a region that is conserved in most Pap A subunit serotypes, it seems likely that this peptide might also confer heterologous protection. However, to date, this possibility has not been thoroughly investigated. The studies discussed so far indicate that a broadly cross-reactive P pili vaccine might be comprised of two kinds of immunogens: (i) a small number of purified P pili representing different serotypes which when administered as a polyvalent vaccine elicit a broadly cross-reactive immune response; or (ii) peptides corresponding to conserved regions of the Pap A sequence that contain cross-reacting protective epitopes.

Pursuant to their work on the heteropolymeric structure and biogenesis of P pili,

Normark and colleagues have proposed the use of tip proteins of the pilus filament (Pap E, Pap F or Pap G) as vaccines (Lund et al 1988b). This is an attractive idea, particularly as it pertains to the Pap G protein, because tip proteins are likely to be surface-exposed (since they interact directly with host glycoconjugate receptor molecules) and their function is critical for the lectin-like. carbohydrate-binding function of the pilus organelle. A priori it was predicted that these proteins would be conserved between different P pilus serotypes because they subserve a common function. As discussed in a previous section, this prediction has not been confirmed. DNA sequence determination and antigenic analysis have now been performed using the Pap E, Pap F and Pap G proteins (Lund et al 1988a) of three P pilus serotypes (F7, F11 and F13). Only the Pap F protein was structurally and antigenically conserved between the three serotypes. The Pap E protein was as structurally and antigenically diverse as the Pap A subunit which, as noted above, is the major repeating polypeptide of the pilus filament and carries both cross-reacting and serotype-specific epitopes. The Pap G proteins, which are comprised of approximately 316 amino acids, are nearly identical between the F11 and F7 pilus serotypes, but these are only 45% homologous with the Pap G protein of the F13 serotype. Moreover, antisera to the F13 Pap G variant does not cross-react with the F7 or F11 Pap G variants. These structural and antigenic differences aside, it seems likely that conserved galabiose-binding amino acids exist within the Pap G protein and that regions of this protein that contain these residues may also encompass cross-reacting, protective epitopes. The recent purification of the Pap G protein (Hoschutzky et al 1989) and the preparation of a monoclonal antibody that blocks galabiose-dependent adherence and binds the F7, F8 and F13 Pap G variants, provides exciting new evidence that this goal can be achieved.

PREVENTION OF PYELONEPHRITIS BY COMPETITIVE INHIBITION OF RECEPTOR BINDING

The specifity and affinity of adhesin receptor-binding systems suggest that inhibition of adherence by soluble analogues of the receptor is achievable in situ and might block mucosal colonization. The prerequisites of this strategy are: (i) the adhesin conferring infectivity is identified; (ii) the chemical structure of its cell surface receptor is determined; (iii) a soluble analogue of the receptor oligosaccharide is synthesized or is produced from natural sources; and (iv) the compound is applied to mucosal surfaces where competitive inhibition of bacterial adherence occurs and renders the organism non-infectious. The feasibility of this approach has been established using the murine urinary tract infection model by simultaneously administering soluble receptor compounds for the P and type 1 pili of uropathogenic *E. coli* with an infectious inoculum. Methyl α-D-mannopyranoside (a receptor analogue for type 1 pili) prevented bacteriuria (Aronson et al 1979), whereas globotetraose (a receptor analogue for P pili) diminished bladder and renal colonization (Svanborg-Eden et al 1982).

The ultimate utility of this approach will depend on two kinds of technical accomplishments. First, analogues of galabiose will need to be synthesized that have high affinity for the Pap G protein and which, when present in low concentrations, can block the adherence properties of P piliated bacteria in vivo. So far, globotetraose is the most effective competitive inhibitor (Leffler & Svanborg-Eden 1980). Studies of this kind are now in progress with the discovery that the affinity of galabiose for the Pap G protein is mediated by hydrogen bonds directed toward five oxygen atoms located on one surface of this disaccharide and by interactions between non-polar surfaces of galabiose and Pap G (Kihlberg et al 1989). This in turn has led to the prediction that hydrophobic extensions in the 3′ position of galabiose should yield analogues with greater affinity for Pap G.

Further refinements in this kind of analysis should come from the crystal structure of a Pap G protein-galaboise complex. Second, it will be necessary to discover how to administer these analogues either orally or transdermally so that they can be systemically absorbed, filtered by the glomeruli and delivered to the urine as active, soluble Pap G protein-binding compounds.

RECURRENT INFECTION OF THE URINARY TRACT AS A MANIFESTATION OF RECEPTOR AVAILABILITY

Urinary tract infections are a common cause of morbidity, especially among otherwise healthy women of childbearing age. Although antibiotic therapy will cure the infection in approximately 80% of such women, additional episodes occur in the rest. Most recurrent infections are not due to inadequate treatment of the original infection. Instead, they are new infections with different bacterial strains, which occur in women without demonstrable structural or neurological abnormalities of the urinary tract. Such women are considered to be 'infection-prone'. The receptor-ligand model of uropathogenesis discussed earlier predicts that infection-prone women either have more adhesin receptors on their genitourinary mucosa and therefore more binding sites for *E. coli*, or they have fewer soluble receptor compounds in their mucosal secretions and urine and therefore have a lower capacity for competitive inhibition of adhesin-mediated colonization.

Present evidence favours the first possibility. Uroepithelial cells from infection-prone women on average bind more *E. coli* organisms than do cells from healthy women. This effect, however, cannot be explained by an increase in the galabiose content of these cells (Lomberg et al 1986). Instead, it appears to be correlated with the secretor status of the women. The cells of women with the non-secretor phenotype are more readily bound by *E. coli* with P pili than the cells of women with the secretor phenotype; moreover, women with recurrent urinary tract infections and renal scarring are more likely to be non-secretors than women who are not infection prone (Sheinfeld et al 1989, Kinane et al 1982, Lomberg et al 1989).

Thus, the non-secretor phenotype, increased epithelial cell receptivity for uropathogenic *E. coli* and recurrent infection of the urinary tract are all strongly associated with each other. The molecular basis for this association has not been examined directly. However, it is known that the epithelial cells of secretors exhibit fucosyltransferase activity. In turn, this activity is associated with the expression of the A, B, and H blood group oligosaccharides on the surfaces of these cells. As a result, these carbohydrates could obscure the less surface-exposed adhesin-receptor oligosaccharides, such as galabiose and related compounds, making them less accessible for interaction with the tip proteins of P pili. In contrast, the epithelial cells of non-secretors lack fucosyltransferase activity; the A, B and H blood group oligosaccharides are not expressed; and as a result, the adhesin receptors are arguably more accessible. These ideas are now being tested experimentally by directly measuring the surface accessibility of adhesin receptors on epithelial cells and in the urine and mucus of normal and infection-prone women.

SUMMARY

The foregoing discussion suggests a possible three-prong strategy that might prove to be superior to antibiotic therapy for the prophylaxis or treatment of urinary tract infection. First, the risk of infection in women and girls could be evaluated by determining their secretor status or by directly measuring adhesin-receptor accessibility on voided uroepithelial cells. Second, infection-prone women could be vaccinated with P and perhaps type 1 pili, with pilus peptides containing cross-reacting protective epitopes or with the functionally critical tip proteins. Third, soluble oligosaccharide analogues of the receptors of P and type 1 pili could be used in vivo to inhibit competitively adhesin-mediated colonization of susceptible mucous membranes.

REFERENCES

Aronson M, Medalia O, Schori L et al 1979 Prevention of colonization of the urinary tract of mice with *Escherichia coli* by blocking of bacterial adherence with methyl α-D-mannopyranoside. Journal of Infectious Diseases 139: 329-332
Breimer M E, Hansson G C, Leffler H 1985 The specific glycosphingolipid composition of human ureteral epithelial cells. Journal of Biochemistry 98: 1169-1180
DeRee J M, Van Den Bosch J F 1987 Serological response to the P fimbriae of uropathogenic *Escherichia coli* in pyelonephritis. Infection and Immunity 55: 2204-2207
Hoschutzky H, Lottspeich F, Jann K 1989 Isolation and characterization of the α-Galactosyl-1, 4-β-Galactosyl-specific adhesin (Padhesin) from fimbriated *Escherichia coli*. Infection and Immunity 57: 76-81
Hultgren S J, Lindberg F, Magnusson G et al 1989 The PapG adhesin of uropathogenic *Escherichia coli* contains separate regions for receptor binding and for incorporation into the pilus. Proceedings of the National Academy of Sciences (USA) 4357-4361
Kallenius G, Mollby R, Svenson S B et al 1980 The p^k antigen as receptor for the haemagglutination of pyelonephritogenic *Escherichia coli*. FEMS Microbiology Letters 7: 297-302
Kihlberg J, Hultgren S J, Normark S et al 1989 Probing of the combining site of the PapG adhesin of uropathogenic *Escherichia coli* bacteria by synthetic analogues of galabiose. Journal of the American Chemistry Society 111: 6364-6368
Kinane D F, Blackwell C, Brettle R P, Weir D M, Winstanley F P, Elton R A 1982 ABO blood group, secretor state and susceptibility to recurrent urinary tract infection in women. British Medical Journal 285: 7-9
Leffler H, Svanborg-Eden C 1980 Chemical identification of a glycolipid receptor for *Escherichia coli* attaching to human urinary tract epithelial cells and agglutinating human erythrocytes. FEMS Microbiology Letters 8: 126-134
Lomberg H, Cedergren B, Leffler H et al 1986 Influence of blood groups on the availability of receptors for attachment of uropathogenic *Escherichia coli*. Infection and Immunity 51: 919-926
Lomberg H, Hellström J, Jodal U, Svanborg-Eden C 1989 Secretor state and renal scarring in girls with recurrent pyelonephritis In: Blackwell C (ed) Disease Markers. FEMS Microbiology and Immunology 47: 371-376
Lomberg H, Hellström J, Jodal U, Orskov I, Svanborg-Eden C 1989 Properties of *Escherichia coli* in patients with renal scarring. Journal of Infectious Diseases 159: 579-582

Lund B, Lindberg F, Normark S 1988a Structure and antigenic properties of the tip-located P pilus proteins of uropathogenic *Escherichia coli.* Journal of Bacteriology 170: 1887-1894

Lund B, Lindberg F, Marklund B I et al 1988b Tip proteins of pili associated with pyelonephritis: new candidates for vaccine development. Vaccine 6: 110-112

O'Hanley P, Low D, Romero I et al 1985a Gal-Gal binding and hemolysin phenotypes and genotypes associated with uropathogenic *Escherichia coli.* New England Journal of Medicine 313: 414-420

O'Hanley P, Lark D, Fallow S et al 1985b Molecular basis of *Escherichia coli* colonization of the upper urinary tract in BALB/c mice. Journal of Clinical Investigation 75: 347-360

Pecha B, Low D, O'Hanley P 1989 Gal-Gal pili vaccines prevent pyelonephritis by piliated *Escherichia coli.* Journal of Clinical Investigation 83: 2102-2108

Roberts J A, Hardaway K, Kaack B et al 1984 Prevention of pyelonephritis by immunization with P-fimbriae. Journal of Neurology 131: 602-607

Schmidt M A, O'Hanley P, Lark D, et al 1988 Synthetic peptides corresponding to protective epitopes of *Escherichia coli* Gal-Gal pilin prevent infection in a murine pyelonephritis model. Proceedings of the National Academy of Sciences (USA) 85: 1247-1251

Schmidt M A, O'Hanley P, Schoolnik G K 1985 Linear immunogenic and antigenic epitopes. Journal of Experimental Medicine 161: 705-717

Sheinfeld J, Schaeffer A J, Cordon-Cardo C et al 1989 Association of Lewis blood group phenotype with recurrent urinary tract infections in women. New England Journal of Medicine 320: 773-777

Svanborg-Eden C, Freter R, Hagberg L et al 1982 Inhibition of experimental ascending urinary tract infection by receptor analogues. Nature 298: 560-562

Väisanen V, Korhonen T, Jokinen M et al 1982 Blood group M specific haemagglutination in pyleonephritogenic *Escherichia coli.* Lancet 1: 1192

Discussion of paper presented by G. Schoolnik

Discussed by C. Svanborg
Reported by H. C. Neu

Dr Svanborg began her comments with the statement that the concept of anti-adherence appears on the surface to be very simple and straightforward as a great deal of information on the subject has been discovered over the last 10 years. She felt that we do not need to develop a vaccine because we have had receptor analogues for almost 10 years and we know that they can competitively inhibit binding. However, clinical trials have not been carried out. Dr Svanborg felt the reasons for this related to the functional consequences of adherence, and some of the problems in our interpretation of what adherence really does. She felt that most workers have thought that adherence is a colonization factor, i.e. it is a way for bacteria to create stable bacteriuria. Adherence, at least the P-fimbriae mediated adherence, is much more of a tissue attack mechanism that induces symptoms, and when considering vaccination therefore it is also important to discuss whether adherence is a tissue damage mechanism. Do we need to block adherence in patients with recurrent infections and renal scarring?

Both P and type 1 fimbriae enhance bacterial persistence in the urinary tract of experimental animals. This has been established by several groups with isogenic strains and it is not really related to whether the bacteria stay better in the bladder if they attach. We also know that in mice receptor analogues or antibodies which block adherence also shortens or decreases the infection. However, the human system is quite different. Strains causing longterm bacteriuria in man, those that persist best, are rarely adhering. The frequency of adhering strains in asymptomatic bacteriuria is 25%. Dr Svanborg also reported that she used recombinant *E. coli* strains of the same kind as Gary Schoolnik illustrated which colonize humans. She started with a wild-type strain from a child with asymptomatic bacteriuria, carried for three years without any symptoms or signs. This strain was O-negative, capsule negative, and had no large plasmids so it could not transmit the DNA that inserted into it. It was also adherence negative. This strain was then transformed with DNA sequences encoding either the Gal-gal or the mannose-specific adhesives. The patients were injected into the bladder via a catheter and the persistence of the three respective types was determined. (Fig. 7.1)

Both of the adhering transformants were eliminated within 24-48 hours, whereas the persisting strain was the non-adhering wild type strain. This result occurred in all of the seven successfully colonized subjects. What this tells us is that the colonization

Bacterial persistence

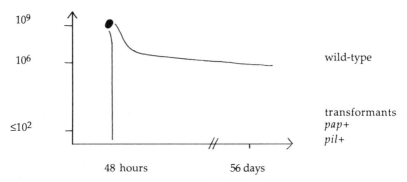

Figure 7.1 Adhering transformants were eliminated within 24-48 hours (Anderson et al in press)

ability of strains persisting in the urinary tract may not necessarily be related to bacterial adherence. Indeed, if adherence is produced in a strain that does not have the additional virulence factors it becomes a suicidal property.

Dr Svanborg has evaluated attachment is a tissue attack mechanism. She found that attaching bacteria and isolated fimbriae directly activate interleukin-6 and were responsible for the recruitment of leucocytes to the urinary tract mucosa. In patients P-fimbriated *E. coli* caused a higher Il-6 mediated inflammatory response that non-attaching strains. The inflammatory response in patients with various types of bacteria and the frequency of Gal-gal binding strains showed a linear relationship between inflammation and binding.

Inflammation leads to tissue damage and renal scarring, thus, is it unrealistic to expect that anti-adherence will prevent this phase of the infection—the chronic phase of the infection? The arguments for anti-adherence are also derived from animal models, where we know that attaching bacteria cause the highest acute inflammatory response. If we block this response we also block the resultant tissue damage. Against this is the finding that the patients who develop renal scarring are very rarely infected with adhering bacteria. Dr Svanborg and colleagues showed that boys aged one year with one episode of acute pyelonephritis were infected most frequently with Gal-gal positive strains, as we expect in this disease. However, if one compared the risk for renal scarring between those infected with Gal-gal positive strains and other strains, there was an inverse relationship of attachment to renal scarring.

Dr Svanborg concluded that it is hard to predict in the human system how a treatment, a vaccine or a receptor analogue that succeeds in blocking attachment, would work. Blocking of colonization may not be the important point, we know the inflammatory response is required for the elimination of bacteria. If one blocks this activation by the attaching organisms, one also decreases the resistance of the host to infection and most importantly chronically infected individuals are not infected with attaching bacteria. Dr Schoolnik replied that Dr Svanborg had illustrated the real life complexities of experiments in humans. Nothing can be as simple as when portrayed in a model system, and how one can reconcile differences in the two systems experimentally is unclear. He felt that a vaccine may establish whether it is possible to obtain protective efficacy.

122

Dr Blaser commented that haemolysin as a pathogenic factor keeps turning up in a variety of extra-intestinal *E. coli* infections and he asked whether haemolysin in the urinary tract model, either through recombinant strains or blocking of the activity, had been studied. Dr Svanborg replied that several groups have evaluated isogenic strains in a rat urinary tract infection model, and it has been shown that the haemolysin increases the tissue attack both on polymorphonuclear and renal tubular cells. Strains with haemolysin persist longer in the kidney than strains without haemolytic capacity. However, the absence of haemolysin, detected both by the phenotype and the genotype, does not correlate with the acute inflammatory response, but there is a reduced blood haemoglobin level in young infants.

Several members of the audience questioned why interleukin-6 was evaluated and whether other interleukins were. Dr Svanborg replied that she selected Il-6 primarily because of the specificity of the assay and the Il-6 spectrum of activity with the pyrogenic effect and the CRP induction. The Il-6 is secreted within minutes to one hour of infection, locally at first and then spreads through the blood stram of the animal. In colonized individuals she saw an increased Il-6 response in urine, but not serum, and patients were not ill.

Dr Lagrange enquired whether a pathogenic strain which is persistent can down-regulate receptors of the production of Il-6. Dr Schoolnik explained in detail the murine model and how he had used dyes as a way of determining whether reflux occurred. He showed experimentally that it is possible to avoid reflux acutely. Dr Schoolnik felt that women with highly recurrent disease are those women that have a larger number of receptors or who have fewer inhibitors in their urine or in their vaginal secretions normally. Patients of the non-secretor phenotype had increased recurrent infections of the urinary tract. Those people who have the secretor pheno-type because of the presence of fucosidal transferases have long oligosaccharides expressing human blood group antigens which physically obscure the receptor glycoconjugates that are much shorter and are less available for interaction with the P-fimbria adhesion molecule because of the presence of these abundant, tall and sterically occlusive blood group substances. Such a theory links three experimental facts, and is a theory that can be easily addressed with some of the anti-receptor antibodies that are available.

Dr Normark stated that it has been known for a long time that there are a number of Gal-gal-containing glycolipids, and the distribution of these Gal-gal-containing glycolipids is different in mice, in rabbits, in dogs and in humans. There are three different types of Gal-gal binding adhesions and the specific type that Schoolnik discussed, strain GA96, has one Gal-gal adhesion that is very rare in human urinary tract infection and seems to bind to a very specific subset of Gal-gal-containing glycolipid. Normark questioned what kind of Gal-gal-containing adhesion was introduced into this non-adhering strain of Dr Svanborg's, and whether that adhesion might recognize Gal-gal but not the typical isoreceptors that would be found in the human urinary tract, or was it that type of adhesion that dominates in human urinary tract infections?

8. The pathogenesis of diarrhoea caused by *Escherichia coli*

T. Wadström and Å. Ljungh

INTRODUCTION

Escherichia coli is the most common facultative anaerobe of the human intestinal flora but may also produce the widest spectrum of disease of any bacterial species (Sussman 1985). *E. coli* causes a variety of extraintestinal and intestinal illnesses. It is responsible for a number of distinct forms of diarrhoeal disease and dysentery. In recent years several specific virulence properties have been described which distinguish these diarrhoeagenic forms of *E. coli* from normal stool flora.

Four categories of *E. coli* which cause diarrhoea are well defined: enterotoxigenic (ETEC), enteropathogenic (EPEC), enteroinvasive (EIEC) and enterohaemorrhagic (EHEC), and one fifth, less well defined, enteroadherent (EAEC). The four main categories exhibit distinct clinical syndromes but still share certain characteristics related to pathogenesis. These include: (i) characteristic interaction with intestinal mucosa, (ii) plasmid-mediated virulence properties, and (iii) production of enterotoxin or cytotoxin.

A great deal of information has accumulated about the pathogenesis and epidemiology of the four main categories of diarrhoeagenic *E. coli* since the late 1960s.

EPIDEMIOLOGICAL PATTERNS OF *Escherichia coli* DIARRHOEA

The high prevalence of many bacterial, viral, protozoal and helminthic enteropathogens is the main cause of endemic intestinal disease in developing countries, particularly in children (Wanke 1988). In the last two decades it has become apparent that rotavirus and enterotoxigenic *E. coli* (ETEC) are major enteropathogens in developing countries with poor sanitation and water quality (Bäck et al 1980, Nicoletti et al 1988) and that water and water-treated vegetables and fruits are major vehicles for transmission of ETEC infections to adult travellers in these areas. Among the approximately 16 million travellers who leave industrialized nations to travel to non-industrialized areas of the world, about one-third will develop diarrhoea (Ericsson 1990, Farthing & Keusch 1989). The major bacterial pathogens besides ETEC in travellers to Mexico and probably also to other nations

Table 8.1 Aetiology of travellers' diarrhoea (data updated from Farthing & Keusch, 1989)

Enterotoxigenic *E. coli* (ETEC)*	40–75%
Enteroadherent *E. coli* (EAEC)	30%
Shigella spp.	5–15%
Salmonella	0–15%
Giardia lamblia	0–3%
Entamoeba histolytica	0–3%

* *Campylobacter jejuni* is the second pathogen to ETEC in many studies. Some recent studies show that enterotoxigenic *Aeromonas hydrophila* and related *Aeromonas* spp. can also be a common cause of travellers' diarrhoea probably related to water and food consumption (Wadström & Ljungh 1988).

are a recently defined class of enteropathogenic *E. coli* called enteroadherent (EAEC) (Table 8.1) (Mathewson & Cravioto 1988, Boedeker 1989, Gomes et al 1989).

Epidemiological studies in Mexico, Nepal (Taylor et al 1988) and other countries showed that ETEC usually accounts for 40 to 75% of travellers' diarrhoea, and EAEC for about one-third in one Mexican study (Ericsson 1990). More recently, a new form of EAEC has been described named enteroaggregative *E. coli* (E-Aggr-EC) (Gomes et al 1989). However, more work is now necessary before we understand the biological relevance of EAEC and E-Aggr-EC as pathogens in both paediatric and travellers' diarrhoea.

Interestingly most of these tissue culture cell-adherent *E. coli* or EAEC tested for O-antigens of the classical enteropathogenic O-groups were found not to belong to these traditional groups (Boedeker 1989). Such EAEC strains were recovered from faecal cultures from American students in Mexico where no other pathogens were isolated, and EAEC were much less commonly isolated from healthy controls (Mathewson & Cravioto 1988). Moreover, treatment of travellers' diarrhoea with antibiotics often gives good response with high curing rates, suggesting that ETEC, EAEC and maybe also other bacterial pathogens such as E-Aggr-EC are major pathogens (Ericsson 1990).

Historically, enteropathogenic *E. coli* (EPEC) were isolated from children with 'summer diarrhoea' in nursery epidemics in Europe and US in the 1940s and 1950s (Wadström 1978, Boedeker 1989). Today EPEC infections around weaning is often a serious enteric disease in developing countries (Senerwa et al 1989a,b) which may be linked to development of epidemics of prolonged diarrhoea (Wanke 1988). It seems most likely that EPEC and EAEC and maybe also E-Aggr-EC are the major pathogens in protracted diarrhoea in children in the tropics and subtropics.

ENTEROTOXIGENIC *E. coli* (ETEC): A BRIEF OVERVIEW

After the pioneer studies by H. W. Smith of ETEC as major causative enteropathogen in young piglets, lambs and calves (Smith 1976) many studies in the late 1970s and early 1980s showed that ETEC producing cholera toxin-like, heat-labile enterotoxin (LT) and heat-stable enterotoxins (named ST_a and ST_b with the original nomenclature of Smith) were also major pathogens in human paediatric diarrhoea (Sussman 1985, Kaper & Tackett 1988).

ST_a or ST_I is a methanol-soluble small peptide toxin active in the infant mouse model. It initiates intestinal secretion by stimulating guanylate cyclase and elevating intracellular cyclic GMP (Evered & Whelan 1985). The methanol-insoluble ST_b or ST_{II} stimulates intestinal secretion by an unknown mechanism probably involving staphylococcal delta-toxin detergent-like destruction of intestinal brush borders.

Heat-labile enterotoxin, LT, is a heterogenous family of toxins with two prototype toxins called human LT (hLT) and porcine LT (pLT) with structural and immunological differences in both the active (A) subunit and the cell-binding (B) subunit.

Interestingly, a second LT (LT II) with biological activity very similar to LT I and cholera toxin (CT) was not cross-neutralized by anti-LT and CT antisera. It does not bind to the common LT_h and CT cell receptor, i.e. the GM_1 ganglioside (see Kaper & Tacket 1988). With the discovery of antigenic variants called LT_a and LT_{II} or LT_b, and of one cytotoxic enterotoxin in *Aeromonas hydrophila*, recently cloned and showing no sequence homology to CT, it seems likely that that the class of heat-labile enterotoxins will be further expanded. Also *Salmonella typhimurium* is able to produce LT-like enterotoxin(s) which (i) do cross-react immunologically, and (ii) do not cross-react with CT (Kaper & Tacket 1988).

Recent epidemiological studies show that ST_b and LT_{II} are not commonly found among human ETEC strains but are probably, by evolution, developed in animal strains. It seems most likely that development of effective vaccines against ETEC infections based on LT subunits may permit selection of new antigenic variants originating among ETEC strains in an animal reservoir. Also, dogs and probably other animals have ETEC diarrhoea with strains producing LT which does not cross-react with CT antiserum or hybridize with LT DNA gene probes (Wasteson et al 1988, Wadström & Hedhammar unpublished).

The pathogenesis of ETEC diarrhoea is further complicated by the fact that human strains, unlike porcine and calf strains, seem to be able to produce a variety of antigenically, structurally and genetically distinct surface hair-like structures called fimbriae, pili, or colonization factor antigens (CFAs) (Table 8.2). The fimbriae of CFA/I (Evans et al 1978) and the three antigens of the CFA/II complex (CS1, CS2 and CS3) (Sjöberg et al 1988) are best characterized, while our knowledge of more recently recognized antigens such as CFA/III and putative colonization factor PCF 8775 (also called CFA/IV) is scanty (Wadström 1988, Wadström & Aleljung 1989).

le 8.2 Putative colonization factors of human enterotoxigenic *E. coli*

nbria	Associated serogroups	Subunit size (kDa)	Haemag glutination	Morphology
A/I	015, 025, 063, 078, 0128, 0153	15.0	+	Filamentous
l	0.6:H16 (biotype A)	16.8	+	Filamentous
		16.3		
2	06:H16 (biotypes B, C, F)	15.3	+	Filamentous
		16.4/17.0		
3	06, 08, 080, 085, 0115, 0139	14.5/15.5	–	Fibrillar
		14.8		
4	025	22.0	+	Filamentous
5	06, 092, 0115, 0167	24.0	–	Filamentous
5	06, 025, 027, 092, 0115, 0148, 0153, 0159, 0167	15.6	–	Fibrillar?
A/III	025	18.0	–	Filamentous
F	0159:H4	19.0	–	Filamentous

127

It seems most likely that ongoing epidemiological studies of ETEC diarrhoea in various countries will permit isolation of novel fimbrial putative colonization factors. Interestingly, recent studies on gene regulation of CFA/I and CFA/II show a complex regulation involving several genes (Hamers et al 1989). This great complexity of variants in a superfamily of CFAs suggests that ETEC organisms can use different strategies to colonize the human small bowel.

However, as shown by Smith (1976) for ETEC diarrhoea in pigs and calves, expression of CFAs is a prerequisite for induction of intestinal colonization and disease lasting for several days up to one week or more with clinical symptoms very similar to classical cholera (Ericsson 1990). These facts make it very attractive to try to construct vaccines to prevent both cholera and ETEC infections based on a combination of LT subunits in gene fusion with ST_I to be combined with CFAs. The great complexity of CFAs will have to be elucidated in order to reveal and define any common antigenic epitope that can be used for vaccine development in genetically designated strains (Kaper & Tacket 1988). However, the complex genetic regulation and expression of these CFAs may require a completely new approach to prevent ETEC diarrhoea based on compounds interfering with regulation. It is interesting that CFA/I as well as CS2 of the CFA/II complex can be defined as sialic acid-specific haemagglutinins or lectins (Lindahl et al 1988, Pieroni et al 1988, Wadström & Aleljung 1989). The cell receptors for these and other CFA structures are yet to be defined in the small bowel mucin and on the enterocyte surface.

ENTEROADHERENT AND ENTEROPATHOGENIC *E. coli*

Mathewson & Cravioto (1988) first showed that *E. coli* adherent to certain tissue culture cells such as HeLa and Hep 2 cells are pathogens in American travellers to Mexico. These EAEC strains are negative in tests for *E. coli* toxins such as LT, ST and Shiga-like toxins (SLT, see later). Based on the tissue culture studies, EAEC could be divided into (i) locally adherent (LA) and (ii) diffusely adherent (DA). Both type of strains can be recovered from patients as well as from healthy controls, as shown in studies in Mexico and Brazil (Nataro et al 1985, Gomes et al 1989).

It is premature to speculate how these non-toxigenic EAEC strains cause diarrhoea. However, in areas of enterocyte attachment the cell membranes lose microvilli and partially surround the *E. coli* organisms with cup-like so-called pedestal projections so that less than 15-20 nm separates the enterocyte and cell membrane (Knutton et al 1989). Thus, this adhesion process is quite different from the 'loose adherence' of ETEC strains. Moreover, in animal experiments these morphological changes were defined as attaching effacement (see later) with destruction of ordinary bundled microfilaments and cytoskeletal elements (Tzipori 1989). Knutton et al (1989) have defined a series of events in this colonization process leading to the late stage of pedestal formation. Okerman and Devriese (1989) further showed that rabbits experimentally colonized with rabbit-specific EAEC of various O:H serotypes were protected against challenge with other EAEC organisms. Thus it is tempting to speculate that further dissecting the adhesion process of human and animal EPEC strains will make it possible to define common features involving specific plasmid as well as chromosomally controlled outer membrane proteins

Table 8.3 Putative enterocyte adhesins produced by enteroadherent and enteropathogenic *E. coli* (EAEC and EPEC)

	Putative adhesin
Hep 2 factor	94 kDa OMP*
	29 and 32 kDa OMPs

*OMP, outer membrane protein.

involved in enterocyte receptor-ligand interactions (Baldini et al 1983, Nataro et al 1985, Wadström et al 1986, Smith et al 1990).

Recent studies by Pal and Ghose (1990) reveal that Hep 2 and HeLa cell adherent strains of classical EPEC O:H serotypes express adherence potential through factors not related to the mannose-resistant (MRHA) cell surface haemagglutinins (Table 8.3). The enterocyte damage may be induced in a similar way as plant lectins induce damage of enterocyte brush borders (Batt et al 1988). It should also be noted that EPEC strains may produce OMPs which, like *Entamoeba*-surface lectins also possess cytolytic membrane-damaging toxins. Interestingly, a number of human as well as animal EPEC strains produce low levels of haemolysin which may allow tissue invasion. Finally, it cannot be excluded that EAEC and certain virulent strains of EPEC of classical O:H serotypes produce surface located or periplasmically located virulence-associated proteins (Adams & Oxende 1989). Further studies are needed to identify such mechanisms as the possible role of locally released endotoxin to trigger enterocyte damage maybe through release of tumour necrosis factors and other cytokines (Barrett et al 1989).

A model for small bowel colonization and tissue penetration of EAEC/EPEC is presented in Table 8.4. Some EAEC strains among EPEC strains have been found to lack the Hep 2 plasmid (Pal & Ghose 1989). Hence, so far the degradation of actin seems to be the common pathogenic trait in EAEC strains (Knutton et al 1989). The use of Hep 2 cell adhesion test (Baldini et al 1983) or EAF-DNA gene probe hybridization (Nataro et al 1985, Levine et al 1987) to detect EAEC will thus not permit detection of all EAEC, and the actin fluorescence test can be an alternative test (Knutton et al 1989). This is an example that it is often premature to develop gene probe diagnostics before the pathogenesis is elucidated.

Human volunteer studies demonstrate that EPEC strains harbouring the EAF plasmid coding for the OMP-determining localized adherence (LA) to Hep 2 cells induce diarrhoea (Kaper & Tacket 1988, Boedeker 1989). EAEC strains lacking the EAF plasmid are also thought to induce diarrhoea (Pal & Ghose 1990). Much more

Table 8.4 Pathogenesis of enteropathogenic *E. coli* diarrhoea: a model

	Mediated by
Interactions with small bowel mucins[1] and surface haemagglutinins	MRHA agglutinins
Two-step binding to enterocyte 'loose and close' adherence	'Hep 2 factor' 29, 32 and 94 OMP[2]
Interactions with actin and the cytoskeleton	
Penetration into subepithelial tissue matrix	
Binding to fibronectin and collagens type I and IV	

[1] Small bowel mucin probably contains fibronectin and other molecules which may interact with human as well as rabbit and porcine EPEC/EAEC (Wadström et al 1986, Wadström 1988, Baloda et al 1985, 1986, Faris et al 1986).
[2] OMP, outer membrane protein.

has to be learnt about the pathogenesis of EAEC and EPEC diarrhoea which has been a challenge to us since the 1950s.

ATTACHING-EFFACING *Escherichia coli*

The term attaching-effacing *E. coli* (AEEC) is used for bacteria which attach closely to the intestinal epithelium at sites where the microvillous brush border is eroded or effaced. Mainly these bacteria belong to EPEC or EHEC groups. The attachment-effacement lesions have been shown to contain filamentous actin (Knutton et al 1989), and the ability to induce these lesions has been suggested to be under chromosomal control. Since EPEC strains mainly colonize the small intestine and EHEC the large intestine, their surface adhesins in which plasmid-born determinants are involved differ (Karch et al 1987, Junkins & Doyle 1989).

ENTEROAGGREGATIVE *Escherichia coli*

EAF-positive EPEC strains were strongly associated with intestinal disease in São Pãolo and in other tropical countries (Mathewson & Cravioto 1988, Gomes et al 1989). Most interestingly, certain *E. coli* strains were shown to form aggregates adhering to Hep 2 cells and glass slides in a 'stacked brick' appearance. Such strains, now defined as enteroadherent-aggregative *E. coli* (EA-Agg-EC), were commonly isolated from Chilean children with diarrhoea and much less commonly from healthy controls (Mathewson & Cravioto 1988). The cell clumping involves cell surface hydrophobicity, as determined by various assays such as hydrophobic interaction chromatography (HIC), cell clumping in the salt aggregation test (SAT) (Wadström et al 1984a,b, Wadström & Trust 1984, Gonzalez et al 1988). We thus speculate today that these strains are related to non-haemagglutinating EPEC strains showing autoagglutination (AA strains) upon growth in various laboratory media. Preliminary studies in our laboratory indicate that E-Agg-EC strains adsorb to HIC gels and permit the isolation of E-Agg-EC-negative variants, which have lost their autoagglutinating properties (Wadström et al 1986, Wadström unpublished).

Screening of 42 isolates of EA-Agg-EC strains showed that 93% harboured a 55-65 MDa plasmid. Apart from the 'stacked brick' adherence pattern, transfer of this plasmid was accompanied by transfer of smooth lipopolysaccharide and expression of fimbriae (see Thorne 1990). These strains further induced pathological changes in rabbit and rat intestinal loops. Inoculation of live EA-Agg-EC caused severe limb paralysis and death of rabbits, indicating the involvement of a toxin. No cytotoxin has so far been detected by screening eight cell lines.

BACTERIAL CELL SURFACE HYDROPHOBICITY

A great number of bacterial pathogens colonizing the small bowel show high surface hydrophobicity and autoaggregating properties. The most well known is virulence plasmid-harbouring *Yersinia enterocolitica* and fimbriae-expressing *Vibrio cholerae*

Table 8.5 High cell surface hydrophobicity is expressed by small bowel pathogens*

Enterotoxigenic *E. coli* (ETEC)	Magnusson 1989
CFA/I > CFA/II > K88 > K99 > Type 1	Wadström 1988
Enteropathogenic *E. coli* (EPEC)	
Haemagglutinating strains	Wadström, unpublished
Non-haemagglutinating strains	Wadström et al 1986
Enteroadherent and aggregative *E. coli*	Wadström, unpublished
(EA-Agg-EC)	-
Vibrio cholerae	Faris et al 1982

* The exception from this rule is probably *Campylobacter jejuni* expressing
hydrophobic cell surface upon growth in various culture media (Trust & Wadström,
unpublished).

(Table 8.5). From these observations one may speculate that these pathogens recognize certain lipids or other hydrophobic (amphiphilic) compounds in the small bowel mucins (Wadström & Baloda 1986) despite the fact that these pathogens are first trapped in the antrum area of the stomach containing mucins expressing a hydrophobic lining to protect the tissue from back-penetration of stomach acids (Spychal et al 1989).

Interestingly, rabbit EPEC strains inducing attaching effacement lesions adhered significantly better to rabbit intestine when grown to express high surface hydrophobicity and poor haemagglutination (Sherman et al 1985). This adhesion was shown to be correlated to non-haemagglutinating fimbriae, and gives further support to the concept that hydrophobic interactions with cell receptors as well as lipids or other hydrophobic compounds in intestinal mucus are important for the colonization of the enterocyte surface.

It cannot be excluded that tissue-invasive pathogens such as *Y. enterocolitica* and various *Salmonella* species can induce close cell adhesion which triggers events to permit the pathogen to penetrate between the cells and cellular tight junctions. We speculate if the common property among EPEC/EAEC strains to interact with fibronectin and various collagens (Ljungh et al 1990) may relate to specific interactions with tissue components between the cells and in connection with cellular receptors for these molecules called integrins (Wadström et al 1985, Wadström 1988). The recent finding that certain EPEC strains and *E. coli* strains isolated from intestinal lesions in patients with ulcerative colitis also bind vitronectin which may down-regulate complement activation indicates that much more has to be learnt about the complex cell surface mosaic of *E. coli* in the indigenous intestinal flora and enterovirulent strains as well as strains that are able to cause various extraintestinal infections. In a later section we speculate on the role of fibronectin and other interactions of mucosal proteins with enteropathogens.

THE INTESTINAL MUCOSA AND FIBRONECTIN

V. cholerae haemagglutinin has a strong protease activity ('fibronectinase'). We showed that certain strains of *V. cholerae* specifically bound ^{125}I-fibronectin (Wiersma et al 1987). Human ETEC strains, enterotoxigenic *Salmonella enteritidis* and *S. typhimurium*, as well as human, porcine and rabbit EPEC strains were also found to bind ^{125}I-fibronectin and its ^{125}I-labelled 29 kDa N-terminal fragment (Table 8.6) (Fröman et al 1984, Faris et al 1986, Wadström & Baloda 1986). On the basis of these findings it seems tempting to speculate that fibronectin in small bowel mucus, released on shedding of villous tip epithelial cells, can provide an initial colonization site for certain organisms expressing binding of fibronectin.

Colonization of epithelial lesions exposing fibronectin and collagens of the subepithelial lamina propria may be a more important intestinal colonization mechanism for EPEC and salmonellae producing cytotoxic enterotoxins. It also seems likely that an infection with rotavirus or other intestinal viruses which induce shedding of epithelial cells may trigger colonization of the exposed subepithelial matrix. This may be compared with a similar situation in the respiratory tract where virus infections often trigger secondary colonization with *Staphylococcus aureus* and other wound pathogens which bind to fibronectin, collagens and laminin (Wadström et al 1985). Since surface hydrophobicity and fibronectin binding do not appear to be correlated in *E. coli* (Ljungh et al 1990) it seems more likely that non-fimbrial surface proteins or carbohydrate structures are involved in the binding process (at least the binding outside the N-terminal domain).

The gene coding for one fibronectin (Fn)-binding novel class of surface organellae was recently cloned (Olsén et al 1989). Since this surface structure is only expressed below 37°C in various culture media the roles of this and at least two other Fn-binding structures have to be further studied. More recently an Fn-binding structure also interacting with collagen type I (Cn I) was defined in one ETEC strain (Visai et al 1990).

SHIGA-LIKE TOXIN-PRODUCING *E. coli* AND ENTEROHAEMORRHAGIC *E. coli* (EHEC)

Cytotoxin-producing *E. coli* associated with human intestinal infections were first reported by Konowalchuk et al in 1977 (see Karmali 1989). The assay used for detection was Vero cells and the toxins were hence described as Vero-cytotoxins. Since

Table 8.6 Fibronectin and collagen binding to enteropathogens

Fibronectin binding	
Escherichia coli[1]	
Enterotoxigenic *E. coli*	Fröman et al 1984
Rabbit enteropathogenic *E. coli*	Faris et al 1986
Porcine enteropathogenic *E. coli*	Baloda 1986[2]
Human enteropathogenic *E. coli*	Wadström & Baloda 1986
Salmonella typhimurium	Baloda et al 1985
Vibrio cholerae	Wiersma et al 1987
Collagen binding	
Human enteropathogenic *E. coli*	Wadström & Baloda 1986
SLT-producing *E. coli*	Ljungh et al 1988
Enterotoxigenic, enterohaemorrhagic,	
enteroadherent and enteroinvasive *E. coli*	Ljungh et al 1990
Yersinia enterocolitica	Emödy et al 1989

[1] The gene for a fibronectin-binding novel class of surface fimbriae (curlin) has been cloned (Olsen et al 1989).
[2] For an extended reference list see Wadström et al (1985), Wadström & Baloda (1986), Wadström (1988).

these toxins are now known to belong to the class of Shiga and Shiga-like toxins the term SLT will be used (Strockbine et al 1986).

Shiga toxin and the corresponding toxin in *E. coli* (SLT-I) have been purified and characterized. The toxin interferes with protein synthesis by inactivating the 60S ribosomal subunit. The toxin is an A-B subunit toxin with five B (binding) subunits to one A subunit. The molecular weights for the subunits are 32.2 kDa (A) and 7.69 kDa (B), respectively, and 70.6 kDa for the holotoxin (Karmali 1989).

The molecular genetics of Shiga and Shiga-like toxins have been extensively studied. The genes encoding the toxin are located on a bacteriophage in *E. coli* (Strockbine et al 1986) but on the chromosome in *Shigella dysenteriae*. The genes for the A and B subunits are arranged in a single transcriptional unit and the complete DNA sequence for SLT genes from *E. coli* has been determined by several investigators. The genes encoding Shiga toxin in *S. dysenteriae* I have been sequenced and shown to differ by very few base pairs from the SLT in *E. coli*. The mature B subunits are identical in amino acid sequence while the A subunits differ by only one of 293 residues. Thus the cytotoxins produced by these species are more like each other than cholera toxins from different *V. cholerae* strains (Kasper & Tacket 1988, Scotland et al 1988).

Strains isolated from patients with haemorrhagic colitis or HUS may also produce a second related toxin which is cytotoxic for HeLa and Vero cells but which is not neutralized by antiserum against Shiga toxin. This toxin has been designated Shiga-like toxin type II (SLT II) (Strockbine et al 1986). *E. coli* strains may produce one or both of these toxins. SLT I and SLT II share 58% overall nucleotide homology and 56% amino acid homology. Despite this divergence, the A and B subunits of both toxins are nearly identical in size and have similar secondary structure and hydropathy plots.

Enterohaemorrhagic *E. coli* (EHEC) were first recognized as human pathogens in 1982 in the USA in a multistate outbreak emanating from hamburger meat (see Martin et al 1986, Ryan et al 1986). The initial studies identified a previously uncommon serotype of *E. coli*, 0157:H7, as the causative agent. This agent has subsequently been implicated in sporadic and outbreak-associated infections. The illness is characterized by severe abdominal cramps, initially watery diarrhoea followed by grossly bloody diarrhoea with little or no fever. The severity of the infection varies, and EHEC strains are also isolated from healthy persons. *E. coli* 0157:H7 can also induce haemolytic uraemic syndrome (HUS) (Griffin et al 1988, Scotland et al 1988).

Strains other than 0157:H7 can also cause haemorrhagic colitis and HUS. These EHEC strains produce high levels of SLT and harbour a typical plasmid (approximately 60 MDa) (Junkins & Doyle 1989, Tooth et al 1990) and include serotypes 026:H11, 0111:H8, 0111:NM, 04:NM, 05:NM, 045:H2, 091:H21, 091:NM, 0103:H2, 0113:H2, 0121:H19, 0125:NM, 0145:NM as well as 0157:NM, and 0 (untypeable):H8 (Karmali 1989). The family of SLTs in *E. coli* is even larger since even wild-type K12 strains have been shown to produce low levels of SLT which can be neutralized by antiserum to SLT I but which shows no homology with DNA sequences encoding SLT I or II (Scotland et al 1988).

A potential adherence factor in EHEC strains is a non-haemagglutinating fimbrial antigen (Karch et al 1987). The genes for this factor are encoded on a plasmid of approximately 60 MDa. Transformation of an *E. coli* K12 strain with this plasmid results in the production of fimbriae by the recipient. Specific antiserum to purified fimbriae reacts with fimbriae in other 0157:H7 strains. Strains with this plasmid adhere to Henle 407 intestinal cells but not to Hep2 cells or erythrocytes. Loss of the plasmid results in loss of adhering ability.

This plasmid has been used to detect *E. coli* of serotype 0157:H7, and of other serotypes which cause haemorrhagic colitis and HUS (Levine et al 1987). A 3.4 kb fragment of this plasmid hybridized with 106 (99%) of 107 0157:H7 strains, and with 34 (77%) of 44 strains of serotype 026:H11 which were SLT-producing and were isolated from patients with colitis, HUS and diarrhoeal disease. The probe also hybridized with 21 (81%) of 26 SLT-positive strains of other serotypes from patients with haemorrhagic colitis and HUS. When 601 other *E. coli* strains of EPEC, EIEC, ETEC and urinary tract infection isolates as well as from normal flora were tested only one strain hybridized.

PATHOGENESIS OF EHEC INFECTIONS

In patients who have undergone colonoscopy during the acute illness the colon may be normal or may appear inflamed, oedematous, haemorrhagic or ulcerated (Karmali 1989). Histopathology of colonic biopsies may be normal or may show low-graded inflammation.

Tzipori and colleagues (1989) showed in gnotobiotic piglets that EHEC attach to and efface enterocytes and destroy the microvilli, a lesion resembling that due to classical EPEC. Unlike EPEC, EHEC proliferate in the lamina propria and glandular crypts. Interestingly, as shown by Knutton and colleagues (1989), EPEC and EHEC induce the same deterioration of actin in the small and large intestine respectively. It may still be justified that EHEC represent a new category of pathogenicity characterized by organisms multiplying in the lamina propria after damaging the surface epithelium (Tzipori et al 1989).

While conclusive evidence for direct involvement of SLT in the pathogenesis of EHEC diarrhoea (as well as of shigellosis) is lacking, substantial epidemiological and experimental evidence support this hypothesis. Since nearly all strains of *E. coli* isolated from patients, healthy controls, animals, and food produce some SLT, the amount of toxin produced may be of importance. Generally, strains isolated from patients with haemorrhagic colitis, HUS or diarrhoea produce moderate to high levels of SLT ($>1\times10^3$ cytotoxic doses per ml of sonic lysate), whereas normal flora *E. coli*, ETEC, EIEC and classical EPEC produce low levels of toxin that are not detected in cell tests (Ljungh & Wadström 1988). Furthermore, the *E. coli* strains that produce low amounts of cytotoxin do not possess DNA sequences homologous to the cloned SLT structural gene, indicating a fundamental difference in the structural genes for these toxins.

Shiga toxin is well known to inhibit protein synthesis in tissue culture cells. It is, however, not clear how these toxins induce fluid secretion in the intestine. One hypothesis holds that Shiga toxin binds to mature absorptive epithelial cells, ultimately resulting in cell death. This concept was supported by studies by Barrett et al (1989) who showed that Shiga toxin and SLT selectively destroy the mature absorptive epithelial cells of the rabbit ileum. Diarrhoea would then result from inhibition of absorption rather than from active secretion.

The role of SLT in EHEC disease was supported by studies in rabbit models, but not in the gnotobiotic piglet model (Tzipori et al 1989). Non-bloody diarrhoea was induced in infant rabbits infected with *E. coli* 0157:H7. When high- and low-level producing strains as well as partially purified toxin were inoculated, only the purified toxin and the high-level toxin producing strains induced diarrhoea. Histological changes were seen in the mid and distal colon with 'individual cell death' of the surface epithelium, increased mitotic activity in the crypts, mucin depletion, and an infiltration of neutrophils into the mucosa. Additional support for the involvement of SLT in disease was provided by using the rabbit pathogen RDEC-1. Bacteriophages encoding SLT 1 were added to the RDEC-1 strain which normally colonizes rabbits and causes diarrhoea. RDEC-1 strains with the SLT gene induced disease with earlier mortality, greater weight loss and more severe inflammatory and degenerative changes in the mucosa than the regular RDEC-1 (Boedeker 1989).

Unlike many enteric pathogens which encode all necessary virulence factors on the chromsome, the known putative virulence factors of EHEC reside on mobile genetic elements, i.e. plasmids and bacteriophage. The plasmids found in different EHEC isolates are highly related and retention of these elements in clinical isolates indicates that they may encode factors essential for virulence.

We have earlier reported the isolation of medium- and high-level SLT-producing strains from patients with relapse of ulcerative colitis in which neutralizing seroantibodies were also detected (Ljungh & Wadström 1988). The possible role of low-level SLT-producing *E. coli* in subchronic colitis has to be further investigated.

Burke and Axon (1988) reported on the isolation of special strains expressing high surface hydrophobicity from patients with inflammatory bowel disease. These studies have not yet been followed up.

Finally, certain *E. coli* with the so-called vir plasmids are able to produce a multinucleating and necrotizing activity (Oswald & de Rycke 1990). The role of these and other cytotoxins in the development of intestinal infections is unknown. Recent studies by Smith et al (1990) confirm that certain EPEC strains produce SLTs. These strains do not express EAF genes typical for most EPEC strains.

More epidemiological studies have to be performed in developing countries to elucidate the role of SLT-producing EAEC, if any, in acute and protracted paediatric diarrhoea.

ENTEROINVASIVE *Escherichia coli*

Certain serotypes of *E. coli* known as EIEC can invade the human colon like *Shigella*. Certain strains of EIEC have many properties in common with *Shigella* but the tissue-invasive properties have not yet been properly defined. The EIEC pose a difficult diagnostic problem since they may be confused with non-pathogenic *E. coli*. There is no one specific biochemical test that can identify these organisms. They belong to a small number of *E. coli* serogroups (Thorne 1990), and these antisera are not readily available in most laboratories. Isolates thought to be EIEC need to be confirmed by their ability to cause keratoconjunctivitis in the guinea-pig eye (Sereny test) or invade and multiply within cultured epithelial cells (Thorne 1990).

Newer techniques such as ELISA and DNA hybridization have been developed for detection of EIEC based on the large-molecular-weight plasmids which encode virulence-associated polypeptides. One single DNA probe (17 kb) was used to detect *Shigella* and EIEC (Taylor et al 1988, Kaper & Tacket 1989). The probe can detect lactose-positive EIEC growing on MacConkey medium more easily than the lactose-negative EIEC and *Shigella* spp. Further development in this area will permit hybridization of stool blots which is a more rapid method than colony blot hybridization. Furthermore, since stool blot hybridization is performed on unselected bacterial growth the detection levels can be expected to be high.

INTERACTION WITH SMALL BOWEL MUCIN

Little is known about the role of intestinal mucins in the pathogenesis of diarrhoeal disease. Lindahl et al (1988) reported that animal ETEC strains show specific binding of radioactively labelled mucin preparations and purified mucin glycopeptides. Moreover, K99 and F41 fimbriated strains bind to small bowel mucins immobilized on Sepharose beads. More recently other investigators have shown that human EPEC strains bind to small bowel mucin preparations as also demonstrated for rabbit EPEC strains producing so-called AF/R1 fimbriae. Interestingly, type I fimbriae were shown to interact with such mucins, suggesting a possible role for type I fimbriae in early step(s) of intestinal colonization. Since both fimbriated and non-fimbriated *E. coli* were shown to interact with mucins, probably several mechanisms are involved including non-specific, hydrophobic interactions (Wanke et al 1990).

INTESTINAL COLONIZATION: WHICH WAY TO GO?

A great complexity of surface appendages on enterotoxigenic organisms (ETEC, *V. cholerae*) and organisms producing cytotoxic toxins such as EPEC make it unlikely that receptor therapy, as proposed by Keusch (Wadström et al 1984, Wadström & Baloda 1986) will work in the gastrointestinal tract. However, further characterization of the fimbrial and non-fimbrial adhesins of enteropathogens seems most important since vaccines against animal ETEC diarrhoea causing K88, K99 and 987P fimbriae have given excellent protection to animals during the first weeks of life. Since vaccination may select for new fimbrial types (such as 987P) it is necessary to try to identify fimbrial as well as non-fimbrial intestinal adhesins. Identification of new adhesion mechanisms is essential for developing procedures to interfere with the colonization of the mucosa by various enteropathogens. Our findings that hydrophobic cellulose fibres and other carbohydrate polymers can prevent intestinal colonization by ETEC strains in a rabbit model indicate that effective prophylactic methods can be developed (Wadström et al 1984, Wadström & Baloda 1986).

CONCLUSIONS

E. coli was once regarded as a harmless microbe of the bowel flora. We now know that it can express a great number of virulence factors. The major types of such enterovirulent *E. coli* have been reviewed: (i) enterotoxigenic *E. coli*, (ii) enteropathogenic and enteroadherent *E. coli*, (iii) enterohaemorrhagic *E. coli*, and (iv) enteroinvasive *E. coli*. The rapid development of simplified screening techniques for these defined virulence factors, such as hybridization techniques and polymerase chain reaction techniques, will help in elucidating epidemiology and prevalence of these factors in the world. However, there are still a large number of *E. coli* strains isolated from intestinal infections where virulence factors probably are yet to be characterized.

ACKNOWLEDGEMENTS

The experimental part of this communication was supported by a grant from the Swedish Medical Research Council (16x-04723).

REFERENCES

Adams M D, Oxende D L 1989 Bacterial periplasmid binding protein tertiary structures. Journal of Biological Chemistry 264: 15739-15742

Bäck E, Möllby R, Kaijser B, Stintzing G, Wadström T, Habte D 1980 Enterotoxigenic *Escherichia coli* and other gram-negative bacteria of infantile diarrhea: surface antigens, hemagglutinins, colonization factor antigen and loss of enterotoxigenicity. Journal of Infectious Diseases 142: 318-327

Baldini M M, Kaper J B, Levine M M, Candy D C A, Moon H W 1983 Plasmid-mediated adhesion in enteropathogenic *Escherichia coli*. Journal of Pediatric Gastroenterology and Nutrition 2: 534-538

Baloda S B, Faris A, Fröman G, Wadström T 1985 Fibronectin binding to Salmonella strains. FEMS Microbiology Letters 28: 1-5

Baloda S B, Fröman G, Peeters J E, Wadström T 1986 Fibronectin binding and cell surface hydrophobicity of attaching effacing enteropathogenic *Escherichia coli* strains isolated from newborn and weanling rabbits with diarrhoea. FEMS Microbiology Letters 34: 225-229

Barrett T J, Potter M E, Wachsmuth I K 1989 Bacterial endotoxin both enhances and inhibits the toxicity of Shiga-like toxin II in rabbits and mice. Infection and Immunity 557: 3434-3437

Batt R M, Sauders J R, Getty B 1988 Lectin-induced damage to the enterocyte brush border. Scandinavian Journal of Gastroenterology 23: 1153-1159

Boedeker EC 1989 Enteroadherent (enteropathogenic) *Escherichia coli*. In: Farti M J G, Kesusch G T (eds) Enteric infections. Raven Press, New York, pp 123-139

Burke D A, Axon A T R 1987 HeLa cell and buccal epithelial cell adhesion assays for detecting intestinal *Escherichia coli* with adhesive properties in ulcerative colitis. Journal of Clinical Pathology 40: 1402-1404

Emödy L, Heesemann J, Wolf-Watz H, Skurnik M, Kapperud G, O'Toole P, Wadström T 1989 Binding to collagen by *Yersinia enterocolitica* and *Yersinia pseudotuberculosis*: Evidence for yopA-mediated and chromosmally encoded mechanisms. Journal of Bacteriology 171: 6674-6679

Ericsson C D 1990 Travellers diarrhoea. Current Science in Gastroenterology 6: 100-104

Evans D G, Evans J D Jr, Tjoa W S, DuPont H L 1978 Detection and characterization of colonization factor of enterotoxigenic *Escherichia coli* isolated from adults with diarrhoea. Infection and Immunity 19: 727-736

Evered D, Wheland J 1985 Microbial Toxins and Diarrhoea disease (Ciba Foundation Symposium No. 112) Pitman, London, 286 pp

Faris A, Lindahl M, Wadström T 1982 High surface hydrophobicity of haemagglutinating *Vibrio cholerae* and other vibrios. Current Microbiology 7: 357-362

Faris A, Fröman G, Truszczynski M, Wadström T 1986 *Escherichia coli* strains of serogroup 0139 isolated from oedema disease of swine bind fibronectin. FEMS Microbiology Letters 34: 221-224

Farthing M J G, Keusch G T 1989 Enteric Infections, Raven Press, New York

Fröman G, Switalski L M, Faris A, Wadström T, Hook M 1984 Binding of *Escherichia coli* to fibronectin: a mechanism of tissue adherence. Journal of Biological Chemistry 259: 14899-14905

Gomes T A T, Vieira M A M, Wachsmuth I K, Blake P A, Trabulsi L R 1989a Serotype-specific prevalence of *Escherichia coli* strains with EPEC adhesion factor genes in infants with and without diarrhoea in Sao Paulo, Brazil. Journal of Infectious Diseases 160: 131-136

Gomes T A T, Blake P A, Trabulski L R 1989b Prevalence of *Escherichia coli* strains with localized diffuse and aggregative adherence to Hela cells in patient with diarrhoea and matched controls. Journal of Clinical Microbiology 27: 266-269

Gonzalez E A, Baloda S B, Blanco J, Wadström T 1989 Growth conditions for the expression of fibronectin and collagen binding to Salmonella. Zentralblatt für Bakteriologie, Mikrobiologie und Hygiene, Sene A 269: 437-446

Griffin P M, Ostroff S M, Tauxe R V et al 1988 Illnesses associated with *Escherichia coli* 0157:H7 infections. Annals of Internal Medicine 109: 705-712

Hamers A M, Pel H J, Willshaw G A, Kusters J G, van der Zeijst B A M, Gaastra W 1989 The nucleotide sequence of the first two genes of the CFA/I fimbrial operon of human enterotoxigenic *Escherichia coli*. Microbiology and Pathogenesis 6: 297-309

Junkins A D, Doyle M P 1989 Comparison of adherence properties of *Escherichia coli* 0157:H7 and a 60-megadalton plasmid-cured derivative. Current Microbiology 19: 21-27

Kaper J B, Tacket C O 1988 Recent advances in enterotoxigenic enterohaemorrhagic and enteropathogenic *Escherichia coli*. In: Bacterial infections of the respiratory and gastrointestinal mucosae. IRL Press, Oxford, pp 113-132

Karch H, Heesemann J, Laufs R, O'Brien A D, Tacket C O, Levine M M 1987 A plasmid of enterohemorrhagic *Escherichia coli* 0157:H7 is required for expression of a new fimbrial antigen for adhesion to epithelial cells. Infection and Immunity 55: 455-461

Karmali M A 1989 Infection by Verocytotoxin-producing *Escherichia coli*. Clinical Microbiology Reviews 2: 15-38

Knutton S, Balwin P H, McNeison A S 1989 Actin accumulation at site of bacterial adhesion to tissue culture cells. Basis of the new diagnostic bacterial test for enteropathogenic and enterohaemorrhagic *Escherichia coli*. Infection and Immunity 57: 1290-1298

Levine M M, Xu J G, Kaper J B et al 1987 A DNA probe to identify enterohemorrhagic *Escherichia coli* of 0157:H7 and other serotypes that cause hemorrhagic colitis and hemolytic uremic syndrome. Journal of Infectious Diseases 156: 176-182

Lindahl M, Brossmer R, Wadström T 1988 Sialic acid and *N*-acetyl-galactosamine specific bacterial lectins of enterotoxigenic *Escherichica coli* (ETEC). In: Wu A M, Adams L G (eds), Molecular immunology of the complex carbohydrates. Plenum Press, pp 123-152

Ljungh A, Wadström T 1988 Subepithelial connective tissue protein binding of *Escherichia coli* isolated from patients with ulcerative colitis. In: MacDermott R P (ed) Inflammatory bowel disease: current status and future approach. Elsevier Science Publishers B V Amsterdam, pp 571-575

Ljung A, Emödy L, Steinruck H, Sullivan P, West B, Zetterberg E, Wadström T 1990 Fibronectin, vitronectin and collagen binding to *Escherichia coli* of intestinal and extraintestinal origin. Zentrablatt für Bakteriologie 255: 300-306

Magnusson K E 1989 Physiochemical properties of bacterial surfaces. Biochemical Journal 17: 452-458

Martin M L, Shipman L D, Wells J G et al 1986 Isolation of *Escherichia coli* 0157:H7 from dairy cattle associated with two cases of haemolytic uraemic syndrome. Lancet ii: 1043

Mathewson J J, Cravioto A 1988 Hep 2 cell adherence as an assay for virulence among diarrhoeagenic *Escherichia coli*. Journal of Infectious Diseases 159: 1057-1060

Nataro J P, Baldini M M, Kasper J P, Blacke R E, Bravo N, Levine M M 1985 Detection of an adherence factor of enteropathogenic *Escherichia coli* with a DNA probe. Journal of Infectious Diseases 152: 560-565

Nicoletti M, Superti F, Conti C, Calconi A, Zagaglia C 1988 Virulence factors of lactose-negative *Escherichia coli* strains isolated from children with diarrhoea in Somalia. Journal of Clinical Microbiology. 26: 524-529

Okerman L, Deuriesie A 1989 Intestinal colonization with different enteropathogenic *Escherichia coli* biotypes and cross-protection induced by different strains. Microbial Ecology in Health and Disease 2: 61-68

Olsén A, Jonsson A, Normark S 1989 Fibronectin binding mediated by a novel class of surface organelles on *Escherichia coli*. Nature 338: 652-655

138

Oswald E, de Rycke J 1990 A single protein of 140 kDa is associated with multinucleating and necrotizing activity coded by the Vir plasmid of *Escherichia coli*. FEMS Microbiology Letters 68: 279-284

Pal R, Ghose A C 1990 Identification of plasmid-encoded mannose resistant heamagglutinin and HEp-2 and HeLa cell adherence factors of two diarrheagenic *Escherichia coli* strains belonging to an enteropathogenic serogroup. Infection and Immunology 58: 1106-1113

Pieroni P, Wrobec E A, Paranchyc W, Armstrong C D 1988 Identification of a human erythrocyte receptor for colonization factor antigen I pili expressed by H 10407 enterotoxigenic *Escherichia coli*. Infection and Immunity 56: 1334-1338

Ryan C A, Tauxe R V, Hosek G W 1986 *Escherichia coli* 0157:H7 diarrhoea in a nursing home: clinical, epidemiological, and pathological findings. Journal of Infectious Diseases 154: 631-638

Scotland S M, Rowe B, Smith H R, Willshaw G A, Gross R J 1988 Verocytotoxin-producing strains of *Escherichia coli* from children with haemolytic uraemic syndrome and their detection by specific DNA probes. Journal of Medical Microbiology 25: 237-243

Senerwa D, Olsvik Ö, Mutanda L N et al 1989a Enteropathogenic *Escherichia coli* serotype 0111:HNT isolated from preterm neonates in Nairobi, Kenya. Journal of Clinical Microbiology 27: 1305-1311

Senerwa D, Olsvik Ö, Mutanda L N, Gathuma J M, Wachsmuth K 1989b Colonization of neonates in a nursery ward with enteropathogenic *Escherichia coli* and correlation to the clinical histories of the children. Journal of Clinical Microbiology 27: 2539-2543

Sherman P M, Houston W L, Boedeker E C 1985 Functional heterogeneity of intestinal *Escherichia coli* strains expressing type 1 somatic pili (fimbriae): Assessment of bacterial adherence to intestinal membranes and surface hydrophobicity. Infection and Immunity 49: 797-804

Sjöberg P O, Lindahl M, Fröman G, Porath J, Wadstrom T 1988 Isolation and characterization of CS 2 sialic acid specific lectins of enterotoxigenic *Escherichia coli*. Biochemical Journal 255: 105-111

Smith H R, Scotland S M, Stokes N, Rowe R 1990 Examination of strains belonging to the enteropathogenic *Escherichia coli* serogroups for genes encoding EPEC adherence factor and Verocytotoxins. Journal of Medical Microbiology 31: 235-240

Smith H W 1976 Neonatal *Escherichia coli* infections in domestic animals. Transmissibility of pathogenic characteristics. In: Elliot K M (ed) Diarrhoea in childhood (Ciba Foundation Symposium No. 42) Elsevier, Amsterdam, pp 45-72

Spychal R P, Marreo J M, Saverymutto S H, Northfied T C 1989 The surface hydrophobicity of human gastrointestinal mucosal. Gastroenterology 97: 104-111

Strockbine N A, Marques L R M, Newland J W, Smith H W, Homes R K, O'Brian A D 1986 Two toxin-converting phages from *Escherichia coli* 0157:H7, strain 933 encode antigenically distinct toxins with similar biological activities. Infection and Immunity 53: 135-140

Sussman M 1985. The virulence of *Escherichia coli*. Academic Press, London

Taylor D M, Houston R, Shlim D R, Bhaibulaya M, Ungar B L P, Ecceverria P 1988 Etiology of diarrhoea among travellers and foreign residents in Nepal. Journal of American Medical Association 260: 1245-1248

Thorne G M 1990 Diagnostic tests in gastrointestinal infections. Current Opinion in Gastroenterology 6: 79-88

Toth I, Cohen M L, Rumschlag H S et al in press Influence of the 60 MDa plasmid on adherence of *Escherichia coli* 0157:H7 and genetic derivatives. Infection and Immunity 58: 1223-1231

Tzipori, Gibson S R, Montanaro J 1989 Nature and distribution of mucosal lesions associated with enteropathogenic and enterohemorrhagic *Escherichia coli* in piglets and the role of plasmid-mediated factors. Infection and Immunity 57: 1142-1150

Ulshen M H, Rollo J L 1980 Pathogenesis of *Escherichia coli* gastroenteritis in man; another mechanism. New England Journal of Medicine 302: 99-101

Visai L, Speziale P, Bozzini S 1990 Binding of collagens to an enterotoxigenic strain of *Escherichia coli*. Infection and Immunology 58: 449-455

Wadstrom T 1978 Relative importance of enterotoxigenic and invasive enteropathogenic bacteria in infantile diarrhoea. Zentralblatt für Bakteriologie, Mikrobiologie und Hygiene, Sene A 242: 52-62

Wadström T, Adegbola R A, Baloda S B, Ljung A, Sethi S K, Yuk Y R 1986 Non-haemagglutinating fimbriae of enteropathogenic *Escherichia coli* (EPEC). Zentralblatt für Bakteriologie, Mikrobiologie und Hygiene, Sene A 261: 417-424

Wadström T, Trust T J 1984a Bacterial surface lectins. In: Jeljaszewicz J & Easman C S F (eds) Medical Microbiology Vol 4. Academic Press, London pp 287-334

Wadström T, Faris A, Hjertén S 1984b Hydrophobic properties of pili. In: Boedecker E C (ed) Attachment of organisms to the gut mucosa, Vol I. CRC Press, Boca Raton, Florida USA pp 113-120

Wadström T, Sjöberg P O, Lindahl M 1984 Sialic acid specific lectins of enterotoxigenic *Escherichia coli*. In: Bog-Hansen T C, Breborowicz J Lectins, Vol 4. Walter de Gruyter Berlin, pp 417-423

Wadström T, Baloda S B 1986 Molecular aspects on small bowel colonization by enterotoxigenic *Escherichia coli*. Microecology and Therapy 16: 243-255

Wadström T, Switalski L M, Speziale P et al 1985 Binding of microbial pathogens to connective tissue fibronectin: an early step in localized and invasive infections. Heidelberg Bayer-Symposium VIII. Springer-Verlag, Berlin, pp 193-207

Wadström T 1988 Adherence traits and mechanisms of microbial adhesion in the gut. In: Guerrant R A (ed) Bailleres Clinical and Tropical Medicine and Communicable Diseases, Vol 3, No 3, pp 417-434

Wadström T, Aleljung P 1988 Molecular aspects of bowel colonization in the regulation and protective role of the normal microflora. In: Grubb R, Midtvedt M, Norrn E (eds).Stockton Press, Houndsmills, UK pp 35-46

Wadström T, Ljungh A 1988 Correlation between toxin formation and diarrhoea in Aeromonas. International Journal of Diarrhoeal Disturbances 6: 113-119

Wanke C A 1988 Infective causes of prolonged diarrhoea. In: Guerrant R A (ed) Bailleres Clinical and Tropical Medicine and Communicable Diseases, Vol 3, No 3, pp 567-590

Wanke C A, Cronan S, Gross C, Chadee K, Guerrant R L 1990 Characterization of binding of *Escherichia coli*: strains which are enteropathogens to small-bowel mucins. Infection and Immunology 58: 794-800

Wasteson Y, Olsvik Ö, Skancke E, Bopp C A, Fossum K 1988 Heat-stable-enterotoxin producing *Escherichia coli* strains isolated from dogs. Journal of Clinical Microbiology 26: 2564-2566

Wennerås C, Holmgren J, Svennerholm A M 1990 The binding of colonization factor of enterotoxigenic *Escherichia coli* to intestinal cell membrane proteins. FEMS Microbiology Letters 66: 107-112

Wiersma E J, Fröman G, Johansson S, Wadström T 1987 Carbohydrate specific binding of fibronectin to *Vibrio cholerae* cells. FEMS Microbiology Letters 44: 365-369

Discussion of paper presented by T. Wadström

Discussed by G. Keusch
Reported by H. C. Neu

Dr Keusch pointed out that *E. coli* is a wonderful genus because of the extraordinary diversity of the disease syndromes it causes, which are often species specific, and the opportunity that it presents to study pathogenesis at the molecular and genetic level. *E. coli* can truly be portrayed as a cloning vector into which virulence genes have been inserted in nature singly or severally. This package of genes determines its in vivo behaviour. The genetic and physiological background of *E. coli* is better understood than any other in microbiology—almost 50 years ago the first EPEC were identified during a newborn nursery epidemic. Identification was by a particular smell of the patient. The relevance of this organism was proved by the demonstration of agglutinating antibodies occurring in convalescing patients with diarrhoea but not in those who did not develop diarrhoea.

Keusch noted that the pathogenesis of disease is complex and often has several discernible steps. Virulence is polygenic, and a particular virulence gene is not necessarily associated with causation, either because it is truly not associated or because one has not been able to implicate it at this time. He felt that the adherence specificity and colonization potential of these organisms should explain a lot of the target organ specificity in the intestine—the jejunum differs from the ileum, the ascending colon is not a mirror image of the descending colon.

Once established in the host, organisms may or may not invade epithelial cells, the lamina propria or further, systemically. Whether they do or not, they may still alter the intracellular architecture of the epithelial cell, by the alteration of the cytoskeleton and the polymerization of actin in the attaching and effacing lesions caused by EAEC and EPEC strains. The membrane signal of non-invasive or attaching *E. coli* that involves these incredible changes in cytoskeleton is not known. When strains such as EPEC do mutate it is not clear that invasion is either important or necessary. The invasion potential of EPEC, which has classically been considered to be a non-invasive strain, was correlated with the presence of the EPEC adherence factor, EAF. However, a single locus which is capable of transforming the invasive phenotype has not been found. Dr Keusch reported use of the TnPhO$_3$ transporter to search for surface factors involved in invasion. He found that some non-invasive isolates with plasmid inserts had lost the ability to locally adhere at three hours in the Hep2 tissue culture assay, but if one continued the assay for another three hours, they were diffusely adherent. Such strains were fluorescence actin-staining positive, but he did

141

not know if they would cause disease. Some clones lost the LA phenotype but had chromosomal inserts, suggesting that there were accessory, and perhaps regulatory chromosomal genes involved in the localized adherence positive, but fluorescence actin-staining negative, and some were LA positive and FAS positive. There is a whole series of organisms that can be tested in models in animals and humans, and may present an opportunity for identifying the genes that are involved in some of these properties.

Dr Keusch concluded his discussion with reference to the *Shigellae* toxin. The significance of low toxin producers is unknown. *Shigella* toxins in the β-sub unit have a Gal-gal binding site and in the α-sub unit there is the bioactivity of ricin, an RNA n-glycosidase surrounded by other amino acids. We do not know exactly where on the molecule current probes are directed. An organism may probe negative but produce biologically active molecules that are being produced and secreted but are not recognized because one does not have a probe to the right area. Keusch also questioned the dogma that the SLT1 and SLT2 are quite distinct because they are immunologically not cross-reactive. He has shown that there are common epitopes between SLT1 and SLT2.

Dr Levine reported that persistent diarrhoea, i.e. an acute episode of diarrhoea that does not stop at 14 days but keeps on going, identifies a subgroup of children at very high risk of fatality in the short and intermediate terms. Studies done in many parts of the less developed world show that approximately 4 or 5% of infants or young children who come to a health centre with acute diarrhoeal disease will go on to have persistent diarrhoea. Dr Levine commented about entero-aggregated *E. coli* damaging microvilli. In collaboration with workers in Melbourne, Australia, two prototype strains of entero-aggregated *E. coli* including 17-2 were fed to piglets. The piglets developed diarrhoea, they were sacrificed and histology and electron microscopy was done. There were lesions visible and one found aggregative adherents similar to those one sees with the Hep2 assay. One also saw an unusual matrix by which these organisms attached like glue to the surface of the enterocytes. This occurred at the time the animals showed no microvillus dissolution or effacement.

Keusch used the term EAF correctly—it is EPEC Adherence Factor. It was referred to inadvertently as entero-adherent factor and that is not what EAF is; it is EPEC Adherence Factor. This raises the question of exactly what one means by entero-adherent *E. coli*. Levine felt that the term Hep2 cell adherent should be used, dividing *E. coli* into localized adhering, diffuse adhering and aggregative pattern adhering.

9. Pathogenesis of *Helicobacter pylori*-induced gastroduodenal diseases

M. J. Blaser

INTRODUCTION

Helicobacter pylori (formerly called *Campylobacter pylori*), a gram-negative, curved, motile, microaerophilic rod, was first isolated from human stomachs in 1982 (Marshall 1989). From the earliest reports, it has become clear that this organism is not universally identified in the stomach but that its presence is highly associated with the histological lesion variably known as chronic superficial, diffuse antral, or type B gastritis (Marshall & Warren 1984, Dooley et al 1989). Infection by this organism now can be diagnosed by histological examination or culture of gastric biopsy specimens (Dooley et al 1989), by detection of its powerful urease activity in biopsies or using breath tests (Graham et al 1987), or by serological examination (Perez-Perez et al 1988).

Using these methods, it has now become evident that *H. pylori* infection is present in persons in all parts of the world, and that the prevalence of infection rises with age (Dooley et al 1989, Megraud et al 1989, Perez-Perez et al 1990). *H. pylori* infection is acquired earlier and more commonly in developing than in developed countries (Fig. 9.1). In virtually all populations, at least 50% of persons 60 years old or above are infected with this organism. No reservoir for infection other than humans has been identified and transmission is believed to occur from person-to-person (Blaser 1990a). Once acquired, infection persists for years (Langenberg et al 1986), probably for decades, and possibly for life.

A critical question is whether *H. pylori* is merely a very successful commensal or colonizer of the human stomach, or whether it plays any pathological role. Currently, the greatest amount of information relates *H. pylori* infection with type B gastritis. There now exists a wide body of evidence indicating that *H. pylori* plays an aetiological role in this disorder (Blaser 1990b).

As a result of intense investigative effort, all four of Koch's postulates have now been fulfilled, demonstrating the pathogenicity of *H. pylori*. Despite the natural scepticism that accompanies such a novel notion there has been essentially no evidence against this hypothesis.

Of potentially even greater significance is the long-standing observation that type B gastritis is observed in virtually all persons with idiopathic peptic ulcer disease (Wyatt et al 1984). The nearly universal association of *H. pylori* and type B gastritis

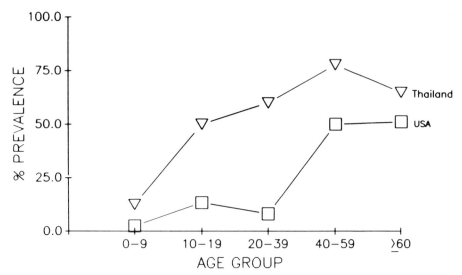

Figure 9.1 Seroprevalence by age (in years) of *H. pylori* infection among healthy persons in two populations in developing and developed countries. One population consists of 194 persons from a village in rural Thailand, as described by Perez-Perez et al (1990). The other population consists of 166 persons from Denver, USA, as described by Perez-Perez et al (1988). Presence of infection was defined as having elevated levels of serum IgG to *H. pylori* antigens (Perez-Perez et al 1988). As represented by the data concerning the Thai population, *H. pylori* infection is acquired earlier and is more common at all ages in the developing countries compared with developed countries.

suggests that most patients with peptic ulcer disease will be infected with this organism. Numerous studies have now shown this prediction to be correct. *H. pylori* infection has been demonstrated in 95 to 100% of patients with duodenal ulceration, and 70 to 95% of those with gastric ulcers; the major exceptions are the Zollinger-Ellison syndrome, and ulceration induced by non-steroidal anti-inflammatory drugs

---

Evidence indicating a role for *Helicobacter pylori* in the pathogenesis of chronic (type B) diffuse antral gastritis is listed below.

1. *Primary evidence*
a. Ingestion of *H. pylori* by human volunteers resulted in gastritis (Marshall et al 1985, Morris & Nicholson 1989).
b. Among *H. pylori*-infected persons, antimicrobial therapy that suppressed infection suppressed gastritis; with recrudescense of infection, gastritis returned. Eradication of infection cleared gastritis (Glupczynski et al 1988, Morgan et al 1988, Rauws et al 1988).
c. Experimental challenge of animals with *H. pylori* resulted in chronic gastritis resembling the lesions seen in humans (Krakowka et al 1987, Lambert et al 1987).

2. *Supporting evidence*
a. *H. pylori* infection is nearly universally present in chronic (type B) diffuse antral gastritis but is not associated with other types of gastritis (Drumm et al 1987, Rauws et al 1988).
b. There is specificity of the tissue tropism; in infected persons, *H. pylori* only overlays gastric-type epithelial cells (Buck et al 1986).
c. Virtually all persons infected with *H. pylori* develop a specific humoral immune response (Perez-Perez et al 1988, Dooley et al 1989, Drumm et al 1990).
d. With antimicrobial therapy that eradicates *H. pylori*, specific antibodies diminish (Van Bohemen et al 1989).
e. Treatment with bismuth salts results in concomitant clearance of organisms and diminution of gastric inflammation (McNulty et al 1986).
f. *H. pylori* infection has been associated with iatrogenic epidemic gastritis and hypochlorhydria (Graham et al 1988, Morris & Nicholson 1989).

(NSAIDS) (Earlam et al 1985, Johnston et al 1986, Wyatt et al 1987, Carrick et al 1989). Although gastric acid has long been considered necessary, it is not sufficient to explain peptic ulceration; a second factor, 'diminished mucosal resistance', has been postulated to play a role. Currently less extensive than the body of evidence for type B gastritis, nonetheless, a large number of investigations point towards *H. pylori* playing an aetiological role in duodenal ulceration.

Evidence indicating a role for *Helicobacter pylori* in the pathogenesis of duodenal ulceration is listed below.

1. Virtually all persons with idiopathic duodenal ulceration are infected with *H. pylori*, a proportion that is significantly greater than in matched controls (Earlam et al 1985, Johnston et al 1986, Wyatt et al 1987, Carrick et al 1989).
2. In the duodenum, *H. pylori* overlays only gastric but not intestinal type epithelial cells (Wyatt et al 1987)
3. Among patients undergoing endoscopy, the presence of *H. pylori* in the duodenum is strongly associated with duodenal ulceration (Carrick et al 1989).
4. Agents with antimicrobial activity heal duodenal ulceration at rates similar to those achieved with H_2-receptor antagonists (Quintero Diaz & Sotto Escobar 1986, Coghlan et al 1987).
5. After ulcer healing due to medical treatment, detection of *H. pylori* in the duodenum is a risk factor for eventual ulcer relapse (Coghlan et al 1987, Marshall et al 1988).
6. Relapse of duodenal ulceration is associated with recolonization with *H. pylori* (Rauws & Tytgat 1990).
7. Cytotoxin production by *H. pylori* strains is associated with presence of duodenal ulceration (Figura et al 1989, Cover et al 1990).

An attractive hypothesis is that, as with gastric acid, *H. pylori* is generally necessary (except for Zollinger-Ellison syndrome, NSAIDs, etc.) but not sufficient to cause ulceration (Wyatt et al 1987, Blaser 1990b). The exact role of *H. pylori* in ulcer disease is now being examined in numerous studies.

PATHOGENESIS OF GASTRODUEDONAL INFLAMMATION

The mechanisms by which *H. pylori* may cause gastroduodenal injury are also undergoing considerable scrutiny. Most importantly, it is clear that *H. pylori* live in the mucous layer overlaying the epithelium (Hazell et al 1986). Most evidence indicates that these organisms do not actually invade tissue, although a variable proportion are adherent to the surface of the epithelial cells (Hessey et al 1990). Several virulence factors have been considered for *H. pylori*, including ammonia generated by its urease, a cytotoxin, lipopolysaccharide (LPS), or urease itself. Since *H. pylori* cells can adhere to the mucosal epithelium, it is possible that adherence itself results in cellular injury (Hessey et al 1990). How an organism that is not generally invasive can result in inflammatory and degenerative lesions in tissue must next be considered.

Bacterial mediators of inflammation
Infection may result in inflammation due to transport of *H. pylori* products into the gastric mucosal tissue (Fig. 9.2). One candidate product is ammonia, which is generated by urease, and which is known to be toxic to eukaryotic cells (Visek 1968). Another possibility is a cytotoxin that produces vacuolation of a wide variety of cell lines (Leunk et al 1988). Yet another possibility is urease itself which is present on the surface of *H. pylori* cells (Dunn et al 1990) and may be secreted. Urense may be found

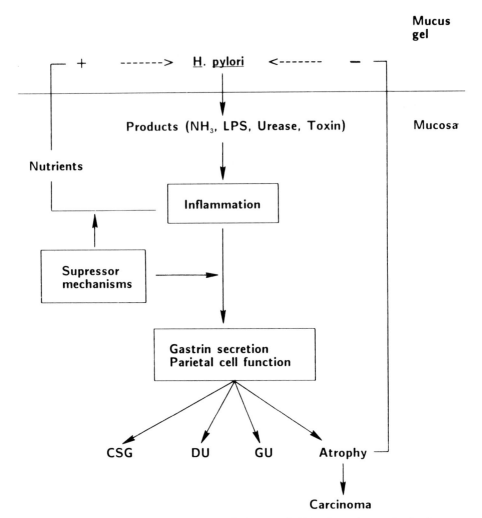

Figure 9.2 Hypothetical relationship between *Helicobacter pylori* infection and gastroduodenal pathology. According to this model, *H. pylori*, which lives in the mucus gel overlaying the gastric epithelium, releases products that result in tissue inflammation; inflammation in turn leads to release of host products into the mucus layer that *H. pylori* can utilize for nutrition. Chronic inflammation has effects on both gastrin secretion and parietal cell function, but host immunological suppressor activity down-regulates this process. The outcome of infection is based on interaction of inflammation and suppression of gastric secretory physiology. Possible outcomes include chronic superficial gastritis (CSG), duodenal ulceration (DU), gastric ulceration (GU), and gastric atrophy, which is a precursor lesion for gastric carcinoma.

within the mucosa of infected humans (Mai et al) showed that urease may be found within the mucosa of infected monkeys. Many Gram-negative bacteria, including the *Campylobacter* species (Blaser et al 1983), overproduce outer membranes and these excesses may form blebs that can be found in culture supernatants. These outer membrane structures are enriched for LPS and other outer membrane antigens. LPS of *H. pylori* is structurally heterogeneous (Perez-Perez & Blaser 1987), and may have variable degrees of endotoxicity. Any of the above products of *H. pylori* growth may serve as inflammatory mediators. It is interesting to speculate that unlike more distal portions of the gastrointestinal tract, the human stomach is poorly equipped to cope with colonizing bacteria. This organ relies on high gastric acidity and peristalsis to clear microbial intruders following ingestion and passage through the oropharynx; however, *H. pylori* is apparently able to overcome such barriers. The very fact of survival of large numbers of Gram-negative organisms in close proximity to 'relatively undefended' mucosa may be sufficient to initiate pathological processes.

Inflammatory and immune responses

H. pylori cells activate both neutrophils and monocyte/macrophages in vitro, but these organisms must be opsonized to activate neutrophils. Serum from infected persons contains specific IgG which performs this function, whereas there is no opsonization by serum from uninfected persons. Monocyte activation has been more extensively studied (Mai et al 1990). *H. pylori* cells, as well as purified LPS and the proteins extracted in water from the bacterial surface, are all capable of this activation. Activated cells express HLA-DR and IL-2 receptors on their surface, as well as to produce superoxide, IL-1, and TNF-α. These in vitro data indicate that *H. pylori* cells and particular components are capable of activating host effector cells. Antigen-presenting monocytes in conjunction with PGE_2, another monokine induced by *H. pylori* antigens, induces a suppressor T-cell response. In vivo, *H. pylori* infection stimulates HLA-DR expression on gastric epithelial cells (Engstrand et al 1989). Gastric mucosal biopsy culture supernatants from infected persons show high-level production of TNF-α (Crabtree et al in press). Supernatants from such biopsies also contain specific IgG and secretory IgA, and *H. pylori* cells in the gastric lumen are coated with secretory IgA (Rathbone & Heatley 1989). Following antimicrobial treatment of *H. pylori* infections, levels of humoral immunity decline (Van Bohemen et al 1989), reflecting elimination of the antigenic focus (Gray & Skarvall 1988). These in vivo studies substantiate that the host is both recognizing *H. pylori* locally and responding to the infection. How *H. pylori* is able to survive despite a host that recognizes its existence is not known, but several possibilities should be considered.

Inflammatory lesions

The hallmarks of *H. pylori* infection are derangements in structure and function of mucosal glands and increased numbers of inflammatory cells in the mucosa (Tricottet et al 1986, Paull & Yardley 1989). Most *H. pylori*-infected persons have neutrophils present in the lamina propria and in the epithelial glands (Paull & Yardley 1989). In addition, in virtually all infected persons there is also an increase in chronic inflammatory cells, including lymphocytes, monocyte/macrophages, eosinophils, and plasma cells. The plasma cells secrete IgG or sIgA. Both B- and T-lymphocytes are present, but among the T-cells, suppressor-type cells appear to predominate. In

---

Mechanisms by which pathogenic microbes may avoid host immune responses is listed below.

1. Antigenic variation
2. Induction of ineffective (blocking) antibodies
3. Shedding of antibody-antigen complexes from the surface of the microbe
4. Release of soluble antigens that bind all available antibodies
5. Non-specific (Fc) binding of immunoglobulins
6. Enzymatic (IgA protease) inactivation of antibodies
7. Suppression of host immune effector mechanisms
8. Residence in immunologically privileged site

some *H. pylori*-infected persons, glandular atrophy occurs. In general, active infection is associated with depletion of mucus from the epithelial cells (Gilman et al 1986). However, mucus production is increased over normal levels (Crabtree et al 1984). Whether or not there is primary involvement of the epithelial glands in the pathological process is uncertain; inflammation per se might cause the lesions observed. Next, it is important to consider how *H. pylori* infection may lead to these particular pathological processes, and their clinical consequences.

SPECULATION ABOUT THE ROLE OF *H. pylori* IN THE PATHOGENESIS OF SPECIFIC UPPER GASTROINTESTINAL PATHOLOGY

Chronic superficial gastritis

Studies of the natural history of superficial gastritis undertaken before *H. pylori* was discovered suggest that this process may persist for decades (Siurala et al 1968, Kekki et al 1977). An important point to consider is whether gastric inflammation is advantageous for the survival of *H. pylori*. To survive and multiply in its location in the mucus gel, *H. pylori* must be provided with a constant supply of nutrients. Inflammation, with disruption of mucosal barriers, may facilitate the release of nutrients into the mucus gel (Hazell et al 1986). Therefore, induction of the release of inflammatory mediators by *H. pylori* may be adaptive. The constitutive production of both LPS and urease are consistent with this hypothesis. However, inflammation disrupts epithelial function, which is therefore deleterious to the host. The predominance of suppressor lymphocytes in inflammatory lesions suggests that the host may be attempting to down-regulate the exuberance of the inflammatory response. Successful down-regulation may be viewed as occurring in persons who no longer have neutrophils in the lesions, since pyogenic infection is a most destructive host-parasite interaction. Superficial gastritis due to *H. pylori*, with or without neutrophils, may persist for years (Langenberg et al 1986). Thus, chronic superficial gastritis may represent a long-term equilibrium between a host unable to remove a noxious stimulus but able to contain the damage. Analogies include the granulomatous process containing but not eliminating *Mycobacterium tuberculosis*, or the oyster creating a pearl. Another possibility is that *H. pylori* may have a resemblance with *Mycobacterium leprae*, another bacterial pathogen that susceptible hosts cannot eliminate and in whom infection persists for years or decades. The exuberant host response to *M. leprae* observed in tuberculoid leprosy results in significant local lesions. In patients with lepromatous leprosy the predominant lymphocyte type is suppressor cells (Van Voorhis et al 1982), which may be appropriate to the high bacillary load that results from inadequate containment of infection by macrophages.

Atrophic gastritis

What might be the outcome of *H. pylori* infection in persons in whom immune suppression is not adequate, or gradually becomes inadequate? Without adequate down-regulation, a florid inflammatory response might lead to continuing destruction of epithelial glandular structure and function. Thus, atrophy of gastric glands may occur in those persons in whom suppressor mechanisms are inadequate. The determinants of the adequacy of this postulated immune-suppression and whether or not suppression may be antigen-specific or non-specific are unknown. Furthermore, longitudinal population-based studies suggest that chronic superficial gastritis may progress to atrophic gastritis in some cases (Siurala et al 1966); and that with ageing atrophic gastritis begins in the antrum and moves proximally into the fundus (Kimura 1972). Whether these processes represent the gradual accumulation of inflammatory insults, or an age-related diminution in immune suppression is not now certain (Steinheber 1985). The familial nature of gastric atrophy suggests that lack of specific immune suppression could be an inherited tendency.

However, gastric atrophy appears to be negatively associated with *H. pylori* infection (Blaser et al in press), an observation suggesting that perhaps the atrophic stomach has become inhospitable to *H. pylori*. Thus, adequate immune suppression could be in the best interest of *H. pylori* as well as the host. Other factors may influence the progression from superficial gastritis to atrophy as well; such factors may include dietary considerations, gastric secretion, and inherited traits not related to immune suppression (Correa 1983). In any event, if progression of *H. pylori* infection to gastric atrophy occurs, this may be of great significance since atrophy is well-recognised to be a risk factor for the development of gastric carcinoma (Howson et al 1986). These speculations lead to the hypothesis that the decline in the incidence of gastric cancer over the past 50 years (Howson et al 1986) may, at least in part, be related to delayed acquisition of *H. pylori* among persons in developed countries (Megraud et al 1989, Blaser 1990a, Perez-Perez et al 1990).

Peptic ulceration
Immediately after initiation of *H. pylori* infection, there is hypersecretion of acid, pepsin, and mucus (Graham et al 1988), but in the next several months hypochlorhydria and decreased pepsin and mucus secretion occurs; restoration of secretion generally occurs within one year (Morris & Nicholson 1989). Subsequently and chronically, *H. pylori* infection induces a chronic hypergastrinaemia, but acid secretion occurs at normal levels (Levi et al 1989, Smith et al 1989, Karnes et al in press). This observation suggests interruption of the physiological mechanisms governing gastrin-hydrochloric acid homoeostasis in at least two loci. First, in *H. pylori*-infected patients the presence of normal acid levels appears not to reduce gastrin production. One possible mechanism for this altered physiology may be that ammonia production by *H. pylori* neutralizes the environment adjacent to the G-cell, or the somatostatin-secreting cell which monitors luminal acidity. Another hypothesis is that chronic antral inflammation up-regulates gastrin production. The factors that normally regulate gastrin production are complex (Calam 1989) (Fig. 9.3). TNF-α and TGF-β are known to increase gastrin production. The second physiological abnormality is that in the face of heightened gastrin levels, production of hydrochloric acid appears not to be increased in most infected hosts. This observation suggests that ability of parietal cells to respond to the gastrin signal may be impaired, possibly due to *H. pylori*-induced inflammation of the fundus (Morris et al 1988, Dooley et al 1989); TGF-α, a product of activated monocytes, suppresses parietal cell acid production. Recent work has indicated a number of ways in which *H. pylori* infection alters the normal physiology of the gastrin-gastric acidity feedback loop, as listed below.

The factors that determine the consequences of the disordered regulation of acid

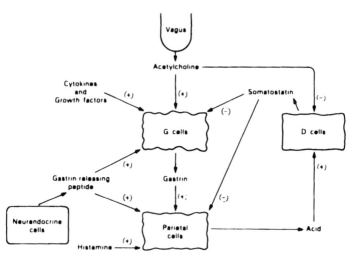

Figure 9.3 Elements involved in control of gastric acidity. Gastrin release is increased by cholinergic innervation, gastrin-releasing peptide (GRP), and cytokines but is diminished by somatostatin. Somatostatin release is diminished by cholinergic stimulation but release and mRNA are increased by low intraluminal pH. Histamine, gastrin, and gastrin-releasing peptide increase while somatostatin decreases acid production by parietal cells.

production are unknown. Differences in *H. pylori* strain characteristics is one possibility, but host genetic factors also could play a role. Those persons with minimal parietal cell destruction may maintain the altered physiology (new 'set-point') indefinitely, if on a functional level, parietal cell (fundal) acid hypoproduction and G-cell (antral) gastrin hyperproduction are roughly in balance. For such persons, the clinical consequences of chronic superficial gastritis may be minimal. In contrast, other infected persons may have more extensive antral inflammation. A subgroup may develop chronic G-cell hyperfunction in the face of a relatively spared fundus, capable of responding to gastrin. This hyperstimulation may result in increased parietal cell mass and acid production, which may then contribute to duodenal (Soll 1990), or prepyloric gastric ulceration. Less commonly, high-intensity antral inflammation may lead to G-cell damage or death, resulting in gastrin hypoproduction. As such, parietal cell stimulation is diminished. This extensive inflammation might result in hypoacidity and independently lead to local (gastric) ulceration (Gear et al 1971). The regulation of the anatomical and functional

---

The relationships between *Helicobacter pylori* infection and gastrin physiology are listed below.

1. *H. pylori* infection results in more severe inflammation of the crypts than the superficial mucosa; G-cells are in highest concentration in the crypts (Price 1988, Paull & Yardley 1989).
2. The absolute number of antral G-cells is apparently preserved during *H. pylori* infection (Sankey et al 1990).
3. *H. pylori* infected-persons have higher levels of immunoreactive gastrin per G-cell than do uninfected persons (Sankey et al 1990).
4. In *H. pylori*-infected persons, the levels of G-cell gastrin are inversely correlated with magnitude of *H. pylori* colonization (Sankey et al 1990).
5. Compared with uninfected persons, *H. pylori*-infected persons have increased levels of fasting and meal-induced hypergastrinaemia (Levi et al 1989, Smith et al 1989, Karnes et al in press).
6. Low pH inhibits gastrin release to the same extent in infected and uninfected persons (Karnes et al in press).

7. Treatment of *H. pylori* infection results in a diminution of the hypergastrinaemia to normal levels (McColl et al 1989).
8. *H. pylori* culture supernatants inhibit parietal cell acid production (Cave & Vargas 1989)

consequences of antral inflammation may have an inherited basis, or may be related to hormonal status; such hypotheses would explain both the familial tendency to duodenal ulceration as well as the male predominance (Soll 1990).

CONCLUSIONS

H. pylori is among the most common of human bacterial pathogens. This organism has developed ways of surviving in the hostile gastric environment. Infection leads to chronic superficial gastritis, and perhaps ultimately to atrophic gastritis or peptic ulcer disease. The regulation of inflammation following *H. pylori* infection may have important consequences for gastric function. Two key factors may be the adequacy of the host to suppress the inflammatory response to *H. pylori* and its products, and the effect of the residual inflammatory process on the physiology of gastrin-mediated production of hydrochloric acid. Careful characterization of the immunology and pathophysiology of gastric acid regulation induced by *H. pylori* infection may enable prediction of its natural history in individual hosts.

REFERENCES

Blaser M J 1990a Epidemiology and pathophysiology of *Campylobacter pylori* infection. Reviews of Infectious Diseases 12: S99-106
Blaser M J 1990b *Helicobacter pylori* and the pathogenesis of gastroduodenal inflammation. Journal of Infectious Diseases 161: 626-633
Blaser M J, Hopkins J A, Berka R M, Vasil M L, Wang W-L L 1983 Identification and characterization of *Campylobacter jejuni* outer membrane proteins. Infection and Immunity 42: 276-284
Blaser M J, Lindenbaum J, Perez-Perez G I, Van Derenter G, Schneidman D, Weinstein WM in press Association of *Campylobacter pylori* with specific upper gastrointestinal pathology. Reviews of Infectious Diseases
Buck G E, Gourlay W K, Lee W K et al 1986 Relation of *Campylobacter pyloridis* to gastritis and peptic ulcer. Journal of Infectious Diseases 153: 664-670
Calam J 1989 Gut hormones. Current Opinion in Gastroenterology 5: 786-790
Carrick J, Lee A, Hazell S, Ralston M, Daskalopoulos G 1989 *Campylobacter pylori*, duodenal ulcer and gastric metaplasia: possible role of functional heterotrophic tissue in ulcerogenesis. Gut 30: 790-797
Cave D R, Vargas M. Effect of a *Campylobacter pylori* protein on acid secretion by parietal cells. Lancet ii: 187-189
Coghlan J G, Gilligan D, Humphreys H et al 1987 *Campylobacter pylori* and recurrence of duodenal ulcers—a 12-month follow-up study. Lancet ii: 1109-1111
Correa P 1983 The gastric precancerous process. Cancer Surveys 2: 437-450
Cover T L, Dooley C P, Blaser M J 1990 Characterization and human serologic response to proteins in *Helicobacter pylori* broth culture supernatants with vacuolizing cytotoxin activity. Infection and Immunity 58: 603-610
Crabtree J E, Rathbone B J, Heatley R V, Wyatt J I, Losowsky M S 1987 In vitro glycoprotein synthesis and secretion in *Campylobacter pyloridis*-associated chronic gastritis. Proceedings of the Fourth International Workshop of Campylobacter Infections. Goteborg, Sweden [Abstract 38]
Crabtree J E, Shalleross T, Wyatt J I, Heatley R V in press Tumour necrosis factor alpha secretion by *Helicobacter pylori* colonized gastric mucosa. Gut
Dooley C P, Fitzgibbons P L, Cohen H, Appleman M D, Perez-Perez G I, Baser M J 1989 Prevalence of *Helicobacter pylori* infection and histologic gastritis in asymptomatic persons. New England Journal of Medicine 321: 1562-1566
Drumm B, Sherman P, Cutz E, Karmali M 1987 Association of *Campylobacter pylori* on the gastric mucosa with antral gastritis in children. New England Journal of Medicine 316: 1557-1561

Drumm B, Perez-Perez G I, Blaser M J, Sherman P 1990 Intrafamilial clustering of *Helicobacter pylori* infection. New England Journal of Medicine 322: 359-363

Dunn B E, Campbell G P, Perez-Perez G I, Blaser M J 1990 Purification and characterization of Helicobacter pylori urease. Journal of Biological Chemistry 265: 9464-9469

Earlam R J, Amerigo J, Kakavoulis T, Pollack D 1985 Histological appearances of oesophagus, antrum and duodenum and their correlation with symptoms in patients with a duodenal ulcer. Gut 26: 95-100

Engstrand L, Scheynius A, Pahlson C, Grimelius L, Schwan A, Gustavsson S 1989 Association of *Campylobacter pylori* with induced expression of class II transplantation antigens on gastric epithelial cells. Infection and Immunity 57: 827-832

Figura N, Guglielmetti P, Rossolini A et al 1989 Cytotoxin production by *Campylobacter pylori* strains isolated from patients with peptic ulcers and from patients with chronic gastritis only. Journal of Clinical Microbiology 27: 225-226

Gear M W L, Truelove S C, Whitehead R 1971 Gastric ulcers and gastritis. Gut 12: 639-645

Gilman R J, Leon-Barua R, Koch J et al 1986 Rapid identification of pyloric campylobacter in Peruvians with gastritis. Digestive Diseases and Sciences 31: 1089-1094

Glupczynski Y, Burette A, Labbe M, Dereuck M, Deltenre M 1988 *Campylobacter pylori* associated gastritis: A double blind, placebo-controlled trial with amoxicillin. American Journal of Gastroenterology 83: 365-372

Graham D Y, Evans D J, Alpert L C et al 1987 *Campylobacter pylori* detected non-invasively by the ^{13}C-urea breath test. Lancet i: 1174-1177

Graham D Y, Alpert L C, Smith J L, Yoshimura HH 1988 Iatrogenic *Campylobacter pylori* infection is a cause of epidemic achlorhydria. American Journal of Gastroenterology 83: 974-980

Gray D, Skarvall H 1988 B-cell memory is short-lived in the absence of antigen. Nature 336: 70-73

Hazell S L, Lee A, Brady L, Hennessey W 1986 *Campylobacter pyloridis* and gastritis: association with intracellular spaces and adaptation to an environment of mucus as important factors in colonization of the gastric epithelium. Journal of Infectious Diseases 153: 658-663

Hessey S J, Spencer J, Wyatt J et al 1990 Bacterial adhesion and disease activity in *Helicobacter* associated chronic gastritis. Gut 31: 134-138

Howson C P, Hiyama T, Wynder E L 1986 The decline in gastric cancer: epidemiology of an unexplained triumph. Epidemiologic Reviews 8: 1-27

Johnston B J, Reed P I, Ali M H 1986 Campylobacter-like organisms in duodenal and antral endoscopic biopsies: relationship to inflammation. Gut 27: 1132-1137

Karnes W E, Ohning G V, Sytnik B, Kim S W R, Walsh J H in press Preservation of pH inhibition of gastrin release in subjects with *Helicobacter pylori*. Reviews of Infectious Diseases

Kekki M, Villako K, Tamm A, Siurala M 1977 Dynamics of antral and fundal gastritis in an Estonian rural population sample. Scandinavian Journal of Gastroenterology 12: 321-324

Kimura K 1972 Chronological transition of the fundic-pyloric border determined by stepwise biopsy of the lesser and greater curvatures of the stomach. Gastroenterology 63: 584-592

Krakowka S, Morgan D P, Kraft W G, Leunk R D 1987 Establishment of gastric *Campylobacter pylori* infection in the neonatal gnotobiotic piglet. Infection and Immunity 55: 2789-2796

Lambert J R, Borromeo M, Pinkard K J, Turner H, Chapman C B, Smith M L 1987 Colonization of gnotobiotic piglets with *Campylobacter pyloridis*—an animal model? Journal of Infectious Diseases 155: 1344

Langenberg W, Rauws E A J, Widjojokusumo A, Tytgat G N J, Zanen H C 1986 Identification of *Campylobacter pyloridis* isolates by restriction endonuclease DNA analysis. Journal of Clinical Microbiology 24: 414-417

Leunk R D, Johnson P T, David B C, Kraft W G, Morgan D R 1988 Cytotoxic activity in broth culture filtrates of *Campylobacter pylori*. Journal of Medical Microbiology 26: 93-99

Levi S, Beardshell K, Haddad G, Playford R, Ghosh P, Calam J 1989 *Campylobacter pylori* and duodenal ulcers: the gastrin link. Lancet i: 1167-1168

Mai U, Smith P D, Perez-Perez C J, Blaser M J Unpublished data

McColl K E L, Fullarton G M, Nujumi A M, MacDonald A M, Brown I L, Hilditch T E 1989 Lowered gastrin and gastric activity after eradication of *Campylobacter pylori* in duodenal ulcer. Lancet ii: 499-500

McNulty C A M, Gearty J C, Crump B et al 1986 *Campylobacter pyloridis* and associated gastritis: investigator blind, placebo controlled trial of bismuth salicylate and erythromycin ethylsuccinate. British Medical Journal 293: 645-649

Mai U E, Perez-Perez G I, Wahl L M, Wahl S M, Blaser M J, Smith P D 1990 Inflammatory and cytoprotective responses by human monocytes are induced by *Helicobacter pylori*: possible role in pathogenesis of type B gastritis. Gastroenterology 98: A662

Marshall B J 1989 History of the discovery of *Campylobacter pylori*. In: Blaser MJ (ed). *Campylobacter pylori* in gastritis and peptic ulcer disease. Igaku Shoin Medical Publishers, New York, pp 7-23

152

Marshall, B J, Warren J R 1984 Unidentified curved bacilli in the stomach of patients with gastritis and peptic ulceration. Lancet i: 1311-1313

Marshall B J, Armstrong J A, McGechie D B, Glancy R J 1985 Attempt to fulfill Koch's postulates for pyloric campylobacter. Medical Journal of Australia 142: 436-439

Marshall B J, Goodwin C S, Warren J R et al 1988 Prospective double-blind trial of duodenal ulcer relapse after eradication of *Campylobacter pylori*. Lancet ii: 1437-1445

Megraud F, Brassens-Rabbe M P, Denis F, Belbouri A, Hoa D Q 1989 Seroepidemiology of *Campylobacter pylori* infection in various populations. Journal of Clinical Microbiology 27: 1870-1873

Morgan D, Kraft W, Bender M, Pearson A 1988 Gastrointestinal Physiology Working Group of Cayetano Heredia and the John Hopkins Universities. Nitrofurans in the treatment of gastritis associated with *Campylobacter pylori*. Gastroenterology 95: 1178-1184

Morris A, Nicholson G 1989 Experimental and accidental *C. pylori* infection of humans. In Blaser M J (ed) *Campylobacter pylori* in gastritis and peptic ulcer disease. Igaku Shoin Medical Publishers, New York, pp 61-72

Morris A, Maher K, Thomsen L, Miller M, Nicholson G, Tasman-Jones C 1988 Distribution of *Campylobacter pylori* in the human stomach obtained at postmortem. Scandinavian Journal of Gastroenterology 23: 257-264

Paull G, Yardley J K 1989 Pathology of *pylori*-associated gastric and esophageal lesions. In: Blaser M J (ed) *Campylobacter pylori* in gastritis and peptic ulcer disease. Igaku Shoin Medical Publishers, New York, pp 73-98

Perez-Perez G I, Blaser M J 1987 Conservation and diversity of *Campylobacter pyloridis* major antigens. Infection and Immunity 55: 1256-1263

Perez-Perez G I, Dworkin B, Chodos J, Blaser M J 1988 *Campylobacter pylori*-specific serum antibodies in humans. Annals of Internal Medicine 109: 11-17

Perez-Perez G I, Bodhidatta L, Wongsrichanalai J et al 1990 Seroprevalance of *Helicobacter pylori* infections in Thailand. Journal of Infectious Diseases 161: 1237-1241

Price A B 1988 Histological aspects of *Campylobacter pylori* colonization and infection of gastric and duodenal mucosa. Scandinavian Journal of Gastroenterology 23: 21-24

Quintero Diaz M, Sotto Escobar A 1986 Metronidazole versus cimetidine in the treatment of gastroduodenal ulcer. Lancet i: 907

Rathbone, B J, Heatley R V 1989 Immunology of *C. pylori* infection. In Blaser M J (ed) *Campylobacter pylori* in gastritis and peptic ulcer disease. Igaku Shoin Medical Publishers New York, pp 135-140

Rauws E A J, Langenberg W, Houthoff H J, Zanen H C, Tytgat G N J 1988 *Campylobacter pyloridis* associated chronic active antral gastritis. A prospective study of its prevalence and the effects of antibacterial and anti-ulcer treatment. Gastroenterology 94: 33-40

Rauws E A J, Tytgat G N J 1990 Cure of duodenal ulcer associated with eradication of *Helicobacter pylori*. Lancet 335: 1233-1235

Sankey E A, Helliwell P A, Dhillon A P 1990 Immunostaining of antral gastrin cells is quantatively increased in *Helicobacter pylori* gastritis. Histopathology 16: 151-156

Siurala M, Varis K, Wiljasalo M 1966 Studies of patients with atrophic gastritis: a 10-15 year follow-up. Scandinavian Journal of Gastroenterology 1: 40-48

Siurala M, Isokoski M, Varis K, Kekki M 1968 Prevalence of gastritis in a rural population. Bioptic study of subjects selected at random. Scandinavian Journal of Gastroenterology 3: 211-223

Smith J T L, Pounder R E, Evans D J, Graham D Y, Evans D G 1989 Inappropriate 24 hour hypergastrinaemia in asymptomatic *C. pylori* infection. Gut 30; A732-733

Soll A H 1990 Pathogenesis of peptic ulcer and implications for therapy. New England Journal of Medicine 322: 909-916

Steinheber F U 1985 Aging and the stomach. Clinical Gastroenterology 14: 657-688

Tricottet V, Bruneval P, Vire O, Camilleri J P 1986 *Campylobacter*-like organisms and surface epithelium abnormalities in active, chronic gastritis in humans: an ultrastructural study. Ultrastructural Pathology 10: 113-122

Van Bohemen C G, Langenberg M L, Rauws E A J, Oudbier J, Weterings E, Zanen H C 1989 Rapidly decreased serum IgG to *Campylobacter* in histological chronic biopsy *Campylobacter*-positive gastritis. Immunology Letters 20: 59-62

Van Voorhis W C, Kaplan G, Sarno E N et al 1982 The cutaneous infiltrates of leprosy: cellular characteristics and the predominant T-cell phenotypes. New England Journal of Medicine 307: 1593-1597

Visek W J 1968 Some aspects of ammonia toxicity in animal cells. Journal of Dairy Science 51: 286-295

Wyatt J I, Rathbone B J, Dixon M F, Heatley R V 1987 *Campylobacter pyloridis* and acid-induced gastric metaplasia in the pathogenesis of duodenitis. Journal of Clinical Pathology 40: 841-848

Discussion of paper presented by M. Blaser

Discussed by N. J. Tytgat
Reported by H. C. Neu

Dr Tytgat stated that there are several virulence factors and we do not know at present which are the most important: the urease, the cytotoxins or the vacuolating toxin, the lipases or phospholipases. There is no longer any question regarding the pathogenicity of these organisms based on various studies. What is unclear is what the most important pathogenic factor is, or whether the tissue damage is caused by the inflammatory response of the host itself. We also do not understand why there are such differences in the clinical expression of the infection. For many individuals the organism is almost commensal, causing no symptoms and at the most some chronic inflammation. In others it causes active chronic gastritis, with a lot of polymorphonuclear cells on the epithelial layer and in some patients it leads to a chronic dyspepsia. In a further minority it causes ulcer disease; mainly duodenal ulcer disease, but also gastric ulcer disease. Why the difference in clinical presentation? Why is it so important to look at the age of onset of infection in the population? Why is it important whether someone is infected as a child or if they become infected as an adult?

In duodenal ulcer disease the inflammation is mainly limited to the distal part of the stomach and to the duodenum, although there is gastric metaplasia. We are still uncertain what the main causes of gastric metaplasia are, and we do not understand why some patient's infection and inflammation is limited mainly to the antrum, whereas in others the inflammation and infection is spread throughout the stomach, also involving the acid-secreting corpus/fundus area. Why are some patients only infected in the antrum and have a normal corpus fundus with acid secreting parietal cells? Is that genetically based or is there another reason? Helicobacter can be eradicated, is the gastric metaplasia in the bulb reversible? Can it return to the low level present in any normal human being?

In some individuals after 20 or 30 years gastritis evolves as atrophic gastritis leading to gastric cancer. What determines the transition from Helicobacter-related infection into atrophic gastritis? Is this organism related? Is it host-related? Does it depend on the intensity or the distribution of the inflammation in the stomach? These questions need to be answered. The next question relates to the difficulty in eradicating this organism. Monotherapy, no matter what the drug, is unhelpful and it eradicates the organism in only 20 or maximally 30% of patients. Double therapy, which is usually bismuth with amoxycillin or with metronidazole eradicates 50%, but the best is triply therapy with the combination of bismuth, metronidazole and tetracycline giving a high eradication rate and the fewest side effects. These triple therapies must be given for one or two weeks.

An important and increasing problem is whether there is resistance to metronidazole. We believe that in Africa, almost 100% of the strains are resistant to metronidazole. This is because some organisms deep in the pits in the foveolae are out of reach of the antimicrobial agents, either from the lumen or from the tissue side. What does one do with patients that resist triple therapy? Will such patients, through inadequately sterilized equipment, infect other patients? Iatrogenic transmission is a true possibility.

Why is it so difficult to have an animal model to study Helicobacter? Many workers have tried to find something which really mimics the human situation and have given up, because there are always weaknesses in the animal models. Tytgat stated that he believed that Helicobacter is the leading cause of gastritis. There is no question that it is the dominant factor in duodenal ulcer disease. Eradication of Helicobacter means that there will be no further relapse, and we now have several patients worldwide up to four years after true eradication without relapse. The literature is full of recurrence, but that means ineffective therapy—in many hundreds of patients he has followed, recurrence has not been seen. If Helicobacter is properly eradicated, the only recurrences are reinfections.

Dr Blaser commented that people have looked for *H. pylori* in a variety of sources and no one has found the organism outside human beings. It is not in foods, water or food animals. It is clear that there is an enormous reservoir of *H. pylori* in humans, and at this point the presumption is that humans are the major and only reservoir. Blaser felt that *H. pylori* lives in a very protected niche; the stomach is an organ of rudimentary immunological capabilities and it presumably relies on peristalsis and acid to cleanse itself of bacteria, and in most instances is quite successful—*H. pylori* has figured out a way to live successfully for a long period of time in the stomach, and this is probably due to a variety of factors such as adhesions, urease, motility and microaerophilism. The reason it is so difficult to eradicate Helicobacter is that it is not living in the body. It is mostly living in a mucous layer, and is therefore in a privileged site. This is his belief why it is so difficult to eradicate. The normal host immune mechanisms are present; certainly there is recognition of the organism as indicated by the antibody response, but the antibodies cannot get to the Helicobacter.

It is interesting that in people who have *H. pylori* infection get older and develop atrophic gastritis and decreasing levels of acid production, they begin to get gastric bacterial overgrowth. Most patients in fact start losing their *H. pylori* infection. It may be that *H. pylori* is not such a hearty bug but is living in a very specialized niche. Once that niche is destroyed any other organism can out-compete it. That leads into the question of why it is so difficult to obtain a good animal model. Dr Blaser believes that *H. pylori* is adapted to the human stomach, and in general the only models that one can use are humans and other primates. Pigs have their own Helicobacters, so do ferrets, as do other species. They are interestingly all microaerophilic spiral organisms, which are all urease positive. A lot of organisms are coprophagic, and the normal rodent stomach has a lot of other bacteria which compete for adherence. It is the very specific adaptation to the human subject as well as competition by other organisms that make it difficult for there to be an animal model.

Blaser felt that the most important question is the question of why there are different outcomes to *H. pylori* infection. This is the critical question. There are three possibilities: strain differences, host differences or both. It is probably both. Blaser is investigating virulence factors, i.e. strain differences, but is also investigating host response. It seems likely that there will be different host responses. He believes that the nature of the host immunologic and inflammatory response has some bearing on what the outcome will be. Most studies of early *H. pylori* infection show that both the antrum and the body of the stomach are infected, yet in patients who have duodenal ulcer only the antrum is involved, whereas patients with gastric ulcers have both infected. We know that most patients with duodenal ulcer have high acidity and one speculation may be that if they have extensive inflammation of the fundus, they cannot develop high acidity because of the damage to parietal cells, and that may be why we do not see fundal involvement in duodenal ulcer. In gastric ulcer where we see low acidity, it will correlate with the fact that there is extensive fundal involvement. The paradox is that *H. pylori* infection and inflammation may cause hyperacidity. There may be a stage in which the G-cells and some of the other regulatory cells are stimulated and yet there may be a later, or a consequence of, more severe infection in which there is destruction of these cells and a decrease in their acid production.

There have been studies that have shown that the organism can be present in dental plaque but not in saliva—we know that there are Campylobacters and microaerophilic niches in the oral flora—so this is not surprising. How does an organism get from one person's stomach to another person's stomach? Presumably orally, or faecal-orally? There is very little evidence for oral-oral transmission.

Dr Svanborg noted that there are several obvious parallels between the models of urinary infection with regard to the importance of the inflammatory response. In the mouse urinary model acute inflammation appears to lead to the clearance of infection in an untreated animal. If one blocks this response with either anti-inflammatory agents or genetically the animal becomes hyper-susceptible. In Blaser's system the inflammatory response is really a way for the organism to maintain its nutrient access. But anti-inflammatory agents always cause increased problems in terms of gastritis and ulcer.

Blaser stated that *H. pylori* can stimulate the immune response. He has evidence that *H. pylori* antigens are present in tissue even though the whole organism is not, and so the question is, is this an accident or is *H. pylori* doing this on purpose? Important questions would be what is the pathology in *H. pylori* infected patients who are agammaglobulinaemic? What is the pathology in AIDS patients? Most of the evidence in AIDS patients, at least the preliminary evidence, would suggest that it is similar to the pathology seen in other patients, but this is very preliminary data.

NSAIDS and aspirin can cause gastric injury, but perhaps with a different mechanism. In patients who have non-ulcer dyspepsia, there is a large group who have NSAID-related ulcer disease and also a large group in whom *H. pylori* is present. It is clear that *H. pylori* does not cause dyspepsia in all of them, but it may be that like many disease processes, one or another of several risk factors is needed. NSAIDS may be one, *H. pylori* may be another.

Tytgat stated that there is a very high incidence of *H. pylori* infection in Japan, but that the age of onset is not known. In other parts of the world, China, South America etc, there is a close correlation between the risk of gastric cancer and the *H. pylori* infection rate. The earlier the age of onset, the higher the risk of ultimately developing gastric malignancy. However, we need more data. Blaser noted that with ulcer, *H. pylori* may be necessary but not sufficient. In people who acquire *H. pylori* at a young age, Scandinavian studies have shown that the progression from superficial gastritis to atrophic gastritis to carcinoma may take 40 years. Those who get *H. pylori* when they are 10 have a much greater chance of completing this progression than those who get *H. pylori* at age 40. It is interesting to note that the incidence of gastric cancer is going down all over the developed world, and one correlate is that the age of onset of *H. pylori* has gone up.

Wadstrom commented on the oral cavity reports of Helicobacter. He doubted that Helicobacter can survive in the oral cavity. When mouth hygiene is poor they may stay for a short time, but what is the possibility of oral infections as dormant or resting forms, which may be important in cases of relapse? There could be a faecal-oral route in developing countries if we believe in these dormant forms, which may be outside the body and can be transmitted to children soon after weaning? Blaser reported that studies in Thailand are consistent with faecal-oral transmission. The studies in a Thai village of the seroepidemiology of *H. pylori* infection parallel those for hepatitis A. In an orphanage in Thailand where enteric infection is hyperendemic, 75% of the children are positive for *H. pylori* by age two. He questioned whether there is a dormant form of *H. pylori* or not, and whether that might play a role in either relapse or transmission is not clear. Blaser reported that the studies to date have shown that antibody parallels persistence of organisms. There have been four or five studies now that show that if one treats, antibodies go away, but if one does not treat, antibodies remain stable. The CDC study which evaluated people on average of 7.5 years apart showed a tremendous stability of antibodies. He believes that antibodies in general reflect the persistence of infection.

Section IV: Resistance

Chairman: H. C. Neu

10. The molecular basis of β-lactamase induction in enterobacteria

S. Normark   E. Bartowsky   S. Lindquist
M. Galleni   E. Tuomanen   H. H. Martin and
H Schmidt

INTRODUCTION

The sequencing of the *E. coli ampC* gene (Jaurin & Grundström 1981) revealed that this chromosomal beta-lactamase belonged to a distinct class of serine-β-lactamases denoted class C. It has since become clear that most enterobacterial species and related organisms contain an *ampC* gene coding for a class C β-lactamase (Bergström et al 1982, Bergström et al 1983, Lindberg & Normark 1986a, Galleni et al 1987). In species such as *Citrobacter freundii, Enterobacter clocae, Serratia marcescens*, some of the indole-positive *Proteae* and in *Pseudomonas aeruginosa*, the chromosomal *ampC* β-lactamase is inducible by β-lactam antibiotics, whereas in others such as *E. coli* and *Shigella sonnei* it is not (Sykes & Matthew 1987, Lindberg & Normark 1986b). The basic difference between species with inducible and constitutive β-lactamases is the presence of an additional regulatory gene, *ampR*, present in the inducible ones, however lacking in the non-inducible species (Bergström et al 1983, Lindberg et al 1985). All other components involved are shared between inducible and non-inducible species.

THE AmpR REGULATOR ACTS AS A TRANSCRIPTIONAL ACTIVATOR IN THE PRESENCE OF β-LACTAM INDUCER

The *ampR* gene is transcribed divergently from *ampC*. The *ampR* and *ampC* promoters in *E. cloacae* were defined by Honoré et al (1986) and shown to overlap each other partially (Fig. 10.1). By DNaseI footprinting it was demonstrated that *ampR* encodes a DNA-binding protein which binds to a region located immediately upstream of the *ampC* promoter. The binding site for AmpR overlaps the *ampR* promoter (Fig 10.1). This helped explain why *ampR* transcription, as measured by β-galactosidase activity from an *ampR:lacZ* transcriptional fusion, was repressed by expressing AmpR from a coresident plasmid (Lindquist et al 1989a)

When the *ampR* and *ampC* genes of *C. freundii* were cloned into *E. coli* lacking a native *ampC* gene, the AmpC enzyme was inducible by β-lactam antibiotics (Lindberg et al 1985). However, if *ampR* was deleted, *E. coli* produced twice the basal level of β-lactamase as the wild-type but the *ampC* gene was no longer inducible. The

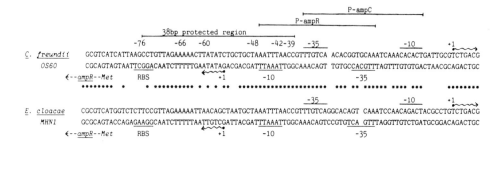

Figure 10.1 Nucleotide sequence of the intercistronic region between *ampR* and *ampC* in *C. freundii* and *E. cloacae*. The DNA-binding site for *ampK* (386p protected region) is indicated as all the respective promoters for *ampC* (P-*ampC*) and *ampR* (P-*ampR*). Reproduced from Lindquist et al 1989a (with permission).

elevated *C. freundii ampC* expression in an *ampR⁻* background suggested that the AmpR protein could occur in an activator state (in the presence of β-lactam inducer) and in a repressor state (no inducer). The in vitro DNase 1 footprints were identical if the AmpR extract was isolated from non-induced or induced cells (Lindquist et al 1989a), implying that AmpR binding to DNA was not affected by β-lactam stimulus. Instead, the activator state of AmpR may facilitate the binding of RNA polymerase.

AmpR belongs to a family of homologous transcriptional activators, referred to as the LysR family (Henikoff et al 1988), encompassing at least twelve proteins: LysR, NodD, TrpI, IlvY, CysB, OxyR, MetR, MerR, MleR, NahR, CatR and AmpR (Table 10.1). Recently Storz et al (1990) demonstrated that OxyR activates transcription of oxidative stress-inducible genes in vitro in the oxidized state but not in the reduced state. This is the only transcriptional activator in this family shown so far to be activated by a mechanism other than binding of a low-molecular-weight ligand. In no case is there evidence for covalent modification such as phosphorylation or methylation.

The AmpR protein contains none of the sequence motifs conserved among β-lactam binding proteins (Honoré et al 1986, Joris 1988, Lindquist et al 1989a) and semipurified AmpR does not bind ³H-benzylpenicillin suggesting that β-lactam induction is not caused by direct interaction with the β-lactam (unpublished data). This in turn implies that conversion of AmpR from its repressor state to its activator state is not due to direct binding of the β-lactam inducer as a ligand.

INACTIVATION OF THE *ampD* GENE CAUSES ACTIVATION OF AmpR AND RESULTS IN CONSTITUTIVE EXPRESSION FROM *ampC*

The hypothesis of a non-β-lactam effector for AmpR is supported by the finding that AmpR may be activated by mutations in chromosomal genes present in *E. coli* and

162

Table 10.1

Bacterial activator proteins of the LysR family

Protein	Bacterial species	Mol. wt (Da)	Inducer	Gene(s) regulated	Target pathway
AmpR	*Citrobacter freundii*	32 537	β-lactam	*ampC*	β-lactamase
AmpR	*Enterobacter cloacae*	32 609	β-lactam	*ampC*	β-lactamase
LysR	*Escherichia coli*	34 318	DAP (diaminopimelate)	*lysR*	lysine biosynthesis
MetR	*Salmonella typhimurium*	30 991	homocysteine	*metJ/H*	methionine biosynthesis
NodD₁	*Rhizobium meliloti*	34 839	flavonoid	*nodABC*	nodulation genes
NodD	*Rhizobium leguminosarum*	34 487	flavonoid	*nodABC*	nodulation genes
Ilvy	*Escherichia coli*	33 200	acetohydroxybutyrate (L-valine) acetolactate (L-isoleucine)	*ilvC*	isoleucine biosynthesis
OxyR	*Escherichia coli*	34 400	oxidative stress	H_2O_2	inducible genes
OxyR	*Salmonella typhimurium*	34 400	oxidative stress	H_2O_2	inducible genes
TrpI	*Pseudomonas aeruginosa*	31 950	indole glycerol phosphate	*trpBA*	tryptophan biosynthesis
CysB	*Salmonella typhimurium*	36 013	O-acetyl-L-serine	*cys*	cysteine biosynthesis
CysB	*Escherichia coli*	36 150	O-acetyl-L-serine	*cys*	cysteine biosynthesis
CatR	*Pseudomonas putida*	32 200	*cis-cis* muconate	*catBC*	benzoate utilization
MerR	*Escherichia coli*	16 000	mercuric salts	*mer*	mercuric ion resistance
MleR	*Lactococcus lactis*	33 813	L-malate		malolactic acid fermentation
NahR	*Pseudomonas putida*	36 000	salicylate	*sal*	degradation of naphthalene

References: AmpR, *C.f* (Lindquist et al 1989), *E.c* (Honore et al 1986); LysR (Stragier et al 1983); MetR (Plamann & Stauffer 1987); NodD, *R.m* (Egelhoff et al 1985), *R.l* (Rossen et al 1985); IlvY (Wek & Hatfield 1986); OxyR (Christman et al 1989); TrpI (Chang et al 1989; CysB (Ostrowski et al 1987); CatR (Rothmel et al 1990); MerR (Lund & Brown 1989); MleR (Renault et al 1989); NahR (Schell & Sukordhaman 1989).

163

that mutants producing elevated levels of AmpC β-lactamase occur spontaneously in *C. freundii (C.f)*, *E. cloacae* and also in *Serratia marcescens* at a frequency of 10^{-6} to 10^{-7} (Findell & Sherris 1976, Gootz et al 1982, Gootz et al 1984, Gutmann & Chabbert 1984, Lindberg et al 1985, Lindberg & Normark 1986b, Hechler et al 1989). To study these 'regulator' genes cefotaxime-resistant mutants of *E. coli* were selected (containing an inactivated native *ampC* gene) carrying the *C.f. ampR*, *ampC* genes on a hybrid plasmid (Lindberg et al 1987). Most of these β-lactam resistant mutations were chromosomal. One of the chromosomal mutations mapped to 2.6 min on the *E. coli* chromosome between the *nadC* and *aroP* genes and defined a new locus denoted *ampD*. The wild-type and the mutant *ampD* alleles were subsequently cloned. While the wild-type clone complemented all β-lactam resistant mutations were chromosomal. One of the chromosomal mutations mapped to 2.6 min on the *E. coli* chromosome between the *nadC* and *aroP* genes and defined a new locus denoted *ampD*. The wild-type and the mutant *ampD* alleles were subsequently cloned. While the wild-type clone complemented all β-lactam resistant mutants to β lactam sensitivity, the mutant clone *(ampD2)* did not complement any of the mutants. It was therefore argued that most, if not all, β-lactam resistant *E. coli* mutants obtained in this way were mutated in *ampD*. Furthermore, the wild-type *ampD*$^+$ clone but not the *ampD2* mutant clone complemented β-lactam resistant *C. freundii* and *E. cloacae* mutants to β-lactam sensitivity and wild-type inducibility (Lindberg & Normark 1987, Lindberg et al 1987). Hence, most natural β-lactam resistant mutants of inducible species are *ampD* mutants. The *E. coli ampD* mutants only mediated β-lactam resistance in the presence of a functional AmpR regulator, and they could be divided into two classes with respect to basal AmpC β-lactamase expression and with respect to induction by β-lactams (Lindberg et al 1987, Lindquist et al 1989b).

The Class 1 *ampD* mutants produced only twice the basal level of AmpC β-lactamase in the absence of inducer. The high β-lactam resistance of Class 1 mutants is due to the hyperinducible phenotype of these mutants. For example, while 5-10 g/l of cefoxitin is required to induce wild-type *E. coli* harbouring a *C.f. ampC*$^+$, *ampR*$^+$ plasmid, only 1-2 g/l induce a Class 1 *ampD* mutant harbouring the same plasmid. The Class 2 *ampD* mutants showed a 20- to 30-fold elevated basal expression of AmpC β-lactamase and could be further induced 2- to 3-fold by additional of β-lactam inducer. Class 2 mutants were referred to as semiconstitutive.

The wild-type *ampD* gene, one Class 1 *ampD* mutant *(ampD1)*, and one Class 2 *ampD* mutant *(ampD2)* were sequenced (Lindquist et al 1989b). The *ampD* gene encodes for a 183 amino acid protein which, by minicell fractionation, was localized to the cytoplasm. This location was consistent with the absence of a leader sequence within the predicted amino acid sequence. The AmpD primary sequence showed no significant homology to any protein present in the EMBL data base. There was, however, a sequence in the central part of the protein (around the Gly-96) that showed homology to the helix turn helix motifs of DNA binding regulatory proteins (Pabo & Sauer 1984). If AmpD is a DNA-binding protein, its binding site is most likely not present in the intercistronic region between *ampR* and *ampC*; since no differences were found in DNase 1 footprinting experiments using cellular extracts with or without AmpD (Lindquist et al 1989a).

The *ampD1* mutation turned out to be a 52 base-pair out-of-frame deletion after

164

codon 23, with endpoints in 9 of 10 base-pair homologous direct repeats whereas the *ampD2* mutation, leading to a semiconstitutive phenotype, was due to the insertion of an IS1 element after codon 121. Thus, two seemingly 'knock-out' *ampD* mutations caused different basal expression of β-lactamase and led to different induction kinetics.

Insertion of an IS element can cause transcriptional polarity on downstream genes in the same transcriptional unit. It was therefore, hypothesized that *ampD* may be followed by a second gene cotranscribed with it. An open reading frame of 284 codons with its putative initiation codon overlapping the termination codon of *ampD* was detected (Lindquist et al 1989b). This novel gene, denoted *ampE*, codes for a protein with a predicted molecular weight of 32 kDa. When placed downstream from an IPTG- inducible *tac* promoter, the *ampE* gene expresses a 28 kDa protein that fractionates with the cytoplasmic membrane. The nature of this protein as being AmpE was verified by aminoterminal sequencing of gel-purified protein. Having identified *ampE* as a gene distal to *ampD*, it was directly demonstrated in minicells that the *ampD2* but not the *ampD1* allele caused a decreased expression of AmpE. Thus the *ampD2::IS1* allele is polar on *ampE*, implying that *ampD* and *ampE* are in the same operon.

Computer analysis of the AmpE primary amino acid sequence predicts that it is an integral membrane protein with four putative *trans*-membrane helices. AmpE was also analyzed for the presence of sequence motifs found among β-lactam binding proteins. The carboxyterminal region of AmpE contains a Ser-X-X-Lys sequence. Such a motif is present in serine type β-lactam binding proteins and represents part of the active site (Joris 1988). However, none of the other conserved motifs, including the essential Lys-Thr-Gly sequence is present in AmpE. Moreover, AmpE does not covalently bind ^{3}H-benzylpenicillin. It was therefore argued that the Ser-X-X-Lys sequence present in AmpE does not present an acylation site for β-lactams and that AmpE does not belong to the β-lactam binding protein family, i.e. proteins that covalently bind β-lactams (Lindquist et al 1989b). It is, however, possible that AmpE interacts in a non-covalent manner with β-lactams.

The sequence analysis of AmpE showed that it contained the two conserved motifs typical of ATP-binding proteins (Lindquist et al 1989b). These motifs were located between the second and third putative *trans*-membrane region. In a tentative model on how AmpE is arranged in relation to the membrane, it was suggested that the putative ATP-binding region faces the cytoplasm. Several membrane-bound ATP-binding proteins (known or putative) act as energy couplers in different transport systems. Some of these systems are periplasmic protein-dependent uptake systems for carbohydrates, peptides, and amino acids (Ames 1986) whereas others are secretion systems for specific polysaccharides or proteins (Kroll et al 1988).

Honoré et al (1989) independently identified the *ampE* gene from *E. coli* and demonstrated that *ampD* and *ampE* formed an operon. They isolated and sequenced three independent *ampD* mutants. In each case the mutation was a base-pair substitution changing codon seven from TGG to GGG thereby replacing a tryptophan with a glycine at position seven in the AmpD protein (provided the aminoterminal methionine is retained in the protein). The *ampD*[G7] allele caused a constitutive phenotype similar to the Class 2 mutants described by Lindquist et al (1989b). It is unlikely that a single base-pair substitution would be polar on *ampE*.

Consequently, the hyperinducible phenotype observed in the Class 1 mutants and represented by the *ampD*1 allele may not represent the true *ampD* 'null' phenotype. It is possible, that in the *ampD*1 mutant a low degree of translational frameshifting occurs, leading to a low production of a biologically active AmpD protein carrying an internal deletion of 52 amino acids. If this interpretation is correct, then the *ampD* 'null' phenotype should be constitutive and the *ampD* [G7] reported by Honoré et al (1989) should yield an inactive AmpD protein.

Langley and Guest (1977) isolated deletion mutants in the *nadC, aroP* region of the *E. coli* chromosome. One of these mutants (JRG582) turned out to be totally deleted for both *ampD* and *ampE*. When the *ampR* and *ampC* genes from *C. freundii* or *E. cloacae* were introduced into this strain, the cells highly overproduced β-lactamase and no further induction was obtained with β-lactams (Honoré et al 1989, Lindquist et al 1989b). Moreover, the overexpression of β-lactamase was AmpR dependent.

The individual role of *ampD* and *ampE* in β-lactamase regulation was explored by constructing an isogenic set of mutated plasmids and measuring the ability of these

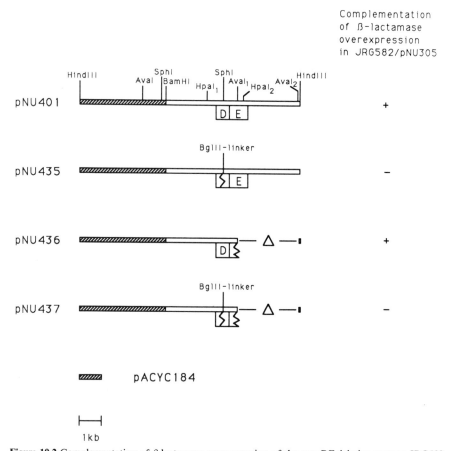

Figure 10.2 Complementation of β-lactamase overexpression of the *ampDE* deletion mutant JRG582 expressing the AmpR and AmpC proteins from plasmid pNU305 by compatible plasmids expressing *AmpD* and/or *AmpE*.+ indicates complementation to β-lactam sensitivity, low level β-lactamase expression and inducibility by β-lactams.

166

plasmid constructs to complement the phenotype mediated by the chromosomal deletion in JRG582.

Introducing *ampD* and *ampE* (Fig. 10.2) on a pACYC184 backbone (pNU401) into JRG582/pNU305 (*ampR⁺*, *ampC⁺*) complemented the β-lactamase hyperproducing phenotype mediated by the chromosomal deletion to β-lactam sensitivity and low basal level of β-lactamase that could be increased by a β-lactam inducer such as cefoxitin. By introducing a synthetic oligonucleotide linker into the single Sph 1 site in *ampD*, we obtained an out-of-frame mutation after codon 96 in *ampD*. Plasmid pNU435 carrying this *ampD* mutation did not complement the phenotype of JRG582 Δ(*ampDE*)/pNU305 to β-lactam sensitivity, though we could still monitor expression of the 28kDa AmpE polypeptide from this construct in *E. coli* minicells. In fact the expression of β-lactamase was the same as in JRG582/pNU305 carrying pNU437 mutated for both *ampD* and *ampE*. A deletion of the AvaI fragment on pNU401 yielded plasmid pNU436 carrying *ampD* and a deletion of the 3′ half of *ampE*. Plasmid pNU436 complemented JRG582/pNU305. The basal level of β-lactamase in JRG582/pNU305 + pNU436 was twice that of JRG582/pNU305 + pNU401 implying that the *ampE* gene has a role in regulating the basal level of *ampC* β-lactamase. The major conclusion, however, is that primarily *ampD* and not *ampE* acts as a negative regulator for *ampC* expression.

MUTATIONS IN THE *ampD* LOCUS AFFECT COMPOSITION OF PEPTIDOGLYCAN

The *amp* regulon has been characterized by its ability to influence β-lactamase expression. However, the *ampD* and *ampE* genes are chromosomal genes present also in species without inducible β-lactamases. Thus it is of major importance to determine what the natural function(s) of this regulon is. The initial hint that *ampD* may be involved in peptidoglycan metabolism was the observation that *E. coli* in the absence of AmpD and β-lactamase are more β-lactam sensitive than isogenic bacteria expressing AmpD (Lindquist et al 1989b).

E. coli strain SN03 (*ampD⁺E⁺*) and its mutant derivatives SN0301 (*ampD1*) and SN0302 (*ampD2*) were analysed for specific changes in peptidoglycan composition. Reverse-phase high performance liquid chromatography (HPLC) analysis was performed on reduced total peptidoglycan hydrolysate (Tuomanen et al 1989). Peaks were identified by comparison of retention times with known *E. coli* standards and the relative abundance of individual peaks was calculated. The most striking difference between the two patterns was the absence of one peak from the analyses of both *ampD* mutant strains that was present in the isogenic *ampD⁺* strain (Tuomanen et al submitted for publication). When this peak was collected, desalted by HPLC and subjected to fast atom bombardment collision activated dissociated mass spectrometry, the mass and fragmentation pattern unambiguously identified the peak as the disaccharide pentapeptide monomer, i.e., *N*-acetylglucosamine-*N*-acetylmuramic acid-L-alanine-D-glutamic acid-*meso*-diaminopimelic acid-D-alanine-D-alanine. We interpret these findings to mean that the *ampD* gene product affects the amount of pentapeptide in the cell wall.

The monomer pentapeptide is the intact peptidoglycan precursor. Most commonly, this precursor is incorporated into the cell wall by transglycosylation of the disaccharide to the glycan backbone and transpeptidation of the peptide side-chain to its neighbour, resulting in loss of the terminal D-alanine. To be detected intact in the cell wall sacculus, the pentapeptide side-chain must remain unmodified by transpeptidase, carboxypeptidase, or endopeptidase activity. Since the change found in the cell wall was not accompanied by distortion of the overall ratio of dimeric (i.e. crosslinked peptides) versus monomeric wall fragments, major distortions in transpeptidase and endopeptidase activities are unlikely. Rather, the simplest hypothesis is that *ampD* fulfills either of two functions: it enhances the activity of a cell wall synthetic enzyme which preferentially inserts pentapeptides into the growing cell wall or it represses a carboxypeptidase which normally trims D-alanine off the cell wall as it matures.

Two approaches were taken to determine if *ampD* affects the synthetic or degradative arms of peptidoglycan metabolism. The penicillin-binding protein profile of the SN03, SN0301 and SN0302 strains were compared, looking for differences in the number or size of cell wall synthetic enzymes. All normal PBPs are present in the parent as well as in the mutants, suggesting that *ampD* does not affect the synthetic arm of peptidoglycan metabolism. *E. coli* normally releases over 30% of its cell wall per generation as the cell wall is modified during maturation. This turnover is largely hidden from standard assays since a very efficient form of recapture of the released species exists (Goodell & Higgins 1987). Thus, net loss of radiolabelled species from the cell wall (turnover rate) is maximally around 10%. If recycling of cell wall turnover products was altered by *ampD* or *ampE*, we reasoned that the mutants might lose more radiolabelled stem peptides into the medium. This proved to be the case. Strains SN0301 and SN0302 lost about twice the amount of radiolabel from the peptidoglycan compared with the wild-type SN03 (Tuomanen et al submitted for publication).

Direct titration of two degradative enzyme activities in parent and mutant cells, the transglycosylase and endopeptidase activities, was also performed. Membrane-bound and soluble degradative enzyme activities in the parent and *ampD*⁻ mutant were not different (unpublished data).

We conclude that the *ampD* locus affects the composition of peptidoglycan. Current evidence is consistent with the hypothesis that the *amp* regulon naturally controls the degradative arm of peptidoglycan metabolism.

THE AmpR REGULATOR EXISTS IN A DIFFERENT FORM IN WILD-TYPE *E. coli* AND IN AN *ampD ampE* DELETION MUTANT

AmpR is a DNA-binding protein and binds to the intercistronic region between *ampR* and *ampC* (Lindquist et al 1989a). AmpR exhibits a similar protein layout to the other members of the LysR family of transcriptional activators. The aminoterminal portion of the protein has the DNA-binding activity and shows the highest degree of homology to the other transcriptional activators. The ligand-responsive region of the protein is located in the carboxyl end where the degree of homology diminishes. This layout is consistent throughout this family of proteins and especially well demonstrated within the NodD protein from the different *Rhizobium* species (Spaink et al 1989). Mutants in AmpR have been isolated in both the DNA-binding and inducer-responsive regions of the protein (unpublished data). The AmpR regulator is constitutively activated in the *E. coli ampD* deletion mutant JRG582 as evidenced by the AmpR-dependent constitutive over-expression from the cloned *C. freundii ampC* gene. To be able to establish the molecular mechanisms for AmpR activation a purification system has been developed for AmpR. AmpR purified according to this scheme retained its ability to bind specifically to the *ampC, ampR* intercistronic region (unpublished data). AmpR was purified from wild-type cells as well as from the isogenic *ampDE* deletion mutant, JRG582. The two protein preparations showed the same molecular weight on SDS-PAGE but migrated differently during isoelectric focusing. This suggests that AmpR activation is caused by binding of an autogenously made effector molecule (autoinducer). It is likely, but not yet shown, that the same effector molecule accumulates during β-lactam induction in wild-type cells. The chemical nature of the autoinducer is yet to be determined.

SENSING OF THE β-LACTAM STIMULUS

The only known cellular targets for β-lactam antibiotics are the penicillin-binding proteins (PBPs). Different β-lactams differ markedly in their ability to induce *ampC* β-lactamase. Hence while imipenem and cefoxitin (and other cephamycins) are highly effective inducers, aztreonam, ceftazidime, piperacillin and others are not. Since these two groups of β-lactams differ in their affinity for PBPs it was hypothesized that one or more of the existing PBPs acts as a sensor in the β-lactamase induction pathway. It was also recently reported that mutations in *pbpA* encoding PBP2 abolished β-lactamase induction (Oliva & Bennett 1989). Induction studies are, however, difficult to interpret when performed on mutants affecting penicillin-binding proteins, since such mutants can be more sensitive to the inducer.

We have performed induction studies on a collection of PBP mutants (obtained by Dr B Spratt) transformed with the *C. freundii ampR* and *ampC* genes. It was clearly established that the 'null' mutant in *ponA* (encoding PBP1A) was still inducible and that a temperature-sensitive PBP2 mutant (*pbp* (ts)45) was inducible at the restrictive temperature. However, it was unclear if a PBP1b 'null' mutant (*ponB::spc*) and a conditional PBP3 mutant (*pbpB*(ts)[R7]) were inducible or not because of the increased β-lactam susceptibility of *E. coli* harbouring these mutant alleles.

To avoid this problem PBP1B and PBP3 mutant derivatives of the minicell producing strain M2141 were constructed by phage transduction. Since *E. coli* minicells are non-growing and therefore resistant to β-lactam antibiotics, induction is not obscured by lysis caused by the β-lactam inducer. Purified minicells carrying the *ponB::spc* or *pbpB*(ts)[R7] alleles and harbouring the *C. freundii ampR* and *ampC* genes on a plasmid were both inducible by 6-aminopenicillanic acid or by imipenem. Hence, none of the known high-molecular-weight PBPs acting as transpeptidases is required for β-lactamase induction.

Single and double mutants in *dacA* and *dacC* encoding PBP5 and PBP6 were still inducible. No mutant is yet available lacking all three of the major carboxypeptidases PBP4, PBP5 and PBP6. It is therefore not yet known if carboxypeptidase activity is required for β-lactam induction.

The data obtained suggest, however, that none of PBP1A, 1B, 2, 3, 5 or 6 act as a sensor in the *ampR*-dependent *ampC* induction system.

It has recently been suggested that AmpE acts as a β-lactam sensor (Honoré et al 1989). An in vitro-generated mutant in the assumed β-lactam acylation site (Ser^{261}→Ala^{261}) was considerably less inducible than the wild-type. This experiment was performed in the *ampDE* deletion mutant JRG582. The induction was monitored in JRG582 harbouring either *ampD, ampE* or *ampD, ampE*^{A261} on a hybrid plasmid and the *E. cloacae ampR* and *ampC* genes on a compatible plasmid. Expression of AmpD from a multicopy plasmid has a negative effect on β-lactamase induction. It is possible that the lower induction observed by Honoré et al (1989) was not caused by the mutation in *ampE* but by gene dosage or other regulatory effects causing a higher expression of AmpD from the mutant construct. Similar experiments performed by us clearly show that cells physically devoid of *ampE* but expressing AmpD are still inducible (Fig. 10.2). Our view is therefore that AmpE is not essential for induction and therefore cannot act as a β-lactam binding sensor protein.

A β-lactam sensitive non-inducible mutant of *E. cloacae* was recently isolated from a β-lactam resistant *E. cloacae* derivative (Korfmann & Sanders 1989). This chromosomal mutation was complemented to β-lactam resistance and β-lactamase hyperproduction by a DNA fragment cloned from *E. cloacae*. The mutation defined a novel locus, *ampG*, required for β-lactamase induction and the cloned fragment was thought to carry the wild-type allele. Similar β-lactam sensitive non-inducible mutants have recently been isolated from the β-lactam resistant hyperinducible *E. coli* mutant SN0301 (*ampD1*)/pNU305 (*C. freundii, ampR,* and *ampC*) (unpublished data).

The cloned wild-type *ampG* allele of *E. cloacae* complemented the *E. coli* mutants to β-lactam resistance and hyperinduction suggesting that the *E. coli* mutants were mutated in *ampG*.

The constitutive β-lactamase activity of an *E. coli ampG* mutant harbouring both *ampR* and *ampC* was lower than for the same mutant harbouring only *ampC*, suggesting that AmpR in the non-inducible mutant is still able to interact with the *ampR, ampC* intercistronic region as a repressor. It is therefore thought that the conversion of AmpR from a repressor into a transcriptional activator is not occurring in an *ampG* mutant.

AmpG may be required to transduce a β-lactam induced stimulus across the cytoplasmic membrane. Another possibility is that, it could be involved in the transport into the cells of an autoinducer binding to AmpR. Alternatively, AmpG may be involved in the generation of the autoinducer.

MODEL FOR INDUCTION OF *ampC* β-LACTAMASE IN ENTEROBACTERIA

Our understanding of β-lactamase induction in enterobacteria is still incomplete. A tentative model for induction is presented in Figure 10.3.

β-lactam binding to PBPs will affect peptidoglycan metabolism. As a consequence of this effect a peptidoglycan-derived fragment is thought to be generated. This fragment may be an autoinducer or be a precursor form for the autoinducer. This

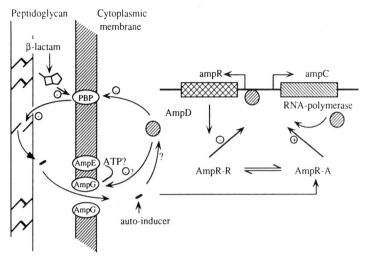

Figure 10.3 Tenative model for β-lactamase induction in enterobacteria. AmpR-R and AmpR-A indicate the regulator in its repressed and activated state respectively.

fragment must be transported across the cytoplasmic membrane in order to interact with AmpR. AmpG and AmpE may be involved in this process. The β-lactam effect in wild-type cells is thought to be down-regulated by AmpD. In *ampD* mutants, however, the autoinducer or its precursor is produced even in the absence of β-lactam. *AmpD* mutants show a changed peptidoglycan composition and exhibit a higher degree of release of radiolabel from peptidoglycan. Therefore, *ampD* may normally regulate peptidoglycan biosynthesis. Our hypothesis is that AmpR 'parasitizes' on a normal regulatory system for peptidoglycan metabolism operating in enterobacteria.

REFERENCES

Ames G F 1986 Bacterial periplasmic transport systems structure, mechanisms and evolution. Annual Review of Biochemistry 55: 397-425
Bergström S, Olsson O, Normark S 1982 Common evolutionary origin of chromosomal β-lactamase genes in enterobacteria. Journal of Bacteriology 150: 528-534
Bergström S, Lindberg F, Olsson O, Normark S 1983 Comparison of the overlapping *frd* and *ampC* operons of *Escherichia coli* with the corresponding DNA sequences in other Gram-negative bacteria. Journal of Bacteriology 155: 1297-1305
Chang M A, Hadero A, Crawford I P 1989 Sequence of the *Pseudomonas aeruginosa trpI* activator gene and relatedness of *trpI* to other procaryotic regulator genes. Journal of Bacteriology 171: 172-183
Christman M F, Storz G, Ames B N 1989 OxyR, a positive regulator of hydrogen peroxide-inducible genes in *Escherichia coli* and *Salmonella typhyimurium* is homologous to a family of bacterial regulatory proteins. Proceedings of the National Academy of Sciences (USA) 86: 3484-3488
Egelhoff T T, Fisher R F, Jacobs T W, Mulligan J T, Long S L 1985 Nucleotide sequence of *Rhizobium meliloti* 1021 nodulation genes: *nodD* is read divergently from *nodABC*. DNA 4: 241-248
Findell C M, Sherris J C 1976 Susceptibility of *Enterobacter* to cefamanodole: evidence for high mutation rate to resistance. Antimicrobial Agents and Chemotherapy 9: 970-974
Galleni M, Lindberg F, Normark S et al 1987 Sequence and comparative analysis of three *Enterobacter cloacea ampC* β-lactamase genes and their products. Biochemistry Journal 250: 753-760
Goodell E W, Higgins C F 1987 Uptake of cell wall peptides by *Salmonella typhimurium* and *Escherichia coli*. Journal of Bacteriology 169: 3861-3865
Gootz T D, Sanders C C, Goering R V 1982 Resistance to cefamandole: derepression of β-lactamases by cefoxitin and mutations in *Enterobacter cloacae*. Journal of Infectious Diseases 146: 34-42

Gootz T D, Jackson D B, Sherris J C 1984 Development of resistance to cephalosporins in clinical strains of *Citribacter* spp. Antimicrobial Agents and Chemotherapy 25: 591-595

Gutmann L, Chabbert 1984 Different mechanisms of resistance to latamoxef in *Serratia marcescens*. Journal of Antimicrobial Chemotherapy 13: 15-22

Hechler U, Van den Weghe M, Martin H H, Frère J M 1989 Overproduced β-lactamase and the outer membrane barrier as resistance factors in *Serratia marcescens* highly resistant to β-lactamase stable β-lactam antibiotics. Journal of General Microbiology 135: 1275-1290

Henikoff S, Haughn G W, Calvo J M, Wallace J C 1988 A large family of bacterial activator proteins. Proceedings of the National Academy of Sciences (USA) 85: 6602-6606

Honoré N, Nicolas M H, Cole S T 1986 Inducible cephalosporinase production in clinical isolates of *Enterobacter cloacae* is controlled by a regulatory gene that has been deleted from *Escherichia coli*. EMBO Journal 5: 3709-3714

Honoré N, Nicolas M H, Cole S T 1989 Regulation of enterobacterial cephalosporinase production; the role of a membrane-bound sensory transducer. Molecular Microbiology 3: 1121-1130

Jaurin B, Grundström T 1981 *ampC* cephalosporinase of *Escherichia coli* K-12 has a different evolutionary origin from that of the β-lactamases of the penicillinase type. Proceedings of the National Academy Sciences (USA 478: 4897-4901

Joris B 1988 The active-site serine penicillin recognizing enzymes as members of the *Streptomyces* R61 DD-peptidase family. Biochemical Journal 250: 313-324

Korfmann G, Sanders C C 1989 *ampG* is essential for high level expression of AmpC β-lactamase in *Enterobacter cloacae*. Antimicrobial Agents and Chemotherapy 33: 1946-1951

Kroll J S, Hopkins I, Moxon E R 1988 Capsule loss in *H. influenzae* type B occurs by recombination-mediated disruption of a gene essential for polysaccharide export. Cell 53: 347-356

Langley D, Guest J R 1977 Biochemical genetics of the α-keto acid dehydrogenase complexes of *Escherichia coli* K12: Isolation and biochemical properties of deletion mutants. Journal of General Microbiology 99: 263-276

Lindberg F, Westman L, Normark S 1985 Regulatory components in *Citrobacter freundii ampC* β-lactamase induction. Proceedings of the National Academy of Sciences (USA) 82: 4620-4624

Lindberg F, Normark S 1986a Sequence of the *Citrobacter freundii* OS60 chromosomal ampC β-lactamase. European Journal of Biochemistry 156: 441-445

Lindberg F, Normark S 1986b Contribution of chromosomal β-lactamases to β-lactam resistance in enterobacteria. Reviews of Infectious Diseases 8: 292-304

Lindberg F, Normark S 1987 Common mechanism of the *ampC* β-lactamase Induction in Enterobacteria: regulation of the cloned *Enterobacter cloacae* P99 β-lactamase gene. Journal of Bacteriology 169: 758-763

Lindberg F, Lindquist S, Normark S 1987 Inactivation of the *ampD* gene causes semi-constitutive overproduction of the inducible *Citrobacter freundii* β-lactamases. Journal of Bacteriology 169: 1923-1928

Lindquist S M, Lindberg F, Normark S 1989a Binding of the *Citrobacter freundii* AmpR regulator to a single DNA site provides both autoregulation and activation of the inducible *ampC* β-lactamase gene. Journal of Bacteriology 171: 3746-3753

Lindquist S, Galleni M, Lindberg F, Normark S 1989b Signalling proteins in enterobacterial β-lactamase regulation. Molecular Microbiology 3: 1091-1102

Lund P A, Brown N L 1989 Regulation of transcription in *Escherichia coli* from the *mer* and *merR* promoters in the transposon Tn501. Journal of Molecular Biology 205: 343-353

Oliva B, Bennett P M, Chopra I 1989 Penicillin-binding protein 2 is required for induction of the *Citrobacter freundii* Class 1 chromosomal β-lactamase in *Escherichia coli*. Antimicrobial Agents and Chemotherapy 33: 1116-1117

Ostrowski J, Jagura-Burdzy G, Kredtich N M 1987 DNA sequences of the *cysB* regions of *Salmonella typhimurium* and *Escherichia coli*. Journal of Biological Chemistry 262: 5999-6005

Pabo C O, Sauer R T 1984 Protein-DNA recognition. Annual Review Biochemistry 53: 293-321

Plamann L S, Stauffer G V 1987 Nucleotide sequence of the *Salmonella typhimurium metR* gene and the *metR—metE* control region. Journal of Bacteriology 169: 3932-3937

Renault P, Gaillardin C, Herlst H 1989 Product of the *Lactococcus lactis* gene required for malolactic fermentation is homologous to a family of positive regulators. Journal of Bacteriology 171: 3108-3114

Rossen L, Shearman C A, Johnston A W B, Downie J A 1985 The *nodD* gene of *Rhizobium leguminosarum* is autoregulatory and in the presence of plant exudate induces the *nodA,B,C* genes. EMBO Journal 4: 3369-3373

Rothmel R K, Aldrich T L, Houghton J E, Coco W M, Ornston L N, Chakrabarty A M 1990 Nucleotide sequencing and characterization of *Pseudomonas putida catR*: a positive regulator of the *catBC* operon is a member of the LysR family. Journal of Bacteriology 172: 922-931

Schell M A, Sukordhaman M 1989 Evidence that the transcription activator encoded by the *Pseudomonas putida nahR* gene is evolutionarily related to the transcription activators encoded by the *Rhizobium nodD* gene. Journal of Bacteriology 171: 1952-1959

Spaink H P, Wijffelman C A, Okker R J H, Lugtenberg B E J 1989 Localization of functional regions of the *Rhizobium nodD* product using hybrid *nodD* genes. Plant Molecular Biology 12: 59-73

Storz G, Tartaglia L A, Ames B N 1990 Transcriptional regulator of oxidative stress-inducible genes: direct activation by oxidation. Science 248: 189-194

Straiger P, Richaud F, Borne F, Patti J C 1983 Regulation of diaminopimelate decarboxylase synthesis in *Escherichia coli*. I. Identification of a *lysR* gene encoding an activator of the *lysA* gene. Journal of Molecular Biology 168: 307-320

Sykes R B, Matthew M 1976 The β-lactamases of gram-negative bacteria and their role in resistance to β-lactam antibiotics. Journal Antimicrobial Chemotherapy 2: 115-157

Tuomanen E, Schwartz J, Sande S, Light K, Gage D 1989 Unusual composition of peptidoglycan in *Bordetella pertussis*. Journal of Biological Chemistry 264: 11093-11098

Wek R C, Hatfield G W 1986 Nucleotide sequence and in vivo expression of the *ilvY* and *ilvC* genes in *Escherichia coli* K12: Transcription from divergent overlapping promoters. Journal of Biological Chemistry 261: 2441-2450

Discussion of paper presented by S. Normark

Discussed by L. Guttmann
Reported by H. C. Neu

Following the presentation by Normark, Gutmann discussed how a molecule or molecules could accumulate in the periplasmic space and be transported across the cytoplasmic membrane to alter the control mechanism for the production of β-lactamase. How a fragment of peptidoglycan would be in the correct location to achieve the induction remains unclear. A weak point to the Normark hypothesis is that diaminopimelic acid and D-alanine are not good inducers. Also, adding a tetrapeptide, which should pass the outer membrane of an *E. coli*, did not induce production of β-lactamase.

A study to demonstrate the inducibility of β-lactamase showed that agents having a high affinity for carboxypeptidases 4, 5 and 6 are good inducers. However, mutants which lack PBPs 3, 4, 5 and 6 can also be induced. Unfortunately, there are no available mutants lacking PBPs 4, 5 and 6. Normark stated that he planned to increase carboxypeptidase activity with cloned carboxypeptidases. This should affect β-lactamase expression if the model is correct. Also if a mutant bacterium lacked PBPs 5 and 6, and had a temperature-sensitive PBP4, it should be possible to dissect the effect of carboxypeptidase activity.

Normark noted that there is 87% homology between the flanking sequences for the *ampR* gene. Thus it would be possible to have horizontal gene transfer from Citrobacter or Enterobacter to *E. coli*, creating strains that would contain the *ampR* gene. Such strains would be inducible, and it would be possible to obtain derepressed mutants, since the *ampD* gene is present in these organisms. Horizontal gene transfer has occurred for PBPs from commensal Neisseria into *Neisseria gonorrhoeae*. It is probable that the resistance level for such *E. coli* strains would be lower than for Citrobacter or Enterobacter due to great permeability in *E. coli*, but for Klebsiella the organisms could be as resistant as the Enterobacter.

Gutmann reviewed in detail what is known about the expanded spectrum β-lactamases that have been found with increasing frequency in clinical specimens in France. In all there are now 18 TEM β-lactamase derivatives and 5 SHV derivatives. All of those enzymes hydrolyse third generation cephalosporins and monobactams. TEM-1 was discovered in 1965, and it was noted that Knowles had produced a point mutation in 1976 of TEM-2 in which alanine at amino acid 235 was replaced by threonine. In 1984, a β-lactamase was found that hydrolysed cefotaxime and was called CTX-1. This enzyme was subsequently shown to be TEM-3, and has been found in Europe, Germany, France, England, Africa, United States, and in Asia. Subsequent enzymes were found that hydrolysed ceftazidime and were called CAZ-1, etc. In fact, all of these enzymes are derivatives of the initial TEM or SHV enzymes and differ by one or two amino acids (Table 10.2).

Table 10.2 AA Substitutions of new expanded spectrum β-lactamases

β-lactamase	Position								
	19	37	102	162	203	235	236	237	261
TEM-1	Leu	Glu	Glu	Arg		Ala	Gly	Glu	Thr
TEM-2		Lys							
TEM-3 (CTX-1)		Lys	Lys				Ser		
TEM-4							Ser		Met
TEM-5 (CAZ-5)	Phe		Lys	Ser		Thr		Lys	
TEM-6			Lys						
TEM-7		Lys		Ser					
TEM-9 (RHH-1)			Lys	Ser					Met
SHV-1					Arg		Gly	Glu	
SHV-2							Ser		
SHV-3					Leu		Ser		
SHV-4 (CAZ-5)					Leu		Ser	Lys	
SHV-5 (CAZ-4)							Ser	Lys	

In the TEM-1 β-lactamase, SHV-1, and even the *Staphylococcus aureus* β-lactamase there are clusters of amino acids which are highly conserved. In essence, the groups of amino acids provide a cavity into which the β-lactam fits so that the serine at the centre can cut the β-lactam bond. The amino acid substitutions occur at a position that allows the β-lactam to fit in the centre cavity of the enzyme. Normally the third generation cephalosporins have a poor affinity for the TEM β-lactamase. The change in amino acids increases the affinity of the enzyme for cefotaxime, ceftazidime, and aztreonam, and the compounds are hydrolysed (see Table 10.3).

In general, it was felt that the selective pressure of high use of the third generation cephalosporins has resulted in the increase of the enzymes. Why they are found most often in Klebsiella is yet to be explained.

Table 10.3 Relative rate[1] of hydrolysis

	Cefotaxime	Ceftazidime	Aztreonam
TEM-2	<0.1	<0.1	<0.1
TEM-3 (CTX-1)	445	40	8.5
TEM-5 (CAZ-1)	150	490	116
SHV-1	<0.1	<0.1	<0.1
SHV-2	70	6.5	1
SHV-3	67	4	<1?
SHV-4	71	19	<1?

1% of benzylpenicillin

11. The molecular basis of quinolone action and resistance

L. M. Fisher   R. Hopewell   M. Oram and
S Sreedharan

INTRODUCTION

Antibacterial 4-quinolones have been widely used in the treatment of infectious diseases (Wolfson & Hooper 1985). Nalidixic acid (Fig. 11.1), the first quinolone, suffered drawbacks including narrow-spectrum activity and rapid emergence of clinical resistance. The new fluoroquinolones, e.g. ciprofloxacin, introduced in the 1980s are much superior both in their inherent potency and antibacterial spectrum being active not only against Gram-negative species including *Pseudomonas* but also Gram-positive bacteria such as *Staphylococcus aureus* (Smith & Eng 1985, Piercy et al 1989). However, problems in certain clinical settings arising from the emergence of fluoroquinolone-resistant strains are beginning to cause medical concern. In this paper, we examine the mode of action of quinolones—their uptake, interaction with their intracellular target DNA gyrase and activation of lethal post-gyrase events; recent identification of resistance pathways in *Escherichia coli*; evidence of similarities in the molecular basis of clinical resistance in *E. coli* and *S. aureus*; and how studies of resistance may shed light on cellular and clinical aspects of quinolone therapy. These topics are approached from a molecular genetics perspective.

MECHANISM AND FREQUENCY OF QUINOLONE RESISTANCE

Many clinically important antibacterial drugs act either by disrupting cell wall biosynthesis (penicillins and cephalosporins) or by interfering with protein synthesis at the ribosome (aminoglycosides, tetracyclines, streptomycin). In contrast, quinolones act by inhibiting bacterial DNA replication (Goss et al 1965). Quinolone resistance arises from mutations in chromosomal genes. With one exception which remains to be confirmed (Munshi et al 1987), there have been no reports of plasmid- or transposon-mediated quinolone resistance. Indeed under laboratory conditions, quinolones promote curing of plasmids from bacteria (Hooper et al 1984). Although some quinolones are metabolized and modified in human cells, there is as yet no evidence for bacterial modification-deactivation as a defence mechanism. The absence of plasmid-borne drug detoxification systems may stem from the fact that quinolones are synthetic agents unlikely to occur in nature.

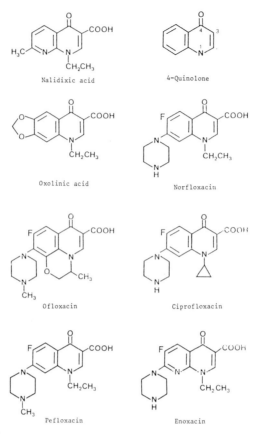

Figure 11.1 Chemical structures of 4-quinolone antimicrobial agents

It is commonly observed that for many bacterial species, it is relatively easy to isolate mutants with high-level resistance to nalidixic acid by a single-step procedure but very difficult to do this for the fluoroquinolones (Piffaretti et al 1983; Hooper et al 1987; Chapman et al 1989). Single-step high-level resistance to nalidixic acid occurs with a frequency of 10^{-7} whereas only low-level resistance ($<10 \times$ MIC) to new quinolones can be obtained with single-step selection at a frequency of $<10^{-9}$. This observation accords with the rapid development of nalidixic acid resistance during therapy which severely curtailed its clinical value. High-level resistance to fluoroquinolones can be engineered in the laboratory by incremental selection procedures producing mutants that are also cross-resistant to other quinolones. The less frequent and low-level resistance observed for the fluoroquinolones in vitro is not understood but indicates that for most pathogens resistance arising from single-step mutations may not be clinically significant. (*Pseudomonas* strains appear to be an exception given their already high intrinsic MICs for quinolones.) However, it is important to note that high-level norfloxacin resistance can be readily selected at a frequency of 10^{-7} in *E. coli* strains that already exhibit the *m*ultiple *a*ntibiotic *r*esistance phenotype due to a prior mutation in the *marA* locus (Cohen et al 1989).

Quinolone-resistant mutants have been studied most intensively in the Gram-negative bacterium *E. coli*. Resistance mutations can be grouped into three classes:

178

Table 11.1 Types of quinolone resistance in *Escherichia coli*, gene locations and phenotypes

Type	Gene and map location (phenotype)
Structural change in DNA gyrase	*gyrA* (48 min): *nfxA*, *ofxA*, *norA*, *cfxA*
	(resistance to quinolones)
	gyrB (83 min): *nalC*, *nalD*
	(resistance to nalidixic acid, new quinolones (*nalD*), hypersusceptibility to new quinolones (*nalC*)
Reduced permeation	*nfxB* (19 min), *cfxB* (34 min), *norB* (34 min)
	(resistance to quinolones and other agents, lowered ompF porin)
	norC (8 min)
	(altered lipopolysaccharides)
Other?	*nalB*, *icd*, *cya*, *crp*

those affecting DNA gyrase—the intracellular target for the 4-quinolones, those decreasing drug permeability, and those whose function is still to be assigned (Table 11.1). We consider first resistance in *E. coli* and then turn to clinical resistance.

QUINOLONE RESISTANCE: STRUCTURAL CHANGES IN DNA GYRASE

Mutations in the *gyrA* (formerly *nalA*) and *gyrB* (*cou*) genes encoding the gyrase A and B subunits have been selected using ciprofloxacin (*cfxA*), nalidixic acid (*nalA*, *nalC*, *nalD*), norfloxacin (*nfxA*, *norA*) and ofloxacin (*ofxA*) (Table 11.1) (Hane & Wood 1969, Hirai et al 1986a, Hooper et al 1986, 1987). Mutations in *gyrA* confer resistance specific to quinolones and cause cross-resistance to quinolones other than the selecting agent. Gellert et al (1977) were the first to show that in *E. coli*, DNA gyrase is the target for quinolones. To appreciate the effects of *gyrA* and *gyrB* mutations in resistance we need to consider the mechanism and cellular functions of DNA gyrase.

Gyrase catalyses ATP-dependent introduction of negative supercoils into bacterial DNA (Gellert et al 1976). The enzyme, a 400 000 mol. wt A_2B_2 tetramer is required for many DNA transactions including gene expression, recombination, transposition and DNA replication (Wang 1985, 1987). Gyrase promotes DNA supercoiling and relaxation, DNA unknotting and the linking/unlinking of DNA rings by passing a DNA segment through an enzyme-bridged transient double-strand break (Fig. 11.2). The 100 000 mol. wt subunits encoded by the *gyrA* gene engage in transient DNA breakage-reunion, and the B subunits from the *gyrB* gene hydrolyse ATP (Higgins et al 1978, Mizuuchi et al 1978).

Quinolones inhibit ATP-dependent DNA supercoiling and ATP-independent DNA relaxation by purified *E. coli* DNA gyrase and in vivo rapidly inhibit DNA replication. Detergent treatment of gyrase-DNA complexes formed in the presence of a quinolone results in double-stranded DNA breakage at specific sites arising from the trapping of the presumptive enzyme-DNA intermediate (Fig. 11.3) Cleavage occurs with a stagger of four base pairs and each newly formed 5′ end of the break is linked by a 5′ covalent phosphotyrosine (Tyr) bond to Tyr-122 of a gyrase A subunit.

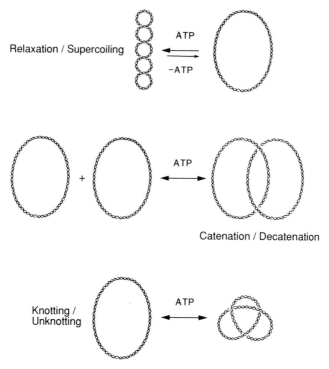

Figure 11.2 Reactions catalysed by DNA gyrase

Similar experiments performed on *E. coli* cells treated with a quinolone result in chromosome fragmentation and the production of DNA fragments about 100 kilobases in size (Snyder & Drlica 1979). This result is consistent with the presence of 50-100 gyrase binding sites on the chromosome which coincidentally matches the number of independent chromosomal loops or domains revealed by nuclease digestion studies. Gyrase cleavage arises from the trapping of a covalent reaction intermediate in the gyrase reaction. These studies identify Tyr-122 as the catalytic residue in the 875 amino acid gyrase A protein responsible for DNA breakage. The nature of the gyrase-quinolone complex is not well understood at the molecular level. However, Shen et al (1989) have proposed a model whereby four quinolone molecules bind and stabilize the transiently broken DNA in the enzyme complex by forming

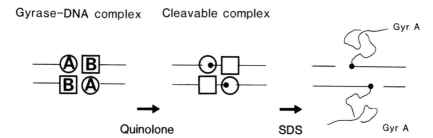

Figure 11.3 Mechanism of DNA breakage by gyrase promoted by the quinolones. A, B denote gyrase subunits; SDS, sodium dodecyl sulphate

hydrogen bonds to DNA, hydrophobic bonds with each other, and by forming side-chain interactions with the enzyme.

How do quinolone resistance mutations affect the gyrase complex? When complemented with B subunit, mutant gyrase A subunits reconstitute a DNA gyrase supercoiling activity that is resistant to quinolone inhibition. Moreover, such gyrase complexes do not promote quinolone-mediated DNA cleavage either in vitro or in bacteria. The nature of mutations in *gyrA* responsible for quinolone resistance has been determined for four resistant *E. coli* K12 strains, two selected with nalidixic acid and two with pipemidic acid (Yoshida et al 1988). High-level resistance to the drugs arose from a single substitution of serine (Ser)-83 to tryptophan (Trp) or leucine (Leu) (Fig.11.4). Low-level resistance arose from an alanine (Ala)-67 to Ser or a glutamine (Glu)-106 to histidine substitution. Thus, the mutations all map to a region of the gyrase A protein close to the catalytic Tyr-122 residue whose function is antagonized by quinolones (Horowitz & Wang 1987). This *N*-terminal region of the gyrase A protein forms a compact protease-resistant domain and appears to carry the active site for DNA breakage and quinolone action (Reece & Maxwell 1989).

Gyrase B subunit mutations conferring low-level nalidixic acid resistance have been assigned to residues 426 and 447 (Yamagishi et al 1986) (Fig.11.4). These mutations lie in a domain of the B subunit that interacts to activate the topoisomerase functions of the A subunits (Gellert et al 1979). It not clear whether these gyrase B residues interact directly with quinolone or act indirectly by modifying the conformation of the A subunits. *NalC* mutations in *gyrB* merit further study because they confer *hypersusceptibility* to fluoroquinolones (Yamagishi et al 1986). The effects of *gyrB* mutations on gyrase activities have yet to be tested.

It is not clear how inhibition of gyrase by a quinolone signals induction of bactericidal pathways. Quinolone treatment causes bacterial filamentation, alters expression of virulence factors, induces the SOS response involving recA protein and

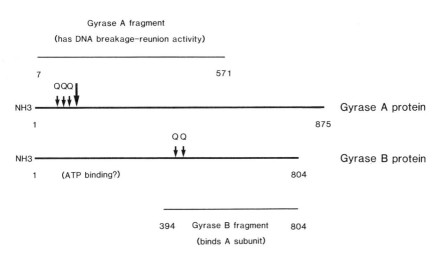

Figure 11.4 Structures of *E. coli* DNA gyrase A and B subunits and locations of known quinolone resistance mutations (Q). The mutations lie within subunit domains that can be isolated as protease-resistant fragments. Numbers indicate amino acid residues, large arrow identifies the position in the gyrase A protein of catalytic tyrosine-122.

results in DNA damage (Drlica & Franco 1988). However, it has been argued that neither SOS nor DNA damage induction is important but that instead *recA*-dependent recombination repair may be implicated (Lewin et al 1989, Lewin & Smith 1990). Whatever the mechanism, killing is greatly stimulated by oxygen and appears to require protein and RNA synthesis. Secondary inhibition of these processes by high levels of quinolones has been invoked to explain the 'paradoxical dose response' whereby increasing quinolone concentrations result in lowered cell kill (Crumplin & Smith 1975). Unlike nalidixic acid, fluoroquinolones such as ciprofloxacin and ofloxacin appear to have an additional killing pathway that is not suppressed by rifampicin, an RNA synthesis inhibitor. One promising approach in unravelling bacteriolytic pathways is the recent isolation of a quinolone-tolerant *E. coli* mutant, i.e. a strain which although inhibited by quinolones is 1000-fold less susceptible to *killing* compared with the wild-type bacterium (Wolfson et al 1989). Mapping of mutations responsible for tolerance may allow the identification of proteins that play a role in cell killing by quinolones. Interestingly, *hipA* mutations in *E. coli* selected for resistance to β-lactams, also show increased resistance to nalidixic acid, suggesting a possible common killing pathway for these drugs, perhaps involving cell division (Scherrer & Moyed 1988).

RESISTANCE THROUGH CHANGES IN QUINOLONE PERMEATION

The second class of mutations selected with ciprofloxacin or norfloxacin confer pleiotropic resistance to quinolones, chloramphenicol and tetracycline (Table 11.1) (Hirai et al 1986a, Hooper et al 1986, 1987). Resistance to quinolones is low-level and involves complex changes that reduce drug permeation (see also Chapman et al 1989).

In Gram-negative bacteria, the outer membrane serves as the major permeability barrier for entry and exit of small hydrophilic compounds, including antibiotics (Hancock 1987, Hancock & Bell 1989) (Fig. 11.5). Many hydrophilic molecules, including quinolones, penetrate the outer membrane through transmembrane water-filled protein pores known as porins. In *E. coli* K12 the major outer membrane porins are OmpF and OmpC whose expression is closely regulated in response to environmental stimuli such as temperature and osmolarity. Uptake of quinolones is a non-saturable diffusive process that does not require energy (Bedard et al 1987). Studies with porin-deficient mutants suggest that relatively hydrophilic quinolones such as ciprofloxacin and norfloxacin permeate via the OmpF porin. However, the reduction in MICs for rough mutants of *Salmonella typhimurium* and the small (several fold) increase in quinolone MIC values for the porin-deficient cells compared with wild-type suggests that additional non-porin uptake pathways operate particularly for hydrophobic quinolones such as nalidixic acid for which the lipopolysaccharide (LPS) layer forms a permeability barrier (Hirai et al 1986b). It has been proposed that quinolones, through their adjacent carbonyls, chelate LPS-associated magnesium ions bridging LPS molecules, thereby destabilizing the outer membrane and revealing an exposed lipid bilayer through which the quinolone is then able to diffuse (Fig.11.5) (Chapman & Georgopapadakou 1988). This mechanism was originally proposed by Hancock for aminoglycosides and is termed 'self-promoted

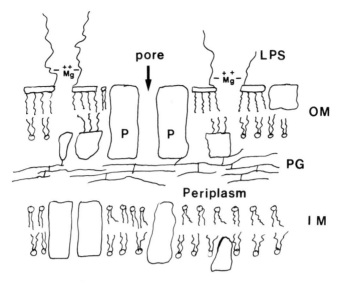

Figure 11.5 Schematic representation of the membrane structure of a gram-negative bacterium. IM and OM are the inner and outer membranes, PG is the peptidoglycan layer, P identifies a porin protein channel. LPS, lipopolysaccharide molecules bridged by the divalent cation Mg^{2+} which in the 'self-promoted uptake' pathway is chelated by quinolones (after Hancock & Bell 1989)

uptake' (Hancock 1987, Hancock & Bell 1989). The relative contributions of porin- and non-porin-mediated pathways appears to depend on extracellular magnesium concentrations and on the relative hydrophobicity of the particular quinolone (Hirai et al 1986b, Chapman & Georgopapadakou 1988).

NfxB and *cfxB* (possibly allelic with *norB*) although mapping at different loci have very similar phenotypes and appear to interact (Hooper et al 1989); both decrease expression of OmpF at the post-transcriptional level and decrease norfloxacin accumulation in cells in an energy-dependent fashion. Reduced quinolone permeation in such mutants has been ascribed to decreased diffusion through porin channels in concert with an energy-requiring saturable drug efflux system recently discovered on the inner membrane (Fig.11.6) (Cohen et al 1988a).

Mutations at the *marA* locus (34 min) selected with chloramphenicol or tetracycline also confer resistance to quinolones by a reduced permeation mechanism involving down-regulation of OmpF (Cohen et al 1988b, 1989). Mar mutants thus share close similarity with *cfxB* and *nfxB* mutants but also exhibit other outer membrane changes in addition to reduced levels of OmpF. Interestingly, *norB* and *cfxB* are closely linked to *marA* and may in fact be alleles of *marA*. It has been found that *marA* mutants can achieve high-level quinolone resistance at high frequency by mutation at the *gyrA* locus (Cohen et al 1989). It may be significant that a number of quinolone-resistant isolates have been described having mutations affecting *both* gyrase and permeation (Hooper et al 1987).

Permeation and gyrase mutations have been described in other bacterial species including *Pseudomonas aeruginosa* and *Citrobacter freundii* (Hirai et al 1987, Inoue et al 1987, Aoyama et al 1988b, Robillard & Scarpa 1988, Celesk & Robillard 1989). None has been identified at the nucleotide level.

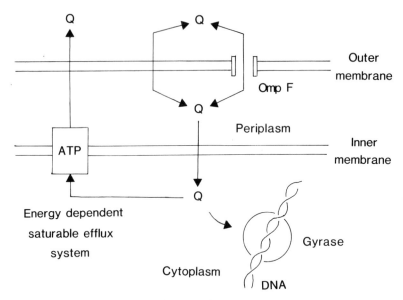

Figure 11.6 Pathways of quinolone permeation and efflux in gram-negative bacteria. Q denotes the quinolone, Omp F porin protein forms a water-filled membrane pore

QUINOLONE RESISTANCE IN CLINICAL ISOLATES

Clinical isolates have received less attention than their laboratory counterparts. Nonetheless, structural changes in DNA gyrase A subunit or reduced permeability were found in quinolone-resistant isolates of *Citrobacter freundii*, *Escherichia coli*, *Pseudomonas aeruginosa* and *Serratia marcescens* (Sanders & Watanakunakorn 1986, Aoyama et al 1987, 1988b, Daikos et al 1988).

Recently, new techniques that circumvent the problems of genetic heterogeneity associated with clinical isolates have given detailed insights into resistance. The known genetic dominance of wild-type *gyrA* and *gyrB* genes over the corresponding resistant alleles has been exploited to examine the proportion of *gyrA* and *gyrB* mutations in quinolone-resistant *E. coli* (Nakamura et al 1989). By introducing wild-type *gyrA* or *gyrB* genes on plasmids and analysing the conferral of quinolone susceptibility, *gyrA* mutations were shown to predominate over *gyrB* mutations in clinical isolates with MICs for nalidixic acid of 200-400 µg/ml (*gyrA* and *gyrB* mutations were equally common in 25 spontaneous mutants of *E. coli* K12). We have focused on eight resistant uropathogenic *E. coli* isolates (MICs for nalidixic acid ranging from 62 to 1000 µg/ml) and showed that several produced a quinolone-resistant gyrase A protein (Cullen et al 1989a). The resistant *gyrA* cloned from one isolate taken from a patient treated with enoxacin was sequenced and found to carry a Ser-83 to Trp codon change responsible for resistance (Cullen et al 1989b). This represents thus far the only reported complete molecular characterization of quinolone resistance in a clinical isolate.

Gyrase A codon 83 mutations eliminate a *Hinf*I restriction site in the *gyrA* gene (Fisher et al 1989). This restriction fragment length polymorphism (RFLP) is readily examined by Southern blotting of chromosomal DNA from clinical isolates and allows for rapid screening of clinical isolates (Southern 1975). Six of the seven uropathogenic clinical isolates had lost the site indicating an amino acid substitution in the gyrase A protein. More recently, we have used the polymerase chain reaction to show that these isolates possess a codon change at Ser-83 to either Leu or Trp (our unpublished results). The predominance of mutations at codon 83 of the gyrase A protein in both clinical and non-clinical strains of *E. coli* strongly suggests a key role for the wild-type Ser-83 residue in quinolone action. In the context of the Shen model, mutation of Ser-83 could either sterically hinder quinolone binding or disrupt a key interaction required for stabilization of the drug-enzyme complex, e.g. a hydrogen-bonding or metal-chelating function of the serine hydroxyl group.

We have also studied molecular aspects of quinolone resistance in clinical isolates of *S. aureus*. Many hospitals are currently witnessing serious difficulties in the management of *S. aureus* infections arising from the recent emergence of ciprofloxacin-resistant methicillin-resistant strains (Lyon & Skurray 1987, Isaacs et al 1988, Schaefler 1989, Shalit et al 1989). The mechanism of quinolone resistance in *S. aureus* is at present unknown. Although *S. aureus* gyrase has been purified by this group and others (Takahata & Nishino 1988), we have experienced difficulties with nuclease contamination. As one approach to this problem, we recently cloned the *S. aureus gyrA* and *gyrB* genes from a methicillin- and ciprofloxacin-susceptible strain (Hopewell et al 1990). The 5′ end of the *gyrA* gene shows remarkable sequence conservation with its *E. coli* counterpart which is even more marked at the protein level. The *S. aureus* gyrase A protein has conserved Ala-68, Ser-84 and Gln-107 residues whose direct counterparts in *E. coli* when mutated confer resistance (Fig. 11.7). By using a *Hin*fI RFLP approach, we have found that several ciprofloxacin-resistant *S. aureus* isolates have amino acid substitutions at codon 84, i.e. analogous to the situation in *E. coli*. It will clearly be important to identify such mutations at the nucleotide level for comparison with the better-defined *E. coli* system. Genetic techniques have allowed cloning of the *norA* gene for norfloxacin resistance in *S. aureus* (Ubukata et al 1989). Interestingly, the resistance gene (like *cfxB*) acts in a dominant fashion to the wild-type allele: it remains to be established whether it is a gyrase allele.

Clinical resistance in *Pseudomonas* is less well understood but is potentially very important, particularly for treating infection in cystic fibrosis patients. Resolution of the molecular nature of such resistance must await the cloning of the gyrase genes from this bacterial species.

PROBLEMS AND PERSPECTIVES

The mechanisms of quinolone action and resistance are understood only in outline. We can identify several areas where progress will be rapid and others where basic essential knowledge is lacking. We focus here on DNA gyrase, resistance pathways and topics of clinical concern.

Much effort has been directed toward understanding the role of DNA gyrase in quinolone resistance. As we have seen, these studies have led to the identification of resistance mutations in *E. coli* gyrase. With the advent of polymerase chain reaction

(PCR) techniques, we can expect rapid progress in the cloning and characterization of drug sensitive and resistant gyrase genes from both clinical and non-clinical bacteria. Consequently, the primary structures of gyrase proteins in most of the clinically important species will soon be known, as will resistance mutations. Indeed, the structures of gyrase A proteins have already been reported for *Escherichia coli*, *Bacillus subtilis*, *Staphylococcus aureus* and *Klebsiella pneumoniae* (Fig.11.7) (Moriya et al 1985, Adachi et al 1987, Swanberg & Wang 1987, Dimri & Das 1990 Hopewell et al 1990). However, a major difficulty in rationalizing the quinolone sensitivities of different gyrases and in interpreting the mode of action of resistance mutations stems from the absence of three-dimensional structural information about the gyrase-quinolone-DNA complex. The model of Shen and coworkers rests on binding studies and must be regarded tentatively in its molecular details. To date several thousand quinolones have been synthesized at random and tested for activity. In terms of optimizing drug design and understanding resistance, it will be essential to have X-ray crystal structure data for gyrase.

Other resistance mechanisms, e.g. reduced permeation, are only now being

```
E. coli      MetSerAspLeuAlaArgGlu---IleThrProValAsnIle
S. aureus    METAlaGluLeuProGlnSerArgIleAsnGluArgAsnIle
B. subtilis  MetSerGluGlnAsnThrProGlnValArgGluIleAsnIle


GluGluGluLeuLysSerSerTyrLeuAspTyrAlaMetSerValIleValGlyArgAla
ThrSerGluMetArgGluSerPheLeuAspTyrAlaMetSerValIleValAlaArgAla
SerGlnGluMetArgThrSerPheLeuAspTyrAlaMetSerValIleValSerArgAla


LeuProAspValArgAspGlyLeuLysProValHisArgArgValLeuTyrAlaMetAsn
LeuProAspValArgAspGlyLeuLysProValHisArgArgIleLeuTyrGlyLeuAsn
LeuProAspValArgAspGlyLeuLysProValHisArgArgIleLeuTyrAlaMetAsn

                                      ▼
ValLeuGlyAsnAspTrpAsnLysAlaTyrLysLysSerAlaArgValValGlyAspVal
GluGlnGlyMetThrProAspLysSerTyrLysLysSerAlaArgIleValGlyAspVal
AspLeuGlyMetThrSerAspLysProTyrLysLysSerAlaArgIleValGlyGluVal

                  ▼
IleGlyLysTyrHisProHisGlyAspSerAlaValTyrAspThrIleValArgMetAla
MetGlyLysTyrHisProHisGlyAspSERSerIleTyrGluAlaMetValArgMetAla
IleGlyLysTyrHisProHisGlyAspSerAlaValTyrGluSerMetValArgMetAla

                              ▼
GlnProPheSerLeuArgTyrMetLeuValAspGlyGlnGlyAsnPheGlySerIleAsp
GlnAspPheSerTyrArgTyrProLeuValAspGlyGlnGlyAsnPheGlySerMetAsp
GlnAspPheAsnTyrArgTyrMetLeuValAspGlyHisGlyAsnPheGlySerValAsp

                  ▽
GlyAspSerAlaAlaAlaMetArgTyrThrGluIleArgLeuAlaLysIleAlaHisGlu
GlyAspGlyAlaAlaAlaMetArgTYRThrGluAlaArgMetThrLysIleThrLeuGlu
GlyAspSerAlaAlaAlaMetArgTyrThrGluAlaArgMetSerLysIleSerMetGlu


LeuMetAlaAspLeuGluLysGluThrValAspPhe.....
LeuLeuArgAspIleAsnLysAspThrIleAspPhe.....
IleLeuArgAspIleThrLysAspThrIleAspTyr.....
```

Figure 11.7 Close sequence homology between the *N*-terminal regions of gyrase A protein from *Escherichia coli*, *Staphylococcus aureus* and *Bacillus subtilis* (indicated by overlining and underlining). Open and filled triangles, the catalytic tyrosine and residues whose substitution confers quinolone resistance in *E. coli*.

186

delineated. More work is needed on the components and control of quinolone uptake and efflux systems, particularly in clinical isolates. It is also conceivable that quinolone resistance mechanisms other than altered gyrase and reduced permeation may be discovered, e.g. affecting DNA repair or cell killing pathways. Furthermore there may be overlap with bacteriocidal events induced by other classes of antibiotics.

Finally, it is possible that clinical resistance may arise by mutation of the same limited set of gyrase A residues. The sequences of gyrase A proteins from different bacterial species appear to be highly conserved in the N-terminal region that interacts with quinolones (Fig. 11.7). Mutation of Ser-83 (or its equivalent) may therefore be commonly implicated constituting a simplifying feature in understanding resistance pathways. In vitro studies suggest that in many situations two or more mutations may be needed for clinically significant resistance. Mutations in *marA* selected in vitro can contribute to this process. It is not known whether *marA* has clinical importance for quinolone resistance and its consequences for multidrug therapy remain to be explored.

SUMMARY

Quinolones are potent broad-spectrum antibacterials used in oral therapy of infection. Resistance arises from mutations in chromosomal genes. Thus far only two classes of resistance have been encountered: altered target (DNA gyrase) and reduced permeation. Molecular genetic techniques have identified the quinolone-resistance mutations in gyrase subunits in clinical and in non-clinical isolates. How these changes modify the association between the gyrase-DNA complex and the drugs is not known and awaits detailed three-dimensional analysis of the enzyme structure. Resistance resulting from reduced permeation points to interesting control mechanisms affecting porin expression and drug efflux. Quinolone permeation mutants selected with unrelated antibacterial agents readily acquire mutations in gyrase that then confer high-level resistance. It remains to be determined whether two-step mutation contributes to resistance in the clinical setting.

ACKNOWLEDGEMENTS

We thank Dr John Wolfson for stimulating and helpful discussion. Work by the authors was supported by the Science and Engineering Research Council under the aegis of the Molecular Recognition Initiative and through SERC CASE (jointly with Glaxo) and SERC Quota Postgraduate Research Studentships.

REFERENCES

Adachi T, Mizuuchi M, Robinson E A et al 1987 DNA sequence of the *E. coli gyrB* gene: application of a new sequencing strategy. Nucleic Acids Research 15: 771-784

Aoyama H, Sato K, Kato T, Hirai K, Mitsuhashi S 1987 Norfloxacin resistance in a clinical isolate of *Escherichia coli*. Antimicrobial Agents and Chemotherapy 31: 1640-1641

Aoyama H, Sato K, Fujii T, Fujimaki K, Inoue M, Mitsuhashi S 1988a Purification of *Citrobacter freundii* DNA gyrase and inhibition by quinolones. Antimicrobial Agents and Chemotherapy 32: 104-109

Aoyama H, Fujimaki K, Sato K et al 1988b Clinical isolate of *Citrobacter freundii* highly resistant to new quinolones. Antimicrobial Agents and Chemotherapy 32: 922-924

Bedard J, Wong S, Bryan L E 1987 Accumulation of enoxacin by *Escherichia coli* and *Bacillus subtilis*. Antimicrobial Agents and Chemotherapy 31:1348-1354

Celesk R A, Robillard N J 1989 Factors influencing the accumulation of ciprofloxacin in *Pseudomonas aeruginosa*. Antimicrobial Agents and Chemotherapy 33: 1921-1926

Chapman J S, Georgopapadakou N H 1988 Routes of quinolone permeation in *Escherichia coli*. Antimicrobial Agents and Chemotherapy 32: 438-442

Chapman J S, Bertasso A, Georgopapadakou N H 1989 Fleroxacin resistance in *Escherichia coli*. Antimicrobial Agents and Chemotherapy 33: 239-241

Cohen S P, Hooper D C, Wolfson J S, Souza K S, McMurray L M, Levy S B 1988a Endogenous active efflux of norfloxacin in susceptible *Escherichia coli*. Antimicrobial Agents and Chemotherapy 32: 1187-1191

Cohen S P, McMurray L M, Levy S B 1988b *MarA* locus causes decreased expression of OmpF porin in multiple-antibiotic-resistant (mar) mutants of *Escherichia coli*. Journal of Bacteriology 170: 5416-5422

Cohen S P, McMurray L M, Hooper D C, Wolfson J S, Levy S B 1989 Cross resistance to fluoroquinolones in multiple-antibiotic-resistant (mar) *Escherichia coli* selected by tetracycline or chloramphenicol: decreased drug accumulation associated with membrane changes in addition to OmpF reduction. Antimicrobial Agents and Chemotherapy 33: 1318-1325

Crumplin G C, Smith J T 1975 Nalidixic acid: an antibacterial paradox. Antimicrobial Agents and Chemotherapy 8: 251-261

Cullen M E, Wyke A W, McEachern F, Austin C A, Fisher L M 1989a Inhibition of DNA gyrase: bacterial sensitivity and clinical resistance to 4-quinolones. In: Jackson G G, Schlumberger H D, Zeiler H-J (eds) Perspectives in antiinfective therapy. Springer-Verlag, Berlin, pp 73-84

Cullen M E, Wyke A W, Kuroda R, Fisher L M 1989b Cloning and characterization of a DNA gyrase A gene from *Escherichia coli* that confers clinical resistance to 4-quinolones. Antimicrobial Agents and Chemotherapy 33: 886-894

Daikos G L, Lolans V T, Jackson G G 1988 Alterations in outer membrane proteins of *Pseudomonas aeruginosa* associated with selective resistance to quinolones. Antimicrobial Agents and Chemotherapy 32: 785-787

Dimri G P, Das H K 1990 Cloning and sequence analysis of the *gyrA* gene of *Klebsiella pneumoniae*. Nucleic Acids Research 18: 151-156

Drlica K, Franco R J 1988 Inhibitors of DNA topoisomerases. Biochemistry 27: 2253-2259

Fisher L M, Lawrence J M, Josty I C, Hopewell R, Margerrison E E C, Cullen M E 1989 Ciprofloxacin and the fluoroquinolones. American Journal of Medicine 87 (suppl 5A): S2-S8

Gellert M, Mizuuchi K, O'Dea M H, Nash H A 1976 DNA gyrase: an enzyme that introduces superhelical turns into DNA. Proceedings of the National Academy of Sciences (USA) 73: 3872-3876

Gellert M, Mizuuchi K, O'Dea M H, Itoh T, Tomizawa J-I 1977 Nalidixic acid resistance: a second genetic character involved in DNA gyrase activity. Proceedings of the National Academy of Sciences (USA) 74: 4772-4776

Gellert M, Fisher L M, O'Dea M H 1979 Purification and catalytic properties of a fragment of gyrase B protein. Proceedings of the National Academy of Sciences (USA) 76: 6289-6293

Goss W A, Deitz W H, Cook T M 1965 Mechanism of action of nalidixic acid on *Escherichia coli*. II. Inhibition of DNA synthesis. Journal of Bacteriology 89: 1068-1074

Hancock R E W 1987 Role of porins in outer membrane permeability. Journal of Bacteriology 169: 929-933

Hancock R E W, Bell A 1989 Antibiotic uptake into gram negative bacteria. In: Jackson G G, Schlumberger H D, Zeiler H-J (eds) Perspectives in antiinfective therapy. Springer-Verlag, Berlin, pp 42-53

Hane M W, Wood T H 1969 *Escherichia coli* K-12 mutants resistant to nalidixic acid: genetic mapping and dominance studies. Journal of Bacteriology 99: 238-241

Higgins N P, Peebles C L, Sugino A, Cozzarelli N R 1978 Purification of subunits of *Escherichia coli* DNA gyrase and reconstitution of enzyme activity. Proceedings of the National Academy of Sciences (USA) 75: 1773-1777

Hirai K, Aoyama H, Suzue S, Irikura T, Iyobe S, Mitsuhashi S 1986a Isolation and characterization of norfloxacin-resistant mutants of *Escherichia coli* K-12. Antimicrobial Agents and Chemotherapy 30: 248-253

Hirai K, Aoyama H, Irikura T, Iyobe S, Mitsuhashi S 1986b Differences in susceptibility to quinolones of outer membrane mutants of *Salmonella typhimurium* and *Escherichia coli*. Antimicrobial Agents and Chemotherapy 29: 535-538

Hirai K, Suzue S, Irikura T, Iyobe S, Mitsuhashi S 1987 Mutations producing resistance to norfloxacin in *Pseudomonas aeruginosa*. Antimicrobial Agents and Chemotherapy 31: 582-586

188

Hooper D C, Wolfson J S, McHugh G L, Swartz M D, Tung C, Swartz M N 1984 Elimination of plasmid pMG110 from *Escherichia coli* by novobiocin and other inhibitors of DNA gyrase. Antimicrobial Agents and Chemotherapy 25: 586-590

Hooper D C, Wolfson J S, Souza K S, Tung C, McHugh G L, Swartz M N 1986 Genetic and biochemical characterization of norfloxacin resistance in *Escherichia coli*. Antimicrobial Agents and Chemotherapy 29: 639-644

Hooper D C, Wolfson J S, Ng E Y, Swartz M N 1987 Mechanisms of action of and resistance to ciprofloxacin. American Journal of Medicine 82 (suppl 4A): 2-11

Hooper D C, Wolfson J S, Souza K S, Ng E Y, McHugh G L, Swartz M N 1989 Mechanisms of quinolone resistance in *Escherichia coli*: characterization of *nfxB* and *cfxB*, two mutant resistance loci decreasing norfloxacin accumulation. Antimicrobial Agents and Chemotherapy 33: 283-290

Hopewell R, Oram M, Briesewitz R, Fisher L M 1990 DNA cloning and organization of the *Staphylococcus aureus gyrA* and *gyrB* genes: close homology between gyrase proteins and implications for 4-quinolone action and resistance. Journal of Bacteriology 172: 3481-3484

Horowitz D S, Wang J C 1987 Mapping the active site tyrosine of *Escherichia coli* DNA gyrase. Journal of Biological Chemistry 262: 5339-5344

Inoue Y, Sato K, Fujii T et al 1987 Some properties of subunits of DNA gyrase from *Pseudomonas aeruginosa* POA1 and its nalidixic acid-resistant mutant. Journal of Bacteriology 169: 2322-2325

Isaacs R D, Kunke P J, Cohen R L, Smith J W 1988 Ciprofloxacin resistance in epidemic methicillin-resistant *Staphylococcus aureus*. Lancet ii: 843

Lewin C S, Smith J T 1990 DNA breakdown by the 4-quinolones and its significance. Journal of Medical Microbiology 31: 65-70

Lewin C S, Howard B M A, Ratcliffe N T, Smith J T 1989 4-quinolones and the SOS response. Journal of Medical Microbiology 29: 139-144

Lyon B R, Skurray R 1987 Antimicrobial resistance of *Staphylococcus aureus*: genetic basis. Microbiological Reviews 51: 88-134

Mizuuchi K, O'Dea M H, Gellert M 1978 DNA gyrase: subunit structure and ATPase activity of the purified enzyme. Proceedings of the National Academy of Sciences (USA) 75: 5960-5963

Moriya A, Ogasawara N, Yoshikawa H 1985 Structure and function of the region of the replication origin of the *Bacillus subtilis* chromosome. Nucleotide sequence of some 10,000 base pairs in the origin region. Nucleic Acids Research 13: 2251-2265

Munshi M H, Sack D A, Haider K, Ahmed Z U, Rahaman M M, Morshed M G 1987 Plasmid mediated resistance to nalidixic acid in *Shigella dysenteriae* type 1. Lancet ii: 419-421

Nakamura S, Nakamura M, Kojima T, Yoshida H 1989 *GyrA* and *gyrB* mutations in quinolone-resistant strains of *Escherichia coli*. Antimicrobial Agents and Chemotherapy 33: 254-255

Piercy E A, Bartaro D, Luby J P, Machowiak P A 1989 Ciprofloxacin for methicillin-resistant *Staphylococcus aureus* infections. Antimicrobial Agents and Chemotherapy 33: 128-130

Piffaretti J C, Demarta A, Leidi-Bulla L, Peduzzi R 1983 In vitro emergence of *Escherichia coli* and *Pseudomonas aeruginosa* strains resistant to norfloxacin and nalidixic acid. European Journal of Clinical Microbiology 2: 600-601

Robillard N J, Scarpa A L 1988 Genetic and physiological characterization of ciprofloxacin resistance in *Pseudomonas aeruginosa* PAO. Antimicrobial Agents and Chemotherapy 32: 535-539

Reece R J, Maxwell A 1989 Tryptic fragments of the *Escherichia coli* DNA gyrase A protein. Journal of Biological Chemistry 264: 19648-19653

Sanders C C, Watanakunakorn C 1986 Emergence of resistance to beta lactams, aminoglycosides and quinolones during combination therapy for infection due to *Serratia marcescens*. Journal of Infectious Diseases 153: 617-619

Schaefler S 1989 Methicillin-resistant strains of *Staphylococcus aureus* resistant to quinolones. Journal of Clinical Microbiology 27: 335-336

Scherrer R, Moyed H S 1988 Conditional impairment of cell division and altered lethality in *hipA* mutants of *E. coli* K 12. Journal of Bacteriology 170: 3321-3326

Shalit I, Berger S A, Gorea A, Frimerman H 1989 Widespread quinolone resistance among methicillin-resistant *Staphylococcus aureus* isolates in a general hospital. Antimicrobial Agents and Chemotherapy 33: 593-594

Shen L L, Mitscher L A, Sharma P N et al 1989 Mechanism of inhibition of DNA gyrase by quinolone anti-bacterials: a cooperative drug-DNA binding model. Biochemistry 28: 3886-3894

Smith S M, Eng R H K 1985 Activity of ciprofloxacin against methicillin-resistant *Staphylococcus aureus*. Antimicrobial Agents and Chemotherapy 27: 688-691

Snyder M, Drlica K 1979 DNA gyrase on the bacterial chromosome: DNA cleavage induced by oxolinic acid. Journal of Molecular Biology 131: 287-302

Southern E M 1975 Detection of specific sequences among DNA fragments separated by gel electrophoresis. Journal of Molecular Biology 98: 503-517

Swanberg S L, Wang J C 1987 Cloning and sequencing of the *Escherichia coli gyrA* gene encoding the A subunit of DNA gyrase. Journal of Molecular Biology 197: 729-736

189

Takahata M, Nishino T 1988 DNA gyrase of *Staphylococcus aureus* and the inhibitory effect of quinolones on its activity. Antimicrobial Agents and Chemotherapy 32: 1192-1195

Ubukata K, Itoh-Yamashita N, Konno M 1989 Cloning and expression of the *norA* gene for fluoroquinolone resistance in *Staphylococcus aureus*. Antimicrobial Agents and Chemotherapy 33: 1535-1539

Wang J C 1985 DNA topoisomerases. Annual Review of Biochemistry 54: 665-697

Wang J C 1987 Recent studies on DNA topoisomerases. Biochimica et Biophysica Acta 909: 1-9

Wolfson J S, Hooper D C 1985 The fluoroquinolones: structures, mechanisms of action and resistance, and spectra of activity in vitro. Antimicrobial Agents and Chemotherapy 28: 581-586

Wolfson J S, Hooper D C, Shih D J, McHugh G L, Swartz M N 1989 Isolation and characterization of an *Escherichia coli* strain exhibiting partial tolerance to quinolones. Antimicrobial Agents and Chemotherapy 33: 705-709

Yamagishi J-I, Yoshida H, Yamayoshi M, Nakamura S 1986 Nalidixic acid mutations of the *gyrB* gene of *Escherichia coli*. Molecular and General Genetics 204: 367-373

Yoshida H, Kojima T, Yamagishi J-I, Nakamura S 1988 Quinolone-resistant mutations of the *gyrA* gene of *Escherichia coli*. Molecular and General Genetics 211: 1-7

Discussion of paper presented by L. M. Fisher

Discussed by B. Weidemann
Reported by H. C. Neu

In his presentation, Fisher provided an excellent overview of the problems with quinolone antimicrobials. Wiedemann, in his discussion, noted that there are a number of important points which should be emphasized. In the literature many of the illustrations of the interaction of quinolones, DNA gyrase, and DNA are inaccurate. We know that there is no RNA core which binds the DNA to form domains and that quinolones do not cause relaxation of the whole DNA molecule in vivo. DNA is in a state of continual rearrangement. Addition of the quinolone to the DNA and DNA gyrase results in a ternary complex that leads to the death of the bacterial cell. Unfortunately we still do not know precisely how this occurs. Electron micrographs of plasmid bound to gyrase always show a three-looped structure. Small DNA molecules bind one gyrase molecule, but with larger plasmids more gyrase molecules are bound. In the small plasmid a twist is introduced into the molecule with the binding of the gyrase, thus preventing a second gyrase from binding. The twist is a result of unwrapping of the DNA around the gyrase molecule.

From studies of small and large plasmids it has been shown that with multiple cut sites gyrase molecules can bind. This would imply that there is not highly specific binding of gyrase to DNA. How quinolones find a binding site of gyrase and DNA is not established; neither is the mechanism by which the mutant gyrase with one amino acid change alters binding of the quinolone. Perhaps it is due to a change in the cavity of the molecule, but it will be necessary to obtain the three-dimensional structure of the enzyme to establish for certain the interaction of quinolone, gyrase and DNA.

Wiedemann pointed out that virtually all nalidixic acid-resistant strains of bacteria have higher MICs to the newer quinolones, but in most cases this microbiological cross-resistance is not of clinical importance. These observations suggest that the mutation frequency is similar for all quinolones and that the differences in mutation frequency reported in the literature are due to use of different concentrations of drugs used for each agent.

It is important to realize that the gene which confers sensitivity to quinolones (gyr-A sensitive gene) is dominant over the resistant one. If a gyr-A resistance gene is cloned, placed on a plasmid, and put into a bacterial cell that has a gyr-A sensitive gene, the organism remains sensitive, irrespective of the number of resistant genes placed into the bacterial cell. Conversely, if a gyr-A sensitive gene is placed on a plasmid and put into a bacterial cell with a resistant gyr-A, the organism becomes susceptible to the quinolones. These experiments show that resistance cannot be plasmid-mediated. Using clinical resistant isolates into which plasmids containing the sensitive gyr-A gene are placed, it is not possible to rescue the MIC to the very low level seen with susceptible wild isolates. This suggests that there are other mutations affecting resistance in the clinical isolates. For example, the ciprofloxacin MIC of *Salmonella typhimurium* can be reduced from 32υg/ml to 0.25υg/ml by introduction of plasmid with a sensitive gyr-A but not to a MIC of 0.06υg/ml.

Wiedemann felt that the data available suggested activity of quinolones to be a 'single hit' event. One molecule forms a ternary DNA-gyrase-quinolone complex that blocks replication, and initiates a cascade of events that ultimately results in bacterial cell death.

In the course of the general discussion, it was pointed out that in nature one can find bacteria, even *E. coli*, with extremely high quinolone MICs, yet in the laboratory these strains were difficult to create. Whether such isolates have multiple mutations in the gyr-A protein has not been established. No explanation was available for the higher quinolone resistance of methicillin-resistant staphylococci. Overall, from the data in Europe, except for increases in quinolone MICs of *Staphylococcus aureus*, *Pseudomonas aeruginosa*, and enterococci, the MICs of most Enterobacteriaceae have remained low. In certain hospital settings one finds quinolone-resistant bacteria. The meeting participants agreed that attempts to reduce cross-contamination in hospitals is extremely important and needs to be emphasized.

Finally, the lack of knowledge of how quinolones cross the cytosplasmic membrane was emphasized. It was suggested that there might be specific permeases involved, but it was apparent from the discussion that much is yet to be learned about resistance of gram-positive species to fluoroquinolones.

192

12. Transport systems and their role in drug resistance in bacteria and mammalian cells

C. F. Higgins

INTRODUCTION

Resistance to an antibiotic is most frequently a result of the acquisition of an enzyme, or set of enzymes, capable of chemically modifying the drug and inactivating it. Resistance can also be achieved by mutations which alter the target and render it insensitive, although this is often less than ideal from the cell's point of view as the target may be altered so as to be less effective in its normal cellular function. A good example of this is streptomycin resistance, achieved only by very specific alterations in the ribosome which still allow the ribosome to function, albeit with reduced efficiency. While such resistance processes are now well understood, it is becoming ever more apparent that resistance to antibacterials, and to drugs targeted against eukaryotic cells, can also be achieved by specific alterations in membrane transport systems, preventing the cell accumulating the agent to sufficient intracellular concentrations to be toxic.

The majority of antibacterial agents, as well as drugs targeted against specific eukaryotic cells, have intracellular targets. Although self-evident, the fact that such agents must be accumulated within the cytoplasm in sufficient quantities to exert their toxic effects, is not often given appropriate consideration. Accumulation of an antibiotic in the cytoplasm not only requires a route into the cell, but also the absence of a route from the cell! Hydrophobic antibacterials may, of course, be soluble in the lipid bilayer and pass passively through the membrane, although unless they are bound by a specific target in the cell this precludes accumulation in the cytoplasm and, in turn necessitates the use of high concentrations of the drug. Most drugs, however, are not lipid soluble and must gain entry into the cell via specific transport systems which have evolved to mediate the uptake of nutrients or other cellular processes. Entry of an antibiotic via an active transport system can permit high-level accumulation of the drug in the cell and, hence, lower the dose which must be provided. A means of obtaining entry into the cell is one of the first requirements that must be met when designing new antibacterials.

Once in the cell an antibacterial must be retained in sufficient concentrations to exert its toxic effect, the drug must be retained in the cell and not pass back out across the membrane. This can be achieved by high-affinity binding to receptors (e.g. many antibiotics which bind tightly to ribosomes) but, unless these receptors are themselves the target for the drug, this does not achieve an increase in the effective concentration of the drug. More importantly, a drug must not be a substrate for a specific export system.

It is becoming increasingly apparent that drug resistance can be achieved either by alterations in uptake systems, preventing the drug ever entering the cell, or by changes in export processes which pump the drug out of the cell and reduce its effective intracellular concentration. It is these mechanisms for achieving drug resistance, involving membrane transport processes, that are the subject of this chapter. Until we understand more about the molecular mechanisms of transport processes we will not be able to devise rational approaches to overcoming these associated problems of resistance.

MECHANISMS OF MEMBRANE TRANSPORT

In recent years a considerable amount of information has accrued concerning the molecular mechanisms of transport across biological membranes. The majority of mechanistic studies have been carried out using bacterial systems. However, one of the most exciting developments in the last few years has been the realization (not unexpected, at least in hindsight) that there is a great deal of similarity between transport systems from bacterial and eukaryotic cell (reviewed in Henderson & Maiden 1990, Higgins et al 1990a,b). The old adage holds: what is true for *E. coli* is also true for an elephant!

Solute transport against a concentration gradient requires energy. In bacterial cells, three basic mechanisms of achieving this have evolved. The phosphotransferase systems (PTS) utilize the high-energy phosphate group of phosphoenol pyruvate to drive transport (reviewed by Postma & Lengeler 1985). The phosphate group is transferred, via a series of phosphorylated protein intermediates, to the substrate as it crosses the membrane. The substrate never enters the cell in a chemically unmodified form and, thus, this class of system cannot be considered as true active transport. While very important for the uptake of certain metabolites by bacteria, specifically many sugars, the chemical limitations of the PTS are such that its substrate specificity is necessarily limited. Furthermore, examples of this class of transporter are not found in eukaryotic cells. This class of transporter is, therefore, unimportant in the context of drug resistance and will not be considered further.

Active transport systems are generally classified as primary systems, driven directly by the hydrolysis of ATP (or other high-energy compound), or secondary systems relying on the generation of transmembrane gradients to energize substrate accumulation. Both primary and secondary transporters play an important role in the development of drug resistance, and are found in prokaryotes and eukaryotes, and both must be considered here.

Primary transport systems

The ABC family of transport systems
Apart from the ion pumps (see later) the primary transport systems from bacteria that have been characterized to date are closely related to each other, not only in terms of their general organization and mechanism but also at the amino acid sequence

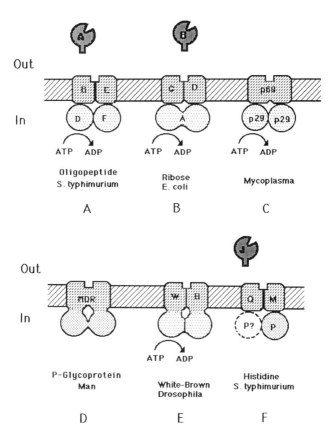

Figure 12.1. Various organizations of ABC transporters. The periplasmic binding proteins of certain bacterial systems are shaded [::::::::] ; the hydrophobic membrane domains [:::::::] ; the ATP-binding domains [:::::::] . The systems illustrated are as follows: A, the oligopeptide permease of *S. typhimurium* (Hiles et al 1987); B, the ribose transporter of *E. coli* (Bell et al 1986); C, the p69 system of mycoplasma (Dudler et al 1988); D, the multidrug resistance P-glycoprotein from man (Chen et al 1986); E, the *white* and *brown* loci of *Drosophila* (O'Hare et al 1984, Dreesen et al 1988); F, the histidine transporter of *S. typhimurium* (Higgins et al 1982). See text for further details.

level. The best characterized of this superfamily of transporters are the bacterial periplasmic-binding protein-dependent uptake systems (reviewed by Ames 1986, Higgins 1990, Higgins et al 1990a,b). However, closely related transporters are now known to mediate export rather than uptake, and increasing numbers of closely related transport systems are being identified in eukaryotic cells. Because the distinguishing feature of this class of transporter is a highly conserved *A*TP-*b*inding *c*assette (Higgins et al 1986, Hyde et al 1990), the class as a whole may be referred to as ABC transporters.

Over 30 such transporters have now been identified (Table 12.1). Regardless of the substrate transported, or the species in which they have been identified, all share a similar basic organization. Essentially, each transport system consists of four membrane-associated domains (Fig.12.1). Two of these domains are highly hydrophobic, integral membrane proteins each consisting of five or six putative α-helices which span the membrane. In a number of cases there is now good

Table 12.1 Members of the superfamily of ABC proteins

Organism	Protein(s)	Function	Transported substrate	Reference
Prokaryotes				
Salmonella typhimurium	OppD/OppF	Import	Oligopeptides	Hiles et al 1987
Streptococcus pneumoniae	AmiE/AmiF	Import (a)	Oligopeptides	Alloing et al 1990
Bacillus subtilis	OppD/OppF	Import (b)	Oligopeptides	Perego et al 1990
S. typhimurium	HisP	Import	Histidine	Higgins et al 1982
Escherichia coli	MalK	Import	Maltose	Gilson et al 1982
E. coli	RbsA	Import	Ribose	Bell et al 1986
E. coli	AraG	Import	Arabinose	Scripture et al 1987
E. coli	LivM/LivG	Import	Leucine/Isoleucine/Valine	Adams et al in press
Pseudomonas aeruginosa	BraF/BraG	Import	Leucine/Isoleucine/Valine	Hoshino & Kose 1989
S. typhimurium	ProV	Import	Glycine betaine	Stirling et al 1989
E. coli	ProV	Import	Glycine betaine	Gowrishankar 1989
E. coli	PstB	Import	Phosphate	Surin et al 1985
E. coli	ChlD	Import	Molybdenum	Johann & Hinton 1987
E. coli	NosF	Import	Copper?	W. G. Zumft, personal communication
E. coli	UgpC	Import	Glycerol 3-phosphate	Overduin et al 1988
E. coli	BtuD	Import	Vitamin B_{12}	Friedrich et al 1986
E. coli	FecE	Import	Iron citrate	Staudenmaier et al 1989
E. coli	FhuC	Import	Iron ferrichrome	Coulton et al 1987
E. coli	FtsE	Cell division	?	Gill et al 1986
Rhizobium leguminosum	NodI	Nodulation	?	Evans & Downie 1986
Mycoplasma hyorhinis	p29	?	?	Dudler et al 1988
E. coli	UvrA	DNA repair	None	Husain et al 1986
Rhizobium melioti	ORF1	?	?	Albright et al 1989
Staphylococcus	MsrA	Export	Antibiotics	Ross et al in press

Organism	Gene	Transport	Substrate	Reference
Haemophilus influenzae	BexA	Export	Capsular polysaccharide	Kroll et al 1988
E. coli	HlyB	Export	Protein (Haemolysin A)	Felmlee et al 1985
Pasturella haemolytica	LtkB	Export	Protein (Leukotoxin A)	Strathdee & Lo 1989
Rhizobium meliloti	NdvA	Export	β-(1→2) glucan	Stanfield et al 1988
Agrobacterium tumifaciens	ChrA	Export	β-(1→2) glucan	Cangelosi et al 1989
Bordatella pertussis	CyaB	Export	Protein (Cyclolysin)	Glaser et al 1988
Yeast				
Saccharomyces cerevisiae	STE6	Export	a-factor polypeptide	McGrath & Varshavsky 1989, Kuchler et al 1989
Saccharomyces cerevisiae	Elongation factor 3	?	?	M. Tuite, 1990 personal communication
Protozoa				
Plasmodium falciparum	pfmdr	Export	Chloroquine (?)	Foote et al 1989
Insects				
Drosophilia	white (c)	Import	Eye pigment	O'Hare et al 1984
	brown (c)	Import	Eye pigment	Dreesen et al 1988
Plants				
Marchantia chloroplast	MbpX	?	?	Ohyama et al 1986
Mammals				
Man	Mdr-1 (d)	Export	Lipophilic drugs	Chen et al 1986
Hamster	Mdr-1 (d)	Export	Lipophilic drugs	Gerlach et al 1986
Mouse	Mdr-1 (d)	Export	Lipophilic drugs	Gros et al 1986
Man	CFTR	?	?	Riordan et al 1989

(a) *ami* mutants have other unexplained phenotypes including sensitivity to branched-chain amino acids, methotrexate resistance and altered transmembrane electric potential.

(b) *opp* mutants of *Bacillus* are also sporulation defective.

(c) white and brown mutations confer different phenotypes.

(d) The *mdr-2* and *mdr-3* genes, present in some mammalian cells, are very closely related to *mdr-1*; they do not confer multidrug resistance and their functions are unknown.

Reproduced and slightly modified from Higgins et al, in press, Journal of Bioenegetics and Biomembranes, with permission.

197

experimental evidence that these 'predicted' helices do indeed span the membrane and that the two-dimensional organization so frequently predicted on the basis of sequence alone, does have a basis in reality (Boyd et al 1987, Higgins et al 1990a, unpublished results). It is these transmembrane proteins that are responsible for mediating the passage of substrate across the membrane. However, because of the difficulties inherent in purifying membrane proteins and analysing their structure, we know little about how they are organized in the membrane in three dimensions. It is assumed that the transmembrane helices are arranged in a barrel-like conformation surrounding a relatively hydrophilic pore, but direct evidence for this is lacking. Nevertheless, it is clear that these components do not simply form a hole in the membrane but confer specificity on the transport process. These transport systems can be highly specific and genetic studies (Shuman 1982, Payne et al 1985, Reyes et al 1986) provide considerable evidence that the membrane proteins themselves possess specific substrate-binding sites. In the case of the multidrug-resistance protein of eukaryotes, a mutation in the membrane-bound domain alters substrate specificity (Choi et al 1988) and it has been shown biochemically that substrate is bound specifically by these components (Cornwall et al 1986a,b, Beck et al 1988). However, until the three-dimensional structure of these membrane proteins is determined, something unlikely to be achieved in the near future, it is unlikely that the nature of the substrate-binding site will be understood in sufficient detail to consider directed manipulations.

The other two domains of each transport system are hydrophilic, located peripherally on the cytoplasmic face of the membrane. These domains share about 30% sequence identity with equivalent domains from other transport systems, regardless of the species (prokaryotic or eukaryotic) from which they come (Higgins et al 1986, Hyde et al 1990). Each domain includes a consensus ATP-binding motif and the proteins have been shown to bind ATP and ATP analogues (Hobson et al 1984, Higgins et al 1985). It must, however, be emphasized that these domains share extensive sequence similarity in addition to that required specifically for ATP-binding; other ATP-binding proteins (e.g. RecA) have the ATP-binding motif but otherwise share little or no sequence similarity with ABC. Although there has been considerable controversy over the energy source used to drive this class of transport system, and many other energy sources have been suggested, it is now clear that direct hydrolysis of ATP provides the driving force (reviewed in Higgins 1990). Not only do the proteins bind ATP specifically (Hobson et al 1984, Higgins et al 1985) but ATP is required for transport in vesicle systems (Horio et al 1988, Dean et al 1989) and hydrolysis of ATP has been measured concomitant with transport (Hamada & Tsuruo 1988, Bishop et al 1989, Mimmack et al 1989). Earlier data purporting to contradict a role for ATP can now be adequately explained (Joshi et al 1989, Higgins 1990). Finally, a stoichiometry of close to two ATP molecules hydrolysed per molecule of substrate transported has been reported (Mimmack et al 1989) consistent with the observation that two ATP-binding subunits are associated with each transport system.

Although each transport system in this superfamily appears to have a similar domain organization, these domains may be fused into multidomain polypeptides in a variety of different ways. In many bacterial systems (e.g. the oligopeptide permease of *S. typhimurium*; Fig.12.1) the four domains are found as four separate polypeptides. However, for example, the two ATP-binding domains are fused into a single, large polypeptide in the ribose system of *E. coli* and in the mycoplasma p69 system the two hydrophobic domains are fused into a single polypeptide. In the HlyB haemolysin secretion system a hydrophobic domain is fused to an ATP-binding domain, and in the mammalian systems identified to date (e.g. the multidrug-resistance protein) all four domains are fused into a single multifunctional polypeptide.

Some transport systems appear to lack domains. For example, the histidine transporter of *S. typhimurium* only has a single gene encoding an ATP-binding protein (Higgins et al 1982). In this case, two identical polypeptides probably function together as a homodimer (Higgins et al 1986, Ames personal communication). The minimalist system is the ProU glycine betaine transporter which only appears, genetically, to have a single membrane component and a single ATP-binding subunit (Gowrishankar 1989, Stirling et al 1989); in this case it is presumed that two molecules of each interact to form a functional transporter of four domains.

Certain transporters have also acquired domains. For example, the bacterial uptake systems require a substrate-binding protein, located in the periplasm, which initially binds the substrate and delivers it to the complex of membrane proteins. However, this protein is not integral to the mechanism of transport across the membrane and exporters or eukaryotic systems do not appear to require a similar component. They are thus best considered as an 'add-on' component specifically adapted to the requirements of these specific transporters (Higgins et al 1990a,b). Other examples of acquired domains, are the R-domain of the cystic fibrosis protein (Riordan et al 1989) which is thought to serve a regulatory role, and the C-terminus of the MalK protein which provides an enzymic function apparently unconnected with transport (Reidl et al 1989). Thus, much of the apparent diversity in organization of this class of transport system does not represent diversity in the mechanism of transport itself but is simply a variation on a common theme.

The ABC transporters can transport a wide variety of substrates although any one system is relatively specific for a single substrate or group of related substrates (Table 12.1). Many handle small molecules, for example the systems specific for an inorganic ion (e.g. phosphate), an amino acid (e.g. histidine), or a sugar (e.g. maltose). However, some systems handle extremely large molecules including polysaccharides and even large polypeptides (e.g. the 107 kDa haemolysin molecule whose export is mediated by the HlyB system). The only transporter in this class which appears to exhibit broad specificity is the P-glycoprotein responsible for multidrug resistance and which handles a variety of apparently unrelated drugs; this is discussed in more detail later. It is important to emphasize that, although this superfamily includes both uptake and export systems, they are not thought to be reversible. Thus, any one system will either export or import substrate, but not both. Attempts to isolate mutations that reverse these transport systems have failed. This is in marked contrast with the secondary transport systems (see later) which are readily reversible and the same system can transport its substrate into or out of the cell depending on external factors.

Ion pumps
Apart from the ABC transporters a number of other ATP-dependent transporters are

known which are unrelated to the ABC systems both in sequence and organization. These are the ion-translocating ATPases which play a central role in cellular bioenergetics and regulation (Pedersen & Carafoli 1987). The vast majority of the ion-translocating ATPases are members of one of two families. The F_0-F_1 family are proton pumps found in bacterial cells and the organelles of eukaryotic cells while the E_1-E_2 family catalyse cation translocation and include the well known Kdp transporter of *E. coli*. Because these transporters are entirely restricted to small inorganic ions they are essentially irrelevant to antibiotic uptake and resistance and will not be considered further. However, there is a third class of ATP-dependent ion translocator whose specificity appears to be restricted to anions (Rosen et al 1990). As many anions are toxic to cells (e.g. arsenate) these systems do play an important role in resistance and, while they may not be relevant as far as designing new drugs are concerned, the principles illustrated by these systems are important.

By far the best characterized of these systems is the arsenical resistance system of *E. coli* (reviewed by Rosen et al 1990). It catalyses extrusion of arsenite, antimonite and arsenate, conferring resistance to these compounds. Three proteins are required for this transporter. ArsB is an integral membrane protein of 45 Kda. The ArsA protein is peripherally located on the cytoplasmic face of the membrane, anchored to the membrane via interactions with ArsB (Chen et al 1986a). ArsA binds and hydrolyses ATP and the hydrolysis of ATP provides the driving force for anion expulsion (Rosen et al 1988). It is important to emphasize that, except for a short ATP-binding motif, ArsA is unrelated to the ABC proteins. However, it may be significant that, like the ABC transporters, two ATP-binding domains are required, both present on a single ArsA polypeptide. Together ArsA and ArsB can mediate the expulsion of arsenite and antimonite. However, in order to transport arsenate the ArsC protein is also required. ArsC is postulated to interact with the ArsA-ArsB complex and alter its substrate specificity. Recently, a homologue of ArsC has been identified as associated with the oligopeptide transport system of *Streptococcus pneumoniae* (Alloing et al 1990). Although the function of this protein (AmiB) is entirely unclear, it may be that such specificity modifiers are rather more widespread than is currently believed.

Besides the Ars system, resistance to many other toxic metal ions probably occurs by efflux in a similar manner (reviewed by Silver & Misra 1988). However, all these systems are specific to metal ions and as they are normally plasmid encoded they are not part of the cell's normal complement of transporters. Thus, other than illustrating certain general principles, they are not directly relevant either to the uptake of antibiotics or to the development of resistance by increased drug efflux, and will not be considered further.

Secondary transport systems

Secondary transport systems are driven by the electrochemical gradient which is generated by respiration or by ATP hydrolysis. The most widely distributed systems, and the most important in the present context, are symporters in which the uptake of a molecule of solute is accompanied by an ion moving down its concentration gradient and providing the energy necessary to drive solute accumulation. The cotransported ion is generally a proton but can be another monovalent cation such as sodium. Alternatively, antiporters are those in which, as an ion passes into the cell down its concentration gradient, a molecule of substrate is translocated outwards. Recently, it has become apparent that, besides these cation-mediated anti- and symporters, there is a class of anion exchangers (Maloney 1990) which can mediate electroneutral 'phosphate-linked' antiport (phosphate in this context refers to either organic or inorganic phosphate). The first direct evidence for the movement of an ion together with a molecule of substrate was obtained almost twenty years ago for the lactose permease (West 1970). However, despite intensive and imaginative studies since, we still do not understand the molecular mechanisms by which transport is mediated: this awaits a three-dimensional structure.

The secondary transport systems are distinguished from the primary transporters by the mechanism of energy coupling but also differ considerably in the number and organization of the protein components. For both antiport and symport the movement of solute and ion is mediated by the same protein (or protein complex). There is probably little mechanistic difference between an antiporter and a symporter, at least for those involving a cation as the counterion. All secondary transporters share a very similar membrane organization and many share sequence similarities and are presumably evolutionarily related (see later). Thus, each secondary system characterized to date consists of a single, highly hydrophobic integral membrane protein, the best characterized of which is the lactose permease of *E. coli*. Many genetic and biochemical studies on the lactose carrier have established a model in which the protein spans the membrane twelve times via hydrophobic α-helices (reviewed by Kaback 1990). Subsequently, the sequences of many other transporters in this class have been determined and all share similar structural characteristics; each involves a single hydrophobic protein with twelve (usually) predicted membrane-spanning helices and small periplasmic or cytoplasmic hydrophilic loops. At least for some of these transporters there is accumulating genetic and biochemical evidence that these transmembrane helices adopt a structure similar to that predicted from the sequence and similar to that known for the lactose permease. Indeed, it appears that the 'rule of twelve' membrane-spanning helices is central to this class of transporter (Maloney 1990).

At the sequence level relationships are also seen. There is extensive sequence similarity between the various anion exchangers (Eiglmeier et al 1987). Even more intriguingly, many of the cation-linked sym- and antiporters share considerable sequence similarities (Maiden et al 1987, Henderson & Maiden 1990). Over a dozen transporters in this class are now known, and include transporters from both prokaryotic and eukaryotic species (Table 12.2). Although most of these are sugar transporters this probably reflects a bias in those selected for study rather than a restriction in the type of substrate that can be handled by this class of transport system. Certainly, the tetracycline transporter is a member of this superfamily and doubtless others will be identified. However, as far as sequence similarity is concerned the lactose and melibiose permeases are distinct from the other transporters. Whether this is simply because they have diverged too far for us to identify conservation (they are structurally related; see earlier) or because they have a different evolutionary origin cannot be ascertained. My prejudice, however, is that all these secondary transporters evolved from a common origin and are mechanistically related. Until we know different they are best considered together in terms of their general mechanism.

It is very clear that the single protein is all that is required to mediate lactose transport (Costello et al 1987) and genetic data indicate the same is true for the other secondary transporters. Furthermore, this single protein binds substrate and mutants in the *lacY* gene which alter substrate specificity of the lactose permease have been obtained. It is also clear that the cotransported ion is also 'bound' by the protein. Whether the ion is a proton, sodium or lithium is probably not mechanistically significant as mutants with altered specificity for the cotransported ion can be isolated and, for the melibiose carrier H^+, Na^+ or Li^+ are all accepted depending on the substrate and ionic environment (Wilson & Wilson 1987). Furthermore, the *D*-glucose transporter of erythrocytes is a passive system, which does not accumulate against a gradient or require a counterion, yet is closely related to bacterial sugar symporters (Henderson & Maiden 1990).

One other point should be emphasized in consideration of possible roles in antibiotic resistance. These secondary transporters can function in either direction depending on the direction of the ion gradient. This is in contrast to the ATP-dependent transporters which are unidirectional. Thus, while most of the characterized transporters are uptake systems, one (the tetracycline carrier) is known to mediate export, tetracycline leaving the cell as a proton (or K^+ ion) enters (see later). Furthermore, this type of system is readily reversible; the possibility that an 'uptake' system may, under certain conditions or following minor mutational changes, reverse and mediate efflux of, say, an antibiotic should not be ignored.

From the previous discussion, it can be seen that, while there is a plethora of transport systems handling all sorts of substrates, sequencing data obtained over the last two or three years have shown that there are actually relatively few classes. Indeed the majority true active transport systems (excluding the ion pumps) whether from prokaryotic or eukaryotic cells, are members of one of two very distinct superfamilies; the ATP-dependent primary transporter systems (ABC transporters) or the ion-linked secondary transporters. Although most of the transporters identified and characterized so far are uptake systems, this probably reflects a bias of investigators; it is historically much easier to study uptake than export. Nevertheless, export systems from both the major classes of transporter have been identified and as studies progress it is likely that many more exporters will be identified. It also seems unlikely that there will be major differences between export systems and

Table 12.2 Members of the secondary (ion-linked) transport superfamily

Organism	Substrate	Function	Reference
Escherichia coli	D-xylose	Import	Maiden et al 1987
Escherichia coli	L-arabinose	Import	Maiden et al 1987
Escherichia coli	Citrate	Import	Sasatsu et al 1985
Escherichia coli	Tetracycline	Efflux	Nguyen et al 1983
Synechocystis	Fructose	Import	Zhang et al 1989
Staphylococcus aureus	Antiseptics	Efflux	Rouch et al, in press
Kluyveromyces lactis	Lactose	Import	Chang & Dickson 1988
Saccharomyces cerevisiae	D-glucose	Import	Celenza et al 1988
Rat brain	D-glucose	Import	Birnbaum et al 1986
Human hepatoma	D-glucose	Import	Mueckler et al 1985
Human erythrocyte	D-glucose	Import	Mueckler et al 1985
Rat liver	D-glucose	Import	Thorens et al 1988
Rat adipocyte	D-glucose	Import	James et al 1989
Rat heart	D-glucose	Import	James et al 1989

importers, at least mechanistically. I suspect that the more we know about bacterial and eukaryotic transport systems the more obvious the similarities between apparently disparate systems will become and the more unified our views on transport mechanisms will become.

TRANSPORT SYSTEMS AND ANTIBIOTIC RESISTANCE

As far as antibiotic resistance is concerned, transport systems must be considered in two ways. First, they provide the route by which antibiotics enter the cell, and second they have the potential to pump antibiotics out of cells, conferring resistance.

Uptake systems

Most antibiotics must enter the cell through specific uptake systems and this is an important consideration in designing new or modified antibiotics. The first potential barrier, at least for Gram-negative species, is the outer membrane. This membrane contains hydrophilic pores formed by the porin proteins which provide an avenue for small hydrophilic molecules to enter the periplasm and gain access to the cytoplasmic membrane. The different porins show general and overlapping specificities and, in the normal course of events it requires elimination of more than one of these porins to increase antibiotic resistance. The fact that the mutations eliminating the porins can reduce sensitivity to certain antibiotics indicates a role in their uptake (e.g. Cohen et al 1989), although loss of the porins does not provide a complete barrier to passage across the outer membrane and can only confer low-level resistance.

It is the cytoplasmic membrane that provides the principal barrier to antibiotic entry into the cell. For many commonly used antibiotics little is known about their route of entry although if they enter via a single transport system then, in principle, a single mutation eliminating the transport system could lead to resistance. As most antibiotics are natural products, or derivatives thereof, evolutionary pressures have presumably selected for those which enter the cell by multiple routes, or for which the transport system is essential and cannot be lost without killing the cell, avoiding the problem of resistance by mutation. This type of consideration must be borne in mind when developing novel antibiotics.

First, for any new antibiotic there must be a route for uptake. Unfortunately, at least so far as antibiotic design is concerned, most of the known transport systems are relatively specific and there is little potential for devising toxic moieties that are sufficiently related to the normally transported substrates (e.g. a sugar or amino acid). At present, only the transport systems for peptides provide an alternative that can be logically exploited. The peptide transport systems handle more or less any small peptide, irrespective of the amino acid side-chains of the individual residues (Payne 1980). Thus potentially toxic molecules can enter the cell, via a peptide transport system when attached to a peptide backbone. Nature, of course, was first to exploit this idea and several natural antibiotics such as bialphos secreted by *Streptomyces* (Mukakami et al 1986) or bacilysin produced by certain bacilli (Kenig & Abraham 1976), have the toxic moieties attached to a small peptide in order that they may gain entry into the cell. This principle of 'illicit transport' was first used in the laboratory many years ago (Ames et al 1973, Fickel & Gilvarg 1973) and, subsequently the concept has been contemplated as a means of targeting new antibiotics. Probably the best example is that of alafosfalin and its chemical relatives (Allen et al 1978). The amino acid derivative aminoethylphosphonic acid (alanine with the COOH group replaced by phosphate), is a very specific inhibitor of D-alanine racemase an essential enzyme in cell wall biosynthesis. Aminoethylphosphonic acid itself is not toxic to Gram-negative bacteria as it cannot enter the cell. However, conjugation into a peptide, alafosfalin (L-alanyl-L-aminoethylphosphonic acid), enables it to enter the cell via a peptide permease where the peptide is cleaved, releasing aminoethylphosphonic acid and killing the cell. Alafosfalin is highly toxic to a wide range of Gram-negative species although the antibiotic never reached the market place because of possible toxicity to mammalian cells and also because resistance to alafosfalin was found to arise too frequently. It turned out that mutations in any one of three genes can confer alafosfalin resistance; *tppB* encoding the tripeptide permease which mediates alafosfalin uptake into the cell, *tppA* which is required for expression of *tppB*, and *pepA* which encodes the peptidase which cleaves alafosfalin intracellularly releasing the toxic moiety (Gibson et al 1984). As spontaneous mutations in any one of these three genes arises at about 1 in 10^5, the antibiotic is unlikely to be useful in clinical terms. However, the principle is relevant. Importantly, at the time of alafosfalin development little was known about the number and specificity of peptide transport systems. In fact there are three genetically distinct peptide transporter systems (Higgins & Gibson 1986) with overlapping specificities. If an aminophosphonic acid peptide derivative had been designed as a substrate for each of the transport systems, resistant mutations would have then arisen at the acceptably low rate of 1 in 10^{15}. Similarly, there are multiple intracellular peptidases of overlapping specificity (Miller 1975); again the right peptide derivative will be cleaved by many of these enzymes and circumvent the problem of resistance.

Other attempts to use the peptide transport systems as a mechanism for smuggling toxic moieties into the cell have also looked promising. For example, the L-ornithine carbamoyltransferase inhibitor N-δ-(phosphonoacetyl)-L-ornithine cannot permeate the cell membrane but becomes highly toxic when conjugated as a tripeptide, entering the cell via the oligopeptide permease (Penninckx & Gigot 1979). A similar system has been used to provide glutamine synthetase inhibitors with access to the cytoplasm (Diddens et al 1976). Non-permeant sulphydryl compounds have gained toxicity when replacing an amino acid side-chain of a peptide. In this case the sulphydryl moiety is released, not by cleavage of a peptide bond, but by a disulphide exchange reaction (Boehm et al 1983). Finally, the most spectacular example is a new class of anti-Gram-negatives designed to inhibit specifically lipopolysaccharide biosynthesis. Chemical modifications were used to develop a highly potent inhibitor of CMP-KDO synthetase but, unfortunately this novel and extremely specific compound could not penetrate the membrane; only when coupled into a peptide could it enter and kill bacterial cells (Hammond et al 1987).

Despite the demonstrated potential of peptide transport systems in circumventing resistance due to transport difficulties, it has to be said that no antibiotic designed on these logical principles has yet reached the market place. Furthermore, we do not yet know enough about the specificities of other transport systems to design antibiotics in this fashion; peptide uptake systems remain the sole route that can be exploited. An important lesson can also be learnt from attempts to design antibiotics based on the concept of illicit transport via the peptide transporters. That is, any antibiotic must cross the membrane by multiple routes, either by virtue of its lipid solubility or by sharing affinity for several genetically distinct transporters, to avoid the problem of resistance by mutation.

Export systems and resistance
Assuming an antibiotic can enter the cell, resistance can arise by increasing its rate of transport from the cell. There are now a number of examples of export systems conferring drug resistance, each of which will be considered in turn.

Tetracycline resistance
In bacteria, the best-known export system responsible for conferring drug resistance is that for tetracycline. It was shown many years ago that cells expressing tetracycline-resistance determinants had reduced intracellular concentrations of the antibiotic due to active expulsion of tetracycline from the cell (McMurry et al 1980). Although the mechanism of resistance is not yet fully understood, efflux is mediated by the TetA protein which, as described above, shares considerable sequence similarity with many bacterial uptake systems and presumably functions by a rather similar mechanism. The TetA protein spans the membrane via twelve putative helices (Eckert & Beck 1989) and exports tetracycline via an antiport mechanism with H^+ or K^+ as the counterion. Until recently, expulsion of tetracycline was considered to be the only mechanism by which resistance to this antibiotic could be achieved. However, it is now apparent that other tetracycline-resistance determinants alter ribosome susceptibility or modify the antibiotic (reviewed by Salyers et al 1990).

Recently, a second example of resistance by efflux has been identified, resistance to intercalating dyes such as ethidium and acriflavin in *Staphylococcus* (Rouch et al in press). Energy-dependent efflux of these dyes is mediated by the *qacA* gene product which shares significant sequence similarity with the tetracycline exporter and with a range of ion-linked sugar uptake systems. It is important, however, to emphasize that although these resistance mechanisms are due to drug efflux, these are export systems that have evolved specifically for this purpose. It is therefore pertinent to ask whether there is potential for transport systems that serve a normal cellular function to be 'sequestered' into a role in drug resistance. There seems little doubt that the answer to this question will turn out to be 'yes' as such a sequestration is seen in the case of multidrug resistance in mammalian cells (see later). Equivalent examples in bacteria are lacking, probably because of the limited effort invested in studying export, although two intriguing systems conferring antibiotic resistance have recently come to light and may provide the first bacterial examples of such a mechanism.

The first is the resistance of *Streptococcus pneumoniae* to aminopterin, methotrexate and celiptium. Resistance to all three of these drugs arises simultaneously as a result of mutations in the *amiA* locus (Sautereau & Trombe 1986). It turns out, from sequencing studies, that the *ami* locus is highly homologous to the ATP-dependent oligopeptide permease of Gram-negative bacteria and, furthermore the Ami system is able to mediate the uptake of peptides (Alloing et al 1990). *opp* mutations in *E. coli* also appear to confer low-level methotrexate resistance

(J-P Claverys 1990, personal communication). *ami* mutants show a two-fold reduction in methotrexate accumulation (Trombe 1985). Although it is not clear how resistance is achieved it is probably by increased efflux. Whether the *ami* system can mediate peptide uptake, but operates in reverse to pump the drugs out, is unclear although this seems unlikely as the ABC transporters are not thought to be reversible (see earlier). The existence, however, of a gene product in the transport operon (AmiB) which is related to the specificity-modifying subunit of the arsenate pump (ArsC: see earlier) may provide a means of reversal. Alternatively, alterations in peptide transport activity might have a 'knock-on' effect on a more specific export system. This intriguing system deserves further investigation.

The second example is the case of erythromycin resistance in staphylococci (Ross et al, in press). Resistance is conferred by a plasmid-encoded *msrA* gene and induction of *msrA* expression results in efflux of erythromycin from the cell. Although, at first sight, this appears to be like tetracycline resistance in that it is mediated by a plasmid-encoded system that has evolved specifically for this purpose, there are peculiarities which imply that a normal cellular transporter may also be involved. Firstly, unlike the tetracycline-resistance determinant, the sequence of MsrA reveals it to be an ATP-binding protein, containing two ATP-binding domains closely related to the ABC transporters. The fact that MsrA is an example of the ABC superfamily of transporters suggests, but does not prove, that the mechanism by which it confers resistance is active efflux. However, unlike the ABC transporters, no hydrophobic membrane proteins are associated with MsrA. Indeed, the *msrA* gene on its own, can confer resistance on a sensitive cell. As there is no sensible possibility of this ATP-binding protein mediating transport on its own, the simplest possibility is that it sequesters the membrane components from a normal chromosomally-encoded transport system. This, of course remains to be proven. However, the possibility that MsrA sequesters and perhaps alters the specificity of components of normal transport systems in order to confer antibiotic resistance is intriguing.

Multidrug resistance

The prototype of drug resistance mediated by a normal cellular protein comes, not from bacteria, but from eukaryotic cells. It has been known for many years that tumours frequently respond to chemotherapy by developing resistance, not only to the agent with which they are being treated but also to a wide variety of apparently unrelated chemotherapeutic agents; the phenomenon of multidrug resistance (reviewed by Endicott & Ling 1989). Multidrug resistance poses a major clinical problem and is responsible for tens of thousands of deaths a year in this country alone. Many lines of evidence showed that presence of a 170 kDa protein, the P-glycoprotein, correlated with multidrug resistance and in 1986 the gene encoding the P-glycoprotein was cloned and sequenced (Chen et al 1986b, Gerlach et al 1986, Gros et al 1986b). The protein is very similar, in sequence and organization, to the ATP-dependent bacterial transporters and a member of the ABC transport superfamily (see earlier). Studies have now demonstrated unambiguously that the protein reduces the internal concentrations of drugs by ATP-dependent active efflux (e.g. Horio et al 1988). Furthermore, simple amplification of the gene resulting in overproduction of the protein, is sufficient to confer multidrug resistance. It is an increase in the activity of a normal cellular component, not an alteration in its function or specificity which is all that is required (Gros et al 1986a). A highly homologous protein is present in *Plasmodium* and is thought to be responsible for chloroquine resistance of the malarial parasite by a similar efflux mechanism (Foote et al 1989). Mdr provides the best example of a normal cellular function playing a role in drug resistance. However, there are some problems. First, we have no idea what the normal cellular substrate for Mdr is. Indeed, its specificity is unusual for ABC transporters in that it handles a wide range of apparently unrelated drugs. The only similarity between them is their lipophilic nature, thought to be necessary for entry into the cell in the first place. The tissue distribution of Mdr has led to suggestions that it may be involved in steroid hormone secretion but this is no more than speculation. Another suggested role is in detoxification, getting rid of molecules that are no longer wanted by the cell. But how does it know which ones to export? A second, not unrelated problem, is the roles of *mdr-2* and *mdr-3*; the proteins encoded by these genes are highly homologous to the P-glycoprotein (Mdr-1) yet amplification of these genes does not confer resistance to any drug tested. A third difficulty is the broadness of the substrate specificity of Mdr. Although the pump recognizes many apparently unrelated drugs it certainly does not pump everything out of the cell. Clearly it does exhibit specificity; we are simply unable to identify the similarities between the various substrates. It is possible that the substrates are modified before export to 'mark' them and provide them with chemical similarity, for example as glutathione conjugates (West 1990). However, this attractive idea is difficult to reconcile with the finding that substrates such as vinblastine can specifically bind to the P-glycoprotein in an unconjugated form (Cornwell et al 1986). Finally, the fact that Mdr substrates are lipid soluble and primarily sequestered in vesicles also poses a problem; Mdr is located principally in the cytoplasmic membrane. Does Mdr aid vesicle fusion with the membrane? Or are substrates 'dissolved' in the lipid bilayer transported, rather than substrates free in the cytoplasm?

To develop treatments that block Mdr it is important to obtain answers to some of these questions. No doubt surprises are in store. Nevertheless, Mdr is a paradigm for drug resistance by export. There is little doubt that similar mechanisms will be uncovered, both in eukaryotic and prokaryotic cells.

CONCLUSION

In this article I have tried to emphasize that, while there is apparently a plethora of different transport systems, they actually fall into a small number of classes of related structure and function. The more we know, the more unified our view of transport processes becomes. One thing is clear: a more complete understanding of the nature and mechanisms of bacterial transport systems is essential to the rational development of new antibiotics and drugs, both in terms of targeting the drug and overcoming drug resistance. Experience suggests that as much emphasis should be placed on the mechanisms of drug entry and exit from the cell as on the target for a given drug. There are accumulating precedents for drug failures due to transport problems rather than the target itself. Trial and error can lead to success but there is no substitute for understanding.

ACKNOWLEDGEMENTS

I am grateful to all members of my laboratory who have contributed significantly to our understanding of transport processes, both experimentally and intellectually. Work in my laboratory is supported by the Imperial Cancer Research Fund.

REFERENCES

Adams M D, Wagner L M, Graddis T J et al 1990 in press Nucleotide sequence and genetic characterization reveal six essential genes for the LIV-I and LS transport systems of *Escherichia coli.* Journal of Biological Chemistry

Albright L M, Ronson C W, Nixon B T, Ausubel F M 1989 Identification of a gene linked to *Rhizobium meliloti ntrA* whose product is homologous to a family of ATP-binding proteins. Journal of Bacteriology 171: 1932-1941

Allen J G, Atherton F R, Hall M J et al 1978 Phosphonopeptides, a new class of synthetic antibacterial agents. Nature 272: 56-58

Alloing G, Trombe M-C, Claverys J-P 1990 Nucleotide sequence of the *ami* locus of *Streptococcus pneumoniae* reveals an organization similar to periplasmic operons of Gram-negative bacteria. Molecular Microbiology 4: 633-644

Ames G F-L 1986 Bacterial periplasmic transport systems: structure mechanism and evolution. Annual Review of Biochemistry 55: 397-425

Ames B N, Ames G F-L, Young J D, Tsuchiya D, Lecocq J 1973 Illicit transport: the oligopeptide permease. Proceedings of the National Academy of Sciences (USA) 70: 456-458

Beck W T, Cirtain M C, Glover C J et al 1988 Effects of indole alkaloids on multidrug resistance and labeling of P-glycoprotein by a photoaffinity analog of vinblastine. Biochemical and Biophysical Research Communications 153: 959-966

Bell A W, Buckel S D, Groarke J M et al 1986 The nucleotide sequence of the *rbsD, rbsA* and *rbsC* genes of Escherichia coli. Journal of Biological Chemistry 261: 7652-7658

Birnbaum M J, Haspel H C, Rosen O M 1986 Cloning and characterization of a cDNA encoding the rat brain glucose-transporter protein. Proceedings of the National Academy of Sciences (USA) 83: 5784-5788

Bishop L, Agbayani R, Ambudkar S V et al 1989 Reconstitution of a bacterial periplasmic permease in proteoliposomes and demonstration of ATP hydrolysis concomitant with transport. Proceedings of the National Academy of Sciences (USA) 86: 6953-6957

Boehm J C, Kingsbury W D, Perry D, Gilvarg C 1983 The use of cysteinyl peptides to effect portage transport of sulfhydryl-containing compounds in *Escherichia coli.* Journal of Biological Chemistry 258: 14850-14855

Boyd D, Manoil C, Beckwith J 1987 Determinants of membrane topology. Proceedings of the National Academy of Sciences (USA) 84: 8525-8529

Cangelosi G A, Martinetti G, Leigh J A et al 1989 Role of *Agrobacterium tumefaciens* ChvA protein in export of β-1,2, glucan. Journal of Bacteriology 171: 1609-1615

Celenza J L, Marshal-Carlson L, Carlson M 1988 The yeast SNF3 gene encodes a glucose transporter homologous to the mammalian protein. Proceedings of the National Academy of Sciences (USA) 85: 2130-2134

Chang Y-D, Dickson R L 1988 Primary structure of the lactose permease from the yeast *Kluyveromyces lactis.* Journal of Biological Chemistry 263: 16696-16703

Chen C, Misra, Silver S, Rosen B P 1986a Nucleotide sequences of the structural genes for an anion pump. Journal of Biological Chemistry 261: 15030-15038

Chen C-J, Chin J E, Ueda K et al 1986b Internal duplication and homology with bacterial transport proteins in the *mdr* 1 (P-glycoprotein) gene from multidrug resistant human cells. Cell 47: 381-389

Choi K, Chen C J, Kriegler M, Roninson I B 1988 An altered pattern of cross-resistance in multidrug resistant human cells results from spontaneous mutation in the *mdr* 1 (P-glycoprotein) gene. Cell 53: 519-529

Cohen S P, McMurry L M, Hooper D C et al 1989 Cross-resistance to fluoroquinolones in multiple antibiotic resistant (Mar) *Escherichia coli.* Antimicrobial Agents and Chemotherapy 33: 1318-1325

Cornwell M M, Gottesman M M, Pastan I 1986a Increased vinblastine binding to membrane vesicles from multidrug resistant KB cells. Journal of Biological Chemistry 261: 7921-7928

Cornwell M M, Safa A R, Felsted R L et al 1986b Membrane vesicles from multidrug resistant human cancer cells contain a specific 150- to 170-kDa protein detected by photoaffinity labeling. Proceedings of the National Academy of Sciences (USA) 83: 3847-3850

Costello M J, Escaig J, Matushita K et al 1987 Purified lac permease and cytochrome o oxidase are functional as monomers. Journal of Biological Chemistry 262: 17072-17082

Coulton J W, Mason P, Allait DD 1987 *fhuC* and *fhuD* genes for iron (III) - fernchrome transport into *Escherichia coli* K-12. Journal of Bacteriology 169: 3844-3849

Dean D A, Fikes J D, Gehring K et al 1989 Actice transport of maltose in membrane vesicles obtained from *Escherichia coli* cells producing tethered maltose-binding proteins. Journal of Bacteriology 171: 503-510

Diddens H, Zahner H, Kraas E et al 1976 On the transport of tripeptide antibiotics in bacteria. European Journal of Biochemistry 66: 11-23

Dreesen T D, Johnson D H, Henikoff S 1988 The brown protein of *Drosophila melanogaster* is similar to the white protein and to components of active transport complexes. Molecular and Cellular Biology 8: 5206-5215

Dudler R, Schmidhauser C, Paris R W et al 1988 A mycoplasma high-affinity transport system and the *in vitro* invasiveness of mouse sarcoma cells. EMBO Journal 7: 3963-3970

Eckbert B, Beck C F 1989 Topology of the transposon *Tn10*-encoded tetracycline resistance protein within the inner membrane of *Escherichia coli*. Journal of Biological Chemistry 264: 11663-11670

Eiglmeier K, Boos W, Cole S T 1987 Nucleotide sequence and transcriptional start point of the glpT gene of *Escherichia coli*: extensive sequence homology of the glycerol-3-phosphate transport protein with components of the hexose-6-phosphate transport system. Molecular Microbiology 1: 251-258

Endicott J A, Ling V 1989 The biochemistry of P-glycoprotein-mediated multidrug resistance. Annual Review of Biochemistry 58: 137-171

Evans I J, Downie J A 1986 The *nodI* gene product of *Rhizobium leguminosarum* is closely related to ATP-binding bacterial transport proteins, nucleotide sequence analysis of the *nodI* and *nodJ* genes. Gene 43: 95-101

Felmlee T, Pellett S, Welch R A 1985 Nucleotide sequence of a *Escherichia coli* chromosomal haemolysin. Journal of Bacteriology 163: 94-105

Fickel T E, Gilvarg 1973 Transport of impermeant substances in E. *coli* by way of the oligopeptide permease. Nature, New Biology 241: 161-163

Foote S J, Thompson J K, Cowman A F, Kemp D J 1989 Amplification of the multidrug resistance gene in some chloroquine-resistant isolates of *P. falciporum*. Cell 57: 921-930

Friedrich M J, Deveaux L C, Kadner R J 1986 Nucleotide sequence of the *btuCED* genes involved in vitamin B_{12} transport in *Escherichia coli* and homology with components of periplasmic-binding-protein-dependent transport systems. Journal of Bacteriology 167: 928-934

Gerlach J H, Endicott J A, Juranka P F et al 1986 Homology between P-glycoprotein and bacterial haemolysin transport protein suggests a model for multidrug resistance. Nature 324: 485-489

Gibson M M, Price M, Higgins C F 1985 Genetic characterization and molecular cloning of the tripeptide permease *(tpp)* genes of *Salmonella typhimurium*. Journal of Bacteriology 160: 122-130

Gill D R, Hatfull G F, Salmond G P C 1986 A new cell division operon in *Escherichia coli*. Molecular and General Genetics 205: 134-145

Gilson E, Higgins C F, Hofnung M et al 1982 Extensive homology between membrane-associated components of histidine and maltose transport systems of *Salmonella typhimurium* and *Escherichia coli*. Journal of Biological Chemistry 257: 9915-9918

Glaser P, Sakamoto H, Bellalou J, Ullmann A, Danchin A 1988 Secretion of cyclolysin, the calmodulin-sensitive adenylate cyclase-haemolysin bifunctional protein of *Bordetella pertussis*. EMBO Journal 7: 3997-4004

Gowrishankar J 1989 Nucleotide sequence of the osmoregulatory *proU* operon in *Escherichia coli*. Journal of Bacteriology 171: 1923-1931

Gros P, Ben Neriah, Croop J M, Housman D E 1986a Isolation and expression of complementary DNA that confers multidrug resistance. Nature 323: 728-731

Gros P, Croop J, Housman D E 1986b Mammalian multidrug resistance gene: Complete cDNA sequence indicates strong homology to bacterial transport protein. Cell 47: 371-380

Hamada H, Tsuruo T 1988 Purification of the 170-to 180-kilodalton membrane glycoprotein associated with multidrug resistance. Journal of Biological Chemistry 263: 1454-1458

Hammond S M, Claesson A, Jansson A M et al 1987 A novel class of synthetic antibacterials acting upon lipopolysaccharide biosynthesis. Nature 317: 730-733

Henderson P J F, Maiden M C J 1990 Homologous sugar transport proteins in *Escherichia coli* and their relatives in both prokaryotes and eukaryotes. Philosophical Transactions of the Royal Society of London B 326: 391-410

Higgins C F 1990 The role of ATP in binding protein-dependent transport systems. Research in Microbiology 141: 353-360

Higgins C F, Hyde S C, Mimmack M M et al 1990a Binding protein-dependent transport systems. Journal of Bioenergetics and Biomembranes 22: 571-592

Higgins C F, Gallagher M P, Hyde S C, Mimmack M L, Pearce S R 1990b Periplasmic binding protein-dependent transport systems: the membrane-associated components. Philosophical Transactions of the Royal Society of London B 326: 353-365

Higgins C F, Gallagher M P, Jamieson D J, Higgins C F 1987 Molecular characterization of the oligopeptide permease of *Salmonella typhimurium*. Journal of Molecular Biology 195: 125-142

Higgins C F, Gibson M M 1986 Peptide transport in bacteria. Methods in Enzymology 125: 365-377

Higgins C F, Haag P D, Nikaido K et al 1982 Complete nucleotide sequence and identification of membrane components of the histidine transport operon of *S. typhimurium*. Nature 298: 723-727

Higgins C F, Hiles I D, Whalley K, Jamieson D J 1985 Nucleotide binding by membrane components of bacterial periplasmic binding protein-dependent transport systems. EMBO Journal 4: 1033-1040

Higgins C F, Hiles I D, Salmond G P C et al 1986 A family of related ATP-binding subunits coupled to many distinct biological processes in bacteria. Nature 323: 448-450

Hiles I D, Gallagher M P, Jamieson D J, Higgins C F 1987 Molecular characterization of the oligopeptide permease of *Salmonella typhimurium*. Journal of Molecular Biology 195: 125-142

Hobson A C, Weatherwax R, Ames G F-L 1984 ATP-binding sites in the membrane components of histidine permease, a periplasmic transport system. Proceedings of the National Academy of Sciences (USA) 81: 7333-7337

Horio M, Gottesman M M, Pastan I 1988 ATP-dependent transport of vinblastine in vesicles from human multidrug resistant cells. Proceedings of the National Academy of Sciences (USA) 85: 3580-3586

Hoshino T, Kose K 1989 Cloning and nucleotide sequence of *braC* the structural gene of the leucine-isoleucine, and valine binding protein of *Pseudomonas aeruginosa* PAO. Journal of Bacteriology 171: 6300-6303

Husain I, Houten B V, Thomas D C, Sancar A 1986 Sequences of *Escherichia coli uvrA* gene and protein reveals two potential ATP-binding sites. Journal of Biological Chemistry 261: 4895-4901

Hyde S C, Emsley P, Hartshorn M J et al 1990 Structural and functional relationship of ATP-binding proteins associated with cystic fibrosis, multidrug resistance and bacterial transport. Nature 346: 362-365

James D E, Strube M, Mueckler M 1989 Molecular cloning and characterization of an insulin-regulatable glucose transporter. Nature 338: 83-87

Johann S, Hinton S M 1987 Cloning and nucleotide sequence of the *chlD* locus. Journal of Bacteriology 169: 1911-1916

Joshi A K, Ahmed S, Ames G F-L 1989 Energy coupling to bacterial periplasmic transport systems. Journal of Biological Chemistry 264: 2126-2133

Kaback H R 1990 *Lac* permease of *Escherichia coli*: on the path of the proton. Philosophical Transactions of the Royal Society of London B 326: 425-436

Kenig M, Abraham E P 1976 Antimicrobial activities and antagonists of bacilysin and anticapsin. Journal of General Microbiology 94: 37-45

Kroll J S, Hopkins I, Moxon E R 1988 Capsule loss in *H. influenzae* type B occurs by recombination-mediated disruption of a gene essential for polysaccharide export. Cell 53: 347-356

Kuchler K, Sterne R E, Thorner J 1989 *Saccaromyces cerevisiae STE6* gene product; a novel pathway for protein export in eukaryotic cells. EMBO Journal 8: 3973-3984

McGrath J P, Varshavsky A 1989 The yeast *STE6* gene encodes a homologue of the mammalian multidrug resistance P-glycoprotein. Nature 340: 400-404

McMurry L M, Petrucci R E, Levy S B 1980 Active efflux of tetracycline encoded by four genetically different tetracycline determinants in *Escherichia coli*. Proceedings of the National Academy of Sciences (USA) 77: 3974-3977

Maiden M C J, Davis E O, Baldwin S A et al 1987 Mammalian and bacterial sugar transport proteins are homologous. Nature 325: 641-643

Maloney P C 1990 Resolution and reconstitution of anion exchange reactions. Philosophical Transactions of the Royal Society of London B 326: 437-454

Miller C G 1975 Peptidases and proteases of *Escherichia coli* and *Salmonella typhimurium*. Annual Reviews of Microbiology 29: 485-504

Mimmack M L, Gallagher M P, Hyde S C et al 1989 Energy-coupling to periplasmic binding protein-dependent transport system: Stoichiometry of ATP hydrolysis during transport. Proceedings of the National Academy of Sciences (USA) 86: 8257-8261

Mueckler M, Caruso C, Baldwin S A 1985 Sequence and structure of a human glucose transporter. Science 229: 941-945

Mukakami T, Anzai H, Imai S et al 1986 The bialaphos biosynthetic genes of *Streptomyces hygroscopicus*: Molecular cloning and characterization of the gene cluster. Molecular and General Genetics 205: 42-50

Nguyen T T, Postle K, Bertrand K P 1983 Sequence homology between the tetracycline-resistance determinants of Tn10 and pBR322. Gene 25: 83-92

O'Hare K, Murphy C, Levis R, Rubin G M 1984 DNA sequence of the white locus of *Drosophila melanogaster*. Journal of Molecular Biology 180: 437-455

Ohyama K, Fukuzana H, Kohchi T et al 1986 Chloroplast gene organization deducted from complete sequence of liverwort *Marchantia polymorpha* chloroplast DNA. Nature 322: 572-574

Overduin P, Boos W, Tommassen J 1988 Nucleotide sequence of the *ugp* genes of *Escherichia coli* K-12; homology to the maltose system. Molecular Microbiology 2: 767-775

Payne G, Spudich E N, Ames G F-L 1985 A mutational hot-spot in the *hisM* gene of the histidine transport operon in *Salmonella typhimurium* is due to deletion of repeated sequences and results in an altered specificity of transport. Molecular and General Genetics 200: 493-496

Payne J W 1980 Transport and utilization of peptides by bacteria. In: Payne J W et al (eds) Microorganisms and nitrogen sources. Wiley, Chichester, UK, pp 211-256

Pedersen P L, Carafoli E 1987 Ion motive ATPases I, Ubiquity properties and significance to cell function. Trends in Biochemical Sciences 12: 146-150

Penninckx M, Gigot D 1979 Synthesis of a peptide form of N-5- (phosphoroacetyl)-L-ornithine. Journal of Biological Chemistry 254: 6392-6396

Postma P W, Lengeler J W 1985 Phosphoenolypyruvate: carbohydrate phosphotransferase systems of bacteria. Microbiology Reviews 49: 232-269

Reidl J, Romisch K, Ehrmann M, Boos W 1989 Mall, a novel protein involved in regulation of the maltose system of *Escherichia coli* is highly homologous to the repressor proteins GalR, CytR and LacI. Journal of Bacteriology 171: 4888-4899

Reyes M, Treptow N A, Shuman H A 1986 Transport of ribophenyl-α-maltosidase by the maltose transport system of *Escherichia coli* and its subsequent hydrolysis by a cytoplasmic α-maltosidase. Journal of Bacteriology 165: 918-922

Riordan J R, Rommens J M, Kerem B-S 1989 Identification of the cystic fibrosis gene: cloning and characterization of complementary DNA. Science 245: 1066-1073

Rosen B P, Weigel W, Karkaria C, Gangola P 1988 Molecular characterization of an anion pump. The *arsA* gene product is an arsenite (antimonite)-stimulated ATPase. Journal of Biological Chemistry 263: 3067-3070

Rosen B P, Hsu C-M, Karkaria C E et al 1990 Molecular analysis of an ATP-dependent anion pump. Philosophical Transactions of the Royal Society of London B 326: 455-463

Ross J I, Eady E A, Cove J H in press Inducible erythromycin resistance in staphylococci is encoded by a member of the ATP-binding transport super-gene family. Molecular Microbiology

Rouch D A, Cram D S, Diberardino D et al in press Efflux-mediated antiseptic resistance gene *qacA* from *Staphylococcus aureus:* common ancestry with tetracycline and sugar transport protein. Molecular Microbiology

Salyers A A, Speer B S, Shoemaker N B 1990 New perspectives in tetracycline resistance. Molecular Microbiology 4: 151-156

Sasatsu M, Misra T K, Chu L et al 1985 Cloning and DNA sequence of a plasmid-determined citrate utilization system in *Escherichia coli*. Journal of Bacteriology 164: 983-993

Sautereau A M, Trombe M C 1986 Electric transmembrane potential mutation and resistance to the cationic and amphiphilic antitumour drugs derived from pyridocarbazole 2-*N*-methylellipticinium and 2-*N*-methyl-9-hydroxyellipticinium, in *Streptococcus pneumoniae*. Journal of General Microbiology 132: 2637-2641

Scripture J B, Voelker C, Miller S et al 1987 High affinity L-arabinose transport operon. Journal of Molecular Biology 197: 37-64

Shuman H A 1982 Active transport of maltose in K12, Role of periplasmic maltose-binding protein and evidence for a substrate recognition site in the cytoplasmic membrane. Journal of Biological Chemistry 257: 5455-5461

Silver S, Misra T K 1988 Plasmid-mediated heavy metal resistances. Annual Reviews of Microbiology 42: 717-743

Stanfield S W. Ielpi L, O'Brochta D et al 1988 The *ndvA* gene product of *Rhizobium meliloti* is required for β-(1-2) glucan production and has homology to the ATP-binding export protein HlyB. Journal of Bacteriology 170: 3523-3550

Staudenmaier H, van Hove B, Yaraghi Z, Braun V 1989 Nucleotide sequences of the *fecBCDE* genes and location of the protein suggest a periplasm-binding-protein-dependent transport mechanism for iron (III) dicitrate in *Escherichia coli*. Journal of Bacteriology 171: 2626-2633

Stirling D A, Hulton C S J, Waddell L et al 1989 Molecular characterization of the *proU* locus of *Salmonella typhimurium* and *Escherichia coli* encoding osmoregulated glycine betaine transport systems. Molecular Microbiology 3: 1025-1038

Strathdee C A, Lo R Y C 1989 Cloning, nucleotide sequence, and characterization of genes encoding the secretion function of the *Pasteurella haemolytica* leukotoxin determinant. Journal of Bacteriology 171: 916-928

Surin B P. Rosenberg H, Cox G B 1985 Phosphate-specific transport system of *Escherichia coli* in nucleotide sequence and gene-polypeptide relationships. Journal of Bacteriology 161: 189-198

Thorens B, Sarkar H K, Kaback H R, Lodish H F 1988 Cloning and functional expression in bacteria and a novel glucose transporter present in liver, intestine, kidney and β-pancreatic islet cells. Cell 55: 281-290

Trombe M C 1985 Entry of methotrexate into *Streptococcus pneumoniae*. Journal of General Microbiology 131: 1273-1278

West I C 1970 Lactose transport coupled to protein movements in *Escherichia coli*. Biochemical and Biophysical Research Communications 41: 655-661

West I C 1990 What determines the specificity of the multidrug resistance pump. Trends in Biological Sciences 15: 42-46

Wilson D M, Wilson T H 1987 Cation specificity for sugar substrates of the melibiose carrier of *E. coli*. Biochimica et Biophysica Acta 904: 191-200

Zhang C-C, Durand M-C, Jeanjean R, Joset F 1989, Molecular and genetic analysis of the froctose-glucose transport system in the cyanobacterium *Synechocystis* PCC6803. Molecular Microbiology 3: 1221-1230

Discussion of paper presented by C. Higgins

Discussed by P. Lambert
Reported by H. C. Neu

In his discussion, Lambert reviewed the experience of the past decades in exploiting the peptide-permease transport systems. Compounds such as alafosfalin could be transferred into bacteria, but the incidence of resistance was high since peptide permeases were non-essential to the bacteria. Studies with KD0 analogues that inhibited the insertion of KD0 into lipopolysaccharide had been developed, but again resistance developed rapidly. Thus although the concept of transferring substances into bacteria is valid, it is unsuccessful due to the rapid development of resistance.

An alternative approach might be to develop agents which inhibit the efflux of antibiotics. The tetA protein causes efflux of tetracyclines from bacterial cells; if this were to be blocked, tetracycline resistance could be overcome. More successful than the aforementioned techniques may be use of the TonB system. Catechol derivatives of penicillins or cephalosporins have enhanced uptake in cells. Since iron uptake is essential, TonB negative mutants would not be viable in vivo. Clearly, TonB should be included in the screening of all new β-lactams.

Lambert also stressed that more knowledge of how to kill bacteria in biofilms is necessary, since bacteria in infections are often in the biofilm stage, at which point we know little about the transport properties and metabolism of bacteria growing as microcolonies.

Higgins was rather sanguine that investigating transport systems might represent a way to find new antibiotics, since as one studies transport systems the high specificity becomes more and more apparent. The difficulty in getting molecules across the cytoplasmic membrane was discussed, the general impression being that targets outside the cytoplasmic membrane or signalling receptor embedded in the membrane are to be preferred. TonB may be an ideal target, since it probably has important relations with virulence properties.

Further research on transport may well provide the ability to overcome transport-based resistance mechanisms and provide alternatives to current antimicrobial agents.

H

Plenary Lecture II

Chairman: J. Verhoef

13. Leprosy: a paradigm for infectious diseases

K. P. W. J. McAdam

INTRODUCTION

Leprosy is a disease 'in slow motion'. The bacillus, *Mycobacterium leprae* divides every 10–15 days, and it is the host immune response, rather than the organism itself which causes the characteristic clinical features of the disease. These intracellular bacilli prefer cooler temperatures (27-30°) and they have a tropism for peripheral nerves, skin and nasal mucous membrane, from which they are thought to be spread by droplet infection. The incubation period is 3–5 years and the cardinal clinical features are anaesthetic skin patches, thickened nerves and the finding of bacilli in the skin and/or nerves. Although most individuals who meet the bacillus mount an effective immune response, the minority develop clinical signs of infection; those with minimal cellular immunity develop multibacillary disease, so called 'lepromatous leprosy' and those who have an enhanced cellular response to the bacillus develop paucibacillary disease or 'tuberculoid leprosy'. This spectrum of clinical manifestations illustrates the battle between the micro-organism and host immunity and leprosy provides a model for other host-microbe interactions. Susceptibility to infections is only partly determined by immune response genes (HLA DR) and there is considerable evidence for an induced immune defect in patients with lepromatous leprosy with decreased production of gamma interferon, IL2 and IL1. The role of the *M. leprae* specific phenolic glycolipid 1 in immunological suppression remains a controversial subject. Cellular immunity has been assessed using T-cell Western blots, defining as many different T-cell specificities as are seen with antibodies on Western blots of *M. leprae* antigens. Some of the dominant antigens are heat shock proteins of molecular weights 70, 65, 18 kDa. Lepromatous leprosy patients, although deficient in T-cell responses, produce a vigorous polyclonal antibody response with many autoantibodies and persistent production of 'starter' IgM antibodies derived from germ line genes.

Animal models for leprosy include the use of mouse foot pad inoculation which takes 6 months for 10^3 organisms to multiply to 10^6. The armadillo supports growth of *M. leprae* and remains the source for vaccine trials. Monkeys have a chronic disease with neuropathy and appear to be the best model of paucibacillary leprosy. The expression of *M. leprae* genes in *E. coli* has permitted expression of the 7–10 main protein antigens recognized by Balb/c mouse monoclonal antibodies. Human

217

immune serum and T-cells pick out additional proteins. The generation of ordered libraries of *M. leprae* will provide better understanding of mycobacterial genetics. Expression in alternate vectors such as Salmonella and *M. bovis* BCG expands the horizons for vaccine development, not only for leprosy and other mycobacteria, but also for other intracellular infectious agents. The inbuilt mycobacterial adjuvant in BCG, the most widely administered vaccine in the world, is an attractive vehicle on which to engineer polyvalent vaccines.

Despite the excitement of immunological and molecular biological advances in leprosy, it is chemotherapeutic advances that offer most hope currently for control of the condition. New bactericidal drugs may now be combined with the best currently available, rifampicin, to allow combination chemotherapy; ofloxacin, clarithromycin and minocycline are showing most promise in experimental trials. In the management of reversal reactions, steroids remain the mainstay, while thalidomide is the drug of preference for erythema nodosum leprosum. A non-teratogenic alternative is required and cyclosporin A analogues are being tried. The stigma of leprosy remains, despite the fact it is a curable infectious disease. The danger of focusing entirely on bacteriological cure is that those who have a neurological deficit may be neglected and develop the stigmatizing disabilities of this historical disease which has already taught us much scientifically about the dynamic interaction between an invading organism and the human host.

EPIDEMIOLOGY

Rough estimates of the number of patients with leprosy in the world suggest 10–15 million cases with the majority being in Asia (64%) and Africa (34%). This proportion is likely to change as control measures in India improve while the situation in Africa deteriorates. In the past patients with leprosy, once diagnosed, have remained on national registers forever; with the institution of short course multidrug therapy, patients will be discharged as 'treated', thus decreasing the national and world figures. This highlights an important problem for the future: bacteriological cure is only part of the treatment of leprosy. The requirement for lifetime care and prevention of handicap remains a vital component of the lifelong responsibility for patients with neurological deficits. However the problem remains: what constitutes a case?

There are marked regional differences in prevalence, with a 1% crude prevalence being high (for a review of epidemiology, see Fine 1982, WHO, 1985). As a rule of thumb, an incidence of 0.001/year leads to a prevalence in the population of 0.02. The disease is now mainly acquired in the Tropics but in the fifteenth century the disease was common in the British Isles and there is excellent documentation of the situation in Norway where peak transmission occurred in the 1850s with 10 000 cases between 1850 and 1950. The disappearance of leprosy transmission from Northern Europe is attributed to social changes including diet, clothing, hygiene, housing, segregation and lack of crowding. In India there is an unexplained gradient in prevalence, with more leprosy being found to the South and East. The best documented epidemic was in the Micronesian island of Nauru where 30% of the inhabitants caught leprosy by 1941 after its introduction in 1911.

There are also differences in the distribution of the clinical types of leprosy with relatively more lepromatous cases in Caucasians (30%) than in Asians (10%) and Africans (5%). Most National Registers contain more males than females, though this may represent biased data resulting from only limited physical examination of women, and the highest incidence is in the 10–20 year olds, with lepromatous cases being older.

TRANSMISSION

Mycobacterium leprae may persist in the soil, like other environmental mycobacteria and polymerase chain reaction should clarify this issue (Hartskeeri et al 1989). It is unlikely to be a zoonosis, except potentially between armadillos and man. Clinical cases therefore represent the major reservoir of infection with multibacillary lepromatous cases being the most important. The risk of acquiring leprosy, if there is a lepromatous case in the household, is about 8-fold increased compared with a 2-fold increase if the case is tuberculoid.

The likely source of infection is by aerosol droplets. The traditional view of transmission by prolonged intimate contact for many years is difficult to sustain. Occasionally short contact in an endemic area has led to infection and the incubation period ranges from less than 1 year to more than 40 years with 95% being between 2–10 years. An untreated lepromatous patient may discharge 10^8 AFBs per nose blow or sneeze and these organisms have been shown to be viable in mouse foot pads (Shepherd 1960).

The site of infection may also be via the upper respiratory tract, particularly via the nose when it is abraded or damaged by other infections, such as perhaps the common cold. Attempts to transmit the infection experimentally via the lungs or gut have not been successful though challenge via these sites could potentially lead to induction of immunological tolerance rather than effective immunity. Again, definition of infection remains a problem. There is no reliable test to monitor whether an individual has met *M. leprae* without developing any stigmata of leprosy. Contacts of leprosy cases frequently develop evidence for immunological sensitisation to *M. leprae* using such markers as antibody to phenolic glycolipid and other mycobacterial antigens (Brennan 1986), in vitro lymphocyte proliferation to *M. leprae* and skin test responses to soluble *M. leprae* antigens (Godal & Negassi 1973). Moreover tuberculoid patches may self-heal. Thus, although many contacts might be 'infected' by a single multibacillary patient sneezing in a crowded place, very few will develop any evidence of disease.

Susceptibility to develop different forms of leprosy may be partly genetic but environmental factors are also important. HLA-DR3 occurs with increased frequency in tuberculoid patients (TT) while HLA-DQWI is associated with a higher frequency of lepromatous (LL) disease (Van Embden & De Vries 1984; De Vries et al 1988).

THE CLINICAL SPECTRUM OF LEPROSY

The clinical hallmarks of leprosy are anaesthetic skin patches, thickened nerves and the detection of acid-fast bacilli. There is frequently an enlarged nerve leading to the patch and other nerve trunks may also be enlarged. The appearances of skin lesions depend on the clinical form of the disease and reflect the degree of cell-mediated immunity to *M. leprae*. The vast majority of people who meet *M. leprae* in their environment develop a sub-clinical infection without any clinical symptoms. A minority develop an 'indeterminate' stage of leprosy in which skin lesions heal in most individuals but, in a small proportion, progress to persisting disease (Ponnighaus et al 1987). Those with persisting disease develop a clinical pattern reflecting their immunological responsiveness to *M. leprae*. Those who develop a hypersensitivity response to *M. leprae*, associated with elimination of bacilli, develop the 'tuberculoid' form of disease, whereas those who have no cell-mediated immunity and large numbers of persisting mycobacteria have the 'lepromatous' form of leprosy. This clinical spectrum was first described by Ridley and Jopling (1966) on a five point scale: from polar lepromatous, LL, through borderline lepromatous, BL, to borderline BB, borderline tuberculoid, BT, to polar tuberculoid, TT. The spectrum represents a clinical, pathological and immunological continuum.

Indeterminate leprosy

Indeterminate leprosy often reflects the uncertainty of the clinician in deciding whether a depigmented patch is leprosy or one of the many other causes of these lesions in the tropics, including fungal infections (e.g. Pityriasis versicolor), syphilis or pinta, vitiligo and the commonest cause of depigmentation probably being post-inflammatory type, sometimes known as pityriasis alba. It is often helpful to document loss of sensation using a standard monofilament nylon for sensory testing and lack of sweating is easily documented after exercise. The diagnosis of leprosy in patients with indeterminate patches frequently requires time to document the evolution of lesions and histological evidence of mycobacteria. Careful clinical examination of peripheral nerve trunks for thickening helps to tip the diagnostic balance in favour of leprosy as the cause of a depigmented skin patch (Boerrighter & Ponnighaus 1986). Histological features that suggest the diagnosis of leprosy include lymphocyte infiltration in the dermis, particularly involving nerves (Lucas 1988). Leprosy is one of the only infections which has a predilection for nerve, although a perivascular lymphocyte infiltration near a nerve can be confused with syphilis and other causes of vasculitis.

Tuberculoid leprosy

Tuberculoid leprosy lesions tend to be few in number, well defined with a raised edge and a healing centre. The cutaneous nerve feeding the lesion is often thickened. No *M. leprae* are found when a split skin smear is performed at the edge of the lesion, but the lepromin test is strongly positive. Many lesions will resolve without treatment, though nerve biopsies, even distant from the tuberculoid skin patch may contain *M. leprae* (Figs. 13.1 and 13.2).

Border tuberculoid leprosy

Borderline tuberculoid leprosy tends to be more disseminated with satellite lesions and less-defined edges to the skin patches. Damage to peripheral nerves is more widespread, with thickening of several nerve trunks. It is important to examine the major peripheral nerves which include greater auricular, ulnar, median, radial, radial

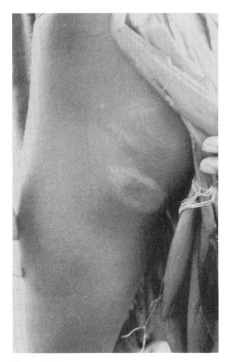

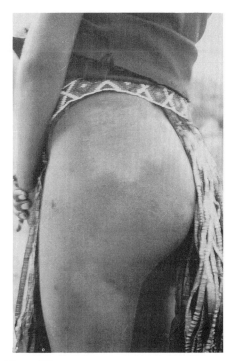

Figure 13.1
Polar tuberculoid (TT) depigmented anaesthetic patch with well demarcated edge and central healing

Figure 13.2
Borderline tuberculoid (BT) depigmented anaesthetic skin lesion showing less defined edges and a satellite lesion lower down the leg.

cutaneous, lateral popliteal and sural. These patients are prone to reversal reactions which can cause nerve damage (Job 1973).

Borderline leprosy
Patients with borderline leprosy are most unstable and may downgrade towards lepromatous leprosy if untreated or upgrade towards tuberculoid disease as part of the reversal reaction. These lesions are usually symmetrical and widespread in the body, with multiple nerves involved. During reversal reactions the edges of lesions become sharply defined or 'punched out' and nerves are tender, often with acute loss of function.

Borderline lepromatous leprosy
Borderline lepromatous leprosy patients show little evidence of immunity, lesions are widespread and macules may be infiltrated. Bacilli are found in the slit skin smears from different sites in the body. Nerves may be enlarged late in the disease and these patients are at risk of developing both reversal and erythema nodosum leprosum reactions (Fig 13.3).

Lepromatous leprosy
Lepromatous leprosy patients express no cellular immunity to the bacillus and may carry 10^{11} organisms in their soft tissues, which it is said, perhaps apocryphally,

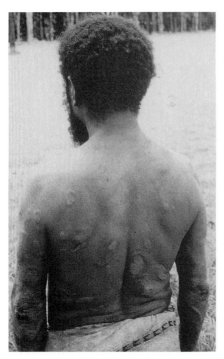

Figure 13.3
Borderline (BB) leprosy with punched out, relatively symmetrical anaesthetic, depigmented skin lesions in reversal reaction with raised edges, associated with tender peripheral nerves.

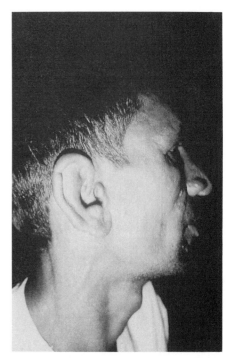

Figure 13.4
Polar lepromatous (LL) multibacillary leprosy with diffusely involved skin. Note especially the ear and nose and loss of eyebrows (madarosis). The nerves are thickened and the greater auricular nerve is clearly visible.

comprises up to one tenth of their soft tissue mass. These patients may be remarkably asymptomatic until late in the course of the disease. The skin is diffusely involved and infiltrated. The first lesions often appear as small nodules on the earlobes and there is evidence for mucosal involvement, with a stuffy nose from which bacilli can easily be identified by nasal swab examination or from a nose blow. In time the skin becomes thickened and the typical leonine faces reflect loss of eyebrows, a saddle nose from destruction of the nasal septum, a waxy skin, pendulous earlobes and extensive involvement of nerves which are thickened late in the disease. Sensory loss of light touch, pain and temperature is in the glove and stocking distribution and spares the axilla, groin and scalp. Compensatory hyperhydrosis tends to occur in these areas to make up for the lack of sweating in the periphery. Some patients develop glomerulonephritis. Testicular atrophy and gynaecomastia are common and those who develop recurrent ENL reactions are at risk of secondary amyoidosis of the Amyloid A protein type (AA) (Fig. 13.4).

Other well-characterised clinical forms of leprosy include neuritic, Lucio and histoid leprosy. These are all clinical descriptions reflecting, in neuritic leprosy, predominant nerve involvement without obvious skin lesions: in histoid leprosy, pruritic nodular lesions resulting from drug resistance and, in Lucio leprosy, a diffuse shiny skin infiltration, seen predominantly in Latin Americans.

REACTIONS

The clinical course of leprosy is complicated by reactions which are difficult to treat and lead to long-term nerve damage and mutilation. Two major varieties are described:

ENL reactions

These are thought to be due to immune complexes liberated from dying *M. leprae*, combining with antibodies to the bacilli and its component parts, complement, C-reactive protein and other constituents (Wemambu et al 1969, Ridley & Ridley 1983). These complexes are deposited either in the skin or in a perivascular distribution around the body, including involvement of kidneys with a glomerulonephritis, in the uveal tract of the eye causing an iritis, in the testis causing an orchitis, in the periosteum causing a periostitis and dactylitis, around nerves causing a neuritis. Skin lesions present as recurrent crops of painful, tender, evanescent, pink nodules lasting three to five days, usually affecting extensor surfaces of the upper arms, thighs, buttocks and back. It is unclear why these sites are affected predominantly. If not managed carefully these lesions can coalesce to form confluent areas of panniculitis affecting the dermis and sub-dermis with severe inflammation and disruption of collagen bundles (Ridley et al 1981). The lesions are predominantly characterized by a neutrophil infiltration associated with a neutrophil leucocytosis in the peripheral blood. Later lymphocyte infiltration is noted and Modlin et al (1986a) suggest that T-cells mediate ENL reactions. Patients are febrile and unwell. ENL reactions affect about 50% of multi-bacillary patients and usually occur after treatment, though reactions may precede diagnosis in some cases.

The earliest indications of ENL reactions are discomfort and pain in the skin, fever associated with a neutrophil leucocytosis and followed a few hours later by elevation of acute phase proteins, including C-reactive protein and serum Amyloid A (SAA) protein. SAA is the precursor of the secondary amyloid fibril protein, AA, and those who suffer recurrent, severe episodes of ENL reactions may go on to develop secondary amyloidosis (McAdam et al 1975). This can occur in as little as three months and the insoluble AA fibrils are difficult to clear from the tissues once they have been deposited. Patients with amyloidosis usually present with proteinuria and later nephrotic syndrome, reflecting their renal involvement.

Lucio reaction is a variant of ENL which occurs in patients of Latin American origin in whom there is dermal necrosis accompanying reactions thought to be due to a necrotising vasculitis (Rea & Ridley 1979) and potentially involving tumour necrosis factor (TNF) production. The marked geographic differences in the clinical features of ENL reactions merit a closer study of genetic factors.

Treatment of ENL reactions depends on their severity. Anti-inflammatory agents such as aspirin, chloroquine and stibophen have been used. Steroids are the mainstay of management, although there is often great difficulty in weaning patients from steroids. No sooner is the dose reduced than the ENL reactions return, and a vicious cycle frequently ends up with steroid-dependent patients. The discovery that thalidomide was effective at treating ENL reactions (Sheskin 1969) has led to its widespread use in males with ENL reactions. However, the danger of teratogeniticy means that it is contraindicated as a treatment for women of childbearing age who end up being managed on steroids. No effective, non-teratogenic analogues of thalidomide have yet been developed. Since steroids induce cytochrome P450 enzymes which metabolize steroids, the dose of steroids often has to be increased for patients on anti-leprosy chemotherapy, which includes rifampicin. Cyclosporin A has been shown to be effective and steroid-sparing in patients with ENL who require steroids to control their ENL reactions (Miller et al 1987).

Reversal reactions

These are in many ways more dangerous than ENL in the short term since they can lead to permanent nerve damage within a few days. As such they should be regarded as a medical emergency. Early symptoms are tenderness in existing skin lesions, particularly around the edges, and pain and tenderness of peripheral nerves. These lesions reflect an increased cellular immunity to the bacillus with T-cell and macrophage infiltration of those tissues that contain bacilli, including skin and nerve (Fig. 13.5). Patients prone to reversal reactions are from the middle of the clinical spectrum including BT, BB and BL classifications and these are the individuals in whom nerve damage predominates. Loss of nerve function can be dramatic, with wrist or foot drop occurring overnight. Patients who have evidence of recent nerve tenderness or functional loss need to be treated with steroids prior to being started on chemotherapy (Kiran et al 1985). All patients should be instructed to return if they develop nerve pain or tenderness. The treatment of choice is steroids and these may be required for 3 to 6 months after an acute episode of reversal reaction.

CHEMOTHERAPY

The major advances in leprosy management have followed the development of drugs

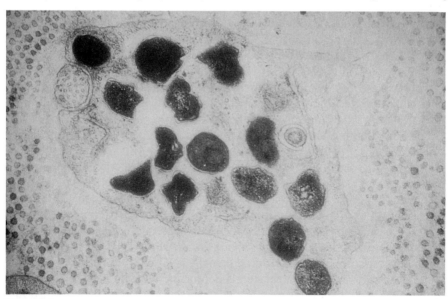

Figure 13.5
Electronmicrograph of peripheral nerve showing Schwann cell packed with electron dense *M. leprae* bacilli

which are effective at controlling the disease (Ellard 1988, WHO 1982, 1988). These include dapsone, a sulphone developed in the 1950s, rifampicin and clofazimine. Resistance to dapsone is common and the drug is only weakly bactericidal, acting by blocking folic acid synthesis. Haemolytic anaemia is a known side effect and patients with G6PD deficiency are particularly at risk. Exfoliative dermatitis, lymphadenopathy, hepatosplenomegaly, fever and hepatitis are recognized side effects. Rifampicin is a potent bactericidal drug which kills bacilli within a few days of starting therapy. Its activity is by inhibiting DNA-dependent RNA polymerase, but resistance to rifampicin develops readily and so the drug should not be used alone. Clofazimine is an anti-inflammatory agent, often used in the management of ENL reactions, but its major problem is discolouration of the skin to a purple or red colour, which is unacceptable to many light-skinned people. However, the pigmentation usually resolves within 6 to 12 months of stopping the drug. Major side effects are gastrointestinal symptoms thought to be due to deposition of clofazimine crystals in the wall of the small bowel.

Exciting new developments include the use of quinolones (ofloxacin), tetracyclines (minocycline) and macrolide antibiotics (clarithromycin). These drugs are all effective against *Mycobacterium leprae* in the mouse footpad model and multidrug therapy trials are currently in progress to assess their effectiveness in killing mycobacteria. The possibility of developing short course regimens to render multibacillary patients non-infectious will be an enormous step forward (Mitchison et al 1988).

The recommended World Health Organisation (1982) regimen employs a 6-month course in paucibacillary patients. This includes monthly supervised rifampicin 600 mg and daily unsupervised dapsone 100 mg. After 6 months, treatment is discontinued and patients observed for a further 2 years. Multibacillary patients are treated for a minimum of 2 years and often until skin smears are negative. They are given monthly supervised rifampicin 600 mg and clofazimine 300 mg together with daily unsupervised dapsone 100 mg and clofazimine 100 mg. After completing the 2 year course patients are kept under surveillance for a further 5 years.

Education remains a vital part of management of leprosy. Patients who have neural deficit have to be trained to prevent damage to their hands and feet. This involves the use of gloves for handling hot objects such as cooking utensils or cups of hot drink. Footwear should be checked regularly for nails and stones and new shoes worn for limited periods of time to avoid blisters; feet should be checked for hyperaemia indicating increased friction and shoes changed, with soft slippers being worn at home.

DEFORMITY

One problem of introducing effective chemotherapy has been that patients with leprosy can be discharged from medical care after they are bacteriologically cured. However, patients who have a neurological deficiency have to live with this for life as it cannot be reversed, except in the acute stage with steroids and/or nerve decompression. If leprosy is going to be managed in a primary health care system, health workers need to be properly educated about the central importance of nerve damage and its management, rather than focusing entirely on the important topic of bacteriological cure. There is a temptation in national statistics to discharge patients who have completed treatment from the national register. Many of these patients, however, require continuing medical contact for management of complications of neuropathy (Keeler & Ryan 1980).

Foot ulcers often require hospital admission to ensure adequate rest. The soaking of dry skin and debridement of thickened ulcer edges can be taught to patients. Plaster casts are often used to protect injured limbs and accelerate healing. Reconstructive surgery can dramatically improve function and appearance in patients with facial paralysis and hand and foot deformities. The role of nerve decompression is currently being re-evaluated as a means of reversing nerve damage (Theuvenet, personal communication). The central role of physiotherapists in rehabilitation and education cannot be underestimated.

Leprosy is still a disease which carries stigma. A classic statement from an AIDS patient recently highlights this unjustified reputation of leprosy: 'I may have HIV infection but at least I do not have leprosy'. In many parts of the world leprosy patients are isolated into colonies and they are often difficult to rehabilitate into their original community. Their deformities make them instantly identifiable and shunned by society. Self-help groups and businesses have been particularly effective at reintroducing these individuals to occupations in which they can earn a living rather than resort to begging and petty crime. Avoiding the term 'leper' in favour of 'leprosy patient' or even 'Hansen's Disease patient' is another step towards reducing stigmatization. The management of patients with leprosy involves a multidisciplinary approach including diagnostic field teams, epidemiologists, microbiologists, physicians, surgeons, psychiatrists, physiotherapists, nurses, occupational therapists and many voluntary workers. Despite the fact that leprosy is a curable disease it remains a demanding problem for society.

THE LEPROSY BACILLUS

Mycobacterium leprae has been known as the causative organism of leprosy since 1873 when Armauer Hansen discovered the bacillus (Hansen 1874). However, Koch's postulates have not been fulfilled to this day, since this acid-fast, Gram positive, intracellular organism cannot be grown on artificial media in vitro. Whereas *E. coli* has a doubling time of about 20 minutes and *M. tuberculosis* about 20 hours, *M. leprae* takes 10–20 days to multiply. It prefers to grow at 27–30°C, which accounts for the clinical observation that *M. leprae* are found in the coolest parts of the body, such as skin, nasal mucosa, earlobes and superficial nerves, while the skin in the warmer parts of the body, including groin, axillae and scalp, tends to be spared.

Shepherd (1960) first demonstrated laboratory growth of *M. leprae* in mouse footpads, and the tedious process of waiting 6 months for 10^3 inoculated organisms to multiply to 10^6 remains the standard method to assess bacterial viability and drug resistance (Rees 1988). The organism multiplies more readily in thymectomised-irradiated or congenitally athymic nude mice, which have been used to identify organisms that persist after chemotherapy, presumably by resting quietly and in a metabolically inert manner (Colston & Hilson 1976). The low core temperature of the banded armadillo is thought to account for its susceptibility to *M. leprae* infection, both in the wild and experimentally, with progressive dissemination to liver, spleen and other tissues 1 year after inoculation. *M. leprae* purified from the armadillo have provided adequate supplies for vaccine trials and for the substantial research efforts of scientists for the last 20 years (Kircheimer & Storrs 1971). The best animal model of leprosy is likely to be the non-human primate. Experimental transmission has been achieved to Mangabey, African green monkeys and most recently to rhesus monkeys, which develop a characteristic neuropathy over several years (Wolf et al 1986).

M. leprae appears to be a single species, regardless of its geographic origin, whether it derives from armadillos or humans and irrespective of type of leprosy. Differences at the genetic level presumably account for drug resistance, but only minor isolate differences have been detected by restriction fragment length polymorphism analysis (Clark-Curtiss et al 1985, Clark-Curtiss & Walsh 1989, Williams & Gillis 1989).

Pathogenicity
The pathogenicity of *M. leprae* is related to its tropism for dermal macrophages and neural Schwann cells. The usual portal of entry is thought to be the respiratory tract (Shepherd 1960) but it is not known how the organism finds its way to the periphery of the body. Mechanisms of receptor binding and bacterial uptake are unknown for *M. leprae*. The bacillus has a thick lipophilic cell envelope (Draper 1984); surrounding its phospholipid cell membrane (containing the mycobacterial phospholipid, phosphatidylinositol mannoside) is the peptidoglycan backbone, typical of Gram positive organisms, linked by a phosphodiester bond to a branched arabinogalactan polymer to which are attached the long chain ($C_{60}-C_{86}$) fatty acids, known as mycolic acids (Wheeler & Routledge 1988).

A major component of the *M. leprae* envelope is an apparently unique phenolic glycolipid (Hunter & Brennan 1981). This is composed of a phenol-phthiocerol core with three sugar units. The terminal sugar 3,6 di-O-methyl glucose, has been identified as the specific epitope involved in antibody recognition (Cho et al 1984). Lepromatous leprosy patients produce IgM antibodies to phenolic glycolipid (PGL-1) (Young et al 1984) which can be detected using a synthetic albumin-disaccharide complex (Brett et al 1986, Fine et al 1988).

There is relatively little known about the essential metabolic pathways in *M. leprae* as evidenced by the continuing inability to grow the organism in vitro. *M. leprae* synthesizes its own ATP but cannot synthesize the purine ring, being dependent on host purines in the form of adenine nucleotides. Its utilization of 6-phosphogluconate as an energy source and ability to oxidize DOPA are unusual characteristics (Wheeler 1984, Wheeler & Routledge 1988). *M. leprae* scavenge iron from the host using two sets of iron chelators, exochelins and mycobactins, whose synthetic pathways are not fully understood, but are potential therapeutic targets (Hall & Routledge 1987).

The survival of *M. leprae* in its hostile environment within cells is attributed to several characteristics (Sibley et al 1987): inhibition of phago-lysosome fusion with escape of the organism into the cytoplasm, away from catabolic lysosomal enzymes (Goren 1978); the oxygen radical scavenging activity of the mycobacterial glycolipid outer coat (Neil & Klebanoff 1988, Launois et al 1989); and the production of superoxide dismutase and peroxidase which help to protect the organism from toxic oxygen metabolites generated during the macrophage respiratory burst (Lowrie & Andrew 1988). However, *M. leprae* appears to lack catalase, making it susceptible to hydrogen peroxide (Klebanoff & Shepard 1984).

MYCOBACTERIAL ANTIGENS

A characteristic feature of *M. leprae* is that it is surrounded by a thick outer coat of lipid which is species specific and has a unique terminal dissacharide component (Hunter & Brennan 1981). This phenolic glycolipid or PGL1 is not only present in large quantities in infected tissues, but finding the antigen in tissue or serum also acts as a marker for multibacillary leprosy. There are elevated titres of antibodies directed against PGL in patients with multibacillary disease, with over 90% of LL patients having PGL antibodies. These antibodies are predominantly of the IgM class (Young et al 1984) which persist beyond the acute phase of the disease. Following treatment, PGL antibody concentrations fall progressively over time. In contrast paucibacillary patients have lower concentrations of PGL antibodies and so in practice PGL antibody detection is not useful for diagnosis of indeterminate skin lesions, but has a place in screening close contacts of leprosy patients (particularly those who are lepromin skin test negative) and in monitoring therapy of multibacillary cases (Cho et al 1984, Brett et al 1983, 1986).

The major carbohydrate antigens of *M. leprae* are lipoarabinomanan (LAM) and the arabinogalactan-peptidoglycan complex (Gaylord & Brennan 1987). Antibodies to LAM are induced in patients with a broad range of mycobacterial infections and are therefore not specific for leprosy, though they are found in paucibacillary as well as multibacillary disease (Brennan 1986). Thus LAM antibodies are a more sensitive indicator of mycobacterial infection than PGL antibodies, but their lack of specificity limits their use in diagnosis of leprosy.

The major protein antigens of *M. leprae* have been the subject of intensive research over the last 5 years since the development of an expression system for *M. leprae* genes, originally cloned into a lambda gt11 bacteriophage expression vector capable of expressing recombinant *M. leprae* antigens in *E. coli* (Young et al 1985, Hopwood et al 1988, Stoker et al 1989). Clark-Curtiss et al (1985) produced a cosmid library containing larger mycobacterial DNA fragments and, in our group, Thompson and Stoker (in preparation) have constructed an ordered DNA library such that overlapping contigs representing the entire mycobacterial genome have been defined and will be available for further studies.

When soluble sonicates of mycobacteria are separated by polyacrylamide gel electrophoresis there are a large number of proteins identified. The relative importance of these proteins as antigens has been assessed by making monoclonal antibodies from mice immunized with *M. leprae* sonicates. These monoclonal antibodies have been made in Balb/c mice which recognize a remarkably small group of seven proteins (70, 65, 36, 30, 28, 18 and 12 kDa) (Engers et al 1986). When other strains of mice have been used, various different antigens were detected and human serum recognizes yet further leprosy antigens (Ivanyi et al 1988, Vega-Lopez et al 1988), but the overall number is still limited. Several of these protein antigens have now been cloned and to date the genes encoding the 65, 18 and 28 kDa proteins have been sequenced. It is extraordinary that in the face of competition by competing antigens, these seven protein antigens are selected regularly as the target for an antibody response. Moreover, three of them have been defined as heat shock proteins (70, 65 and 18 kDa proteins) (Young et al 1987, Booth et al 1988, Nerland et al 1988, Lamb et al 1990). The 36 and 30 kDa proteins are both secreted proteins homologous to *M. tuberculosis* antigens found in the culture media of growing *M. tuberculosis* (Abou-Zeid et al 1986).

Although patients with mycobacterial infections make antibodies to these dominant antigens, an effective immune response depends on T-cell activation and it is now possible to identify antigens recognized by peripheral blood lymphocytes, T-cell clones and to estimate clonal frequency by limiting dilution analysis (Young & Lamb 1986, Abou-Zeid et al 1987, Lee et al 1989). T-cell responses have been identified to many of the proteins from *M. leprae* and in particular, to the 70, 65, 36 and 18 kDa proteins in leprosy patients and their contacts (Watson 1989). In our own laboratory we have concentrated on contacts of long-standing multibacillary patients, believing that these individuals, who have not contracted leprosy despite the prolonged contact, possess an effective immune response against the bacillus, which might be defined by analyzing the T-cell responses to antigens separated by PAGE. In practice, these contacts recognized antigens throughout the molecular range and no single dominant antigen was identified (Dockrell et al 1989a, Lee et al 1989). By cloning T-cells from patients different laboratories have identified clones specific for the major proteins of *M. leprae* (De Vries et al 1986, Modlin et al 1986a, 1989, Mustafa et al 1986, Ottenhof et al 1986, Anderson et al 1988, Lamb et al 1988, Van Schooten et al 1988, Lee et al 1989). Clones have also been particularly useful in mapping T-cell epitopes within defined antigens using synthetic peptides (Lamb et al 1988).

A major focus has centred on the 65 kDa antigen which is highly conserved with amino acid sequences in *M. leprae*, *M. tuberculosis* and *M. bovis* BCG, displaying greater than 95% homology, even though the total genomes of these organisms show only a 20% homology (Shinnick et al 1987). A similar 65 kDa protein known as GroEL has been identified in *E. coli*, *Coxiella burnetii*, *Spirocheles*, *Borrelia*, Legionella and Chlamydia (Young 1990). T-cell reactivity to heat shock proteins have been implicated in the pathogenesis of adjuvant arthritis (Van Eden et al 1988), diabetes and experimental allergic encephalitis (see Cohen I R Chapter 15). Clearly these heat shock proteins provide not only dominant antigens following infection, but are also major epitopes leading to auto-immune disease when the regulatory pathways controlling T-cell reactivity escape the normal network balance (Lamb & Young 1989, Born et al 1990).

IMMUNOLOGY OF LEPROSY

Cell-mediated immunity

The immunological defect of lepromatous leprosy is best highlighted by the lepromin skin response in which a soluble fraction of *M. leprae* is placed intradermally. Within 48 hours a positive skin response reflects a delayed hypersensitivity (Fernandez) reaction which subsides within a few days. Patients with effective immunity to *M.*

leprae and those with paucibacillary disease develop a late Mitsuda reaction at 3−4 weeks, which reflects a granulomatous response locally in the skin. Patients with lepromatous disease recognize none of the *M. leprae* antigens and are lepromin negative, but can still detect the *M. tuberculosis* private antigens, as evidenced by a positive tuberculin skin test. This specific cell-mediated defect to private *M. leprae* antigens as well as to all the shared mycobacterial antigens is difficult to explain. It is unlikely to be due to a single genetic defect, since one would have to postulate non-responsiveness to many different proteins linked to common HLA haplotopes. The genetic susceptibility of mice to various intracellular pathogens (*Salmonella, Leishmania, M. lepraemurium*) has been mapped to a single gene, linked to genes for various adhesion molecules including fibronectin. This gene codes for a resistance mechanism controlling intracellular replication of these pathogens and an active search is in progress to identify the counterpart human gene (Skamene 1989).

Many hypotheses have been put forward to explain an induced tolerance to *M. leprae* antigens (Kaufman 1986, Watson 1989). Waters et al (unpublished) have recently provided evidence that old lepromatous patients after treatment become lepromin positive, suggesting that the immunological defect is related to the presence of mycobacteria.

The route of entry of mycobacteria into the body may induce states of tolerance. Oral ingestion early in life of the environmental mycobacteria which are found in soil and water supplies might induce tolerance to the shared antigens of mycobacteria. It is unclear whether challenge via the lung leads primarily to tolerance or to an effective immune response and this requires further investigation, since *M. leprae* is likely to be spread via the respiratory route.

Mechanisms proposed for the immunological tolerance in lepromatous leprosy include the induction of T-suppressor cells by phenolic glycolipid (PGL1). Reversal of suppression can be achieved by removal of the CD8 T-cell subset in lepromatous patients (Mehra et al 1984), but also in tuberculoid leprosy where there is no specific non-responsiveness (Nath 1983). The finding that antibodies to the terminal sugar of PGL1 abrogated suppression (Bloom & Mehra 1984) provided compelling evidence for a suppressor determinant within this *M. leprae* specific glycolipid. So far CD8 suppressor T-cell clones derived from leprosy patients are not specific for PGL1 (De Vries et al 1986, Modlin et al 1986a, Ab et al 1990). Molloy et al (1990) suggests that this suppression may be mediated by lipopolysaccharide.

The host defence defect in lepromatous leprosy patients is, at its simplest, the inability of macrophages and other phagocytic cells, including Schwann cells, to kill intracellular mycobacteria (see Fig. 13.1; Lowrie & Andrews 1988, Lockwood & McAdam 1990). However, this defect can be corrected by administration either in vivo or in vitro of gamma interferon. Nathan et al (1986) have demonstrated clearing of bacilli locally at the site of injected recombinant gamma interferon in patients with lepromatous leprosy. These studies suggest a defective production of gamma interferon, a major macrophage activating factor, made by activated CD4 cells. The trigger for gamma interferon production is IL2 derived from other CD4 cells which thereby induce higher expression of IL2 receptors and an amplified production of the macrophage activating cytokine, gamma interferon. The stimuli for IL2 production are a number of cytokines derived from macrophages, including IL1, TNF and IL6. Defects have been described at each of the steps of this pathway including decreased

IL1 production (Watson et al 1984), decreased IL2 production (Haregewoin et al 1983) decreased 1L2 receptor expression (Mohaghepour et al 1985) and decreased gamma interferon production in vitro (Nogueria et al 1983). Moreover the pathway can be corrected in vitro by providing exogenous cytokines.

Just as diabetes is now considered the generic name for a disease resulting from defects at different stages in the production of insulin and its binding to receptors, so it seems sensible to suggest that lepromatous leprosy may arise from a variety of different immunological mechanisms, rather than demanding a single unifying defect to account for all patients with lepromatous disease.

Recent concepts on the induction of tolerance are based on the requirements for two separate activation signals for T-cells by antigen-presenting cells: requiring interaction between LFA1, CD2 and T-cell receptor on CD4$^+$ T-cells with ICAM, LFA3 and MHC class II respectively on antigen-presenting cells. Effective adhesion can be blocked by antibody to any one of these proteins (Qin et al 1989). In situations when only one of these signals is provided or one is blocked, then a state of non-responsiveness or tolerance is induced. In leprosy, the cells harbouring mycobacteria are often non-professional antigen-presenting cells such as Schwann cells. These cells might express one of the cell surface molecules (class II MHC), but not the other adhesion molecules required for T-cell activation. Since mycobacterial antigens persist for many years and will be processed by the antigen-presenting cell for presentation in conjunction with MHC II, this might be an ideal situation to induce persistent down-regulation of T-cell responses. It has yet to be determined whether mycobacterial antigens interfere with one of these activation signals, whether there is an auto-antibody response directed at one of the surface molecules and whether the mycobacteria-containing cells are able to express both class II MHC and adhesion molecules. T-cells normally utilize an $\alpha\beta$-heterodimer in the T-cell receptor complex, although in the gut and skin $\gamma\delta$ heterodimer usage is observed. In patients with leprosy there appear to be more T-cells expressing $\gamma\delta$ proteins (Kaufman 1988), and CD4-CD8-T-cells have been cloned from skin expressing $\gamma\delta$ T-cell receptors and reactive with hsp65 (Modlin et al 1986b, Born et al 1990).

Thus at this stage it remains unclear what are the mechanisms for immunological tolerance to specific *M. leprae* antigens in patients with multibacillary disease. It seems likely in the future that immunotherapy with cytokines, in addition to mycobacterial chemotherapy, will be used for optimal treatment of patients with leprosy. Indeed Convit et al (1986) are already using immunotherapy to enhance immunological responses of patients with multibacillary disease during chemotherapy.

Humoral immunity
Although there is an exuberant antibody response in patients with lepromatous disease, this has been assumed to be an irrelevant response. However, many auto-antibodies are produced and we have recently shown that some of these are directed against lymphocytes (Rasheed et al 1989), although the specificity of these auto-antibodies is unclear. In a series of studies (Duggan et al 1988, Locniskar et al 1988, Zumla et al 1988) monoclonal antibodies have been generated from patients with lepromatous disease. These have all been IgM antibodies reactive with self-determinants, including single stranded DNA, mitochondria, and acetyl choline

receptors as well as PGL1 and cardiolipin. Dersimonian et al (1989) has derived a sequence for the light and heavy chain variable regions of several of these polyreactive IgM molecules, showing that these antibodies are encoded in the germ line and are identical in sequence to an anti-DNA antibody from a patient with systemic lupus erythematosus. Using an assay to detect idiotype frequency, we have found this dominant IgM idiotype in patients with mycobacterial disease, other infections and in autoimmune diseases, particularly in patients with rheumatoid arthritis (Williams et al 1989).

It is proposed that these antibodies are designated 'starter antibodies' since they are encoded in the germ line and appear to be expressed at the start of all infections. Since they are polyreactive, they bind to many foreign and auto-antigens. In situations where antigen availability becomes limited, only those B-cells which bind with high affinity to antigens are driven to divide. By a process of somatic mutation, higher and higher affinity antibodies are produced and switched from IgM to other isotypes. In leprosy, mycobacterial antigens persist indefinitely and the drive for somatic mutation is lost. As in autoimmune diseases, there is a persistence of these 'starter antibodies' late in the infection or disease process and lack of down-regulation. We have shown that the PR4 idiotype binds to the dermal-epidermal junction and perhaps accounts for the finding of IgM antibody, even in the apparently normal skin of patients with leprosy (Zumla et al 1988). The role of these autoreactive 'starter antibodies' and anti-idiotypes in immune regulation has yet to be defined (Rees et al 1987).

Amyloidosis
Secondary amyloidosis is one of the only lethal complications of leprosy and occurs in patients who suffer from recurrent acute attacks of ENL reactions. These reactions are accompanied by a neutrophil leucocytosis, inflammation and elevation of the acute phase protein, SAA (Serum Amyloid A protein). SAA is synthesized by hepatocytes in response to IL1 (Selinger et al 1980). It is now known that there are at least six isotypes of SAA encoded by three genes, but it is not yet clear whether those who develop secondary amyloidosis preferentially produce or deposit only one of the isotypes (Bausserman et al 1980). Moreover the site of synthesis of the isotypes is still unclear. At present it is envisaged that deposition of a cleavage product of SAA, known as Amyloid A protein or AA, results from a catabolic enzyme defect. An accumulation of a partially cleaved SAA leads to deposition of insoluble fibrils in the tissues. The pentagonal component of Amyloid (AP) is attached to the fibrils in a calcium-dependent binding reaction and acts as a protease inhibitor for the fibrils, which are remarkably resistant to enzymic cleavage as a result (Vachino et al 1988). Future studies will be directed to understanding the mechanisms of stimulation of SAA synthesis, and strategies for dissolving the fibrils by competitively removing the AP protease inhibitor. By preventing ENL reactions, the stimulus for SAA synthesis and amyloid deposition is removed and reabsorption of the AA amyloid deposits has been documented.

VACCINES

Over the last 30 years BCG has been the standard vaccine used against leprosy with

Table 13.1 A new generation vaccine for leprosy

- a safe, live vector e.g. BCG, Salmonella, Vaccinia
- a good adjuvant
- expressing *M. leprae*-specific antigens (and protective epitopes for other infectious agents)
- not expressing suppressor epitopes

Perhaps
- using a heat shock promoter
- also expressing IL1, IL2 for adjuvanticity

But still requires assessment in mice and human trials

protective efficacies varying between 80 and 20% in four different studies (Dockrell & McAdam 1989b, Fine 1990). The most recent innovation has been to immunize with BCG plus killed *M. leprae* (Convit et al 1986). This seems to induce specific immunity to *M. leprae* with relevant cross-immunity to BCG. Prospective trials of BCG plus killed *M. leprae* vaccine are currently being conducted in Venezuela and in Malawi, while separate trials of *Mycobacterium w* (Zaheer et al 1988) and ICRC bacillus (an *M. avium intracellular* variant) (Chirmule et al 1988) are in progress in India. These vaccine trials are massive undertakings requiring 20 to 30 years of follow up. The capacity to manipulate mycobacterial genes opens up new opportunities for the production of a third generation vaccine. In the experimental mouse model, immunization with *M. habana* has been shown to be protective, and this organism, like *M. leprae* but not other mycobacteria, expresses the 18kDa heat shock protein (Lamb et al 1990). In the past, only live organisms have protected against subsequent *M. leprae* challenge but Gelber et al (1990) have immunized effectively with *M. leprae* subunits. Potential vectors for an *M. leprae* vaccine include *Vaccinia virus*, *Salmonella* and a fast-growing *Mycobacteria*. There are now methods to introduce DNA into mycobacteria (Jacobs et al 1987, Snapper et al 1988) and an attractive concept is to consider introducing a cassette of different genes encoding immunogenic proteins into an established BCG vaccine strain (Bloom 1989, Bloom & Jacobs 1989) (Table 13.1). In this way, immune responses will be generated against both the BCG antigens and the foreign antigens selected for their immunodominance. An inbuilt mycobacterial adjuvant would be provided, inducing both antibody and cell-mediated immunity. A further refinement would be to insert the cassette adjacent to a heat shock protein promoter, thereby expressing part of a heat shock protein which might act as a carrier molecule for the vaccine complex, all of which would be induced when the recombinant BCG organism arrives at its harsh intracellular location in the lysosome. The possibility of including cytokine genes such as IL1 and IL2 in the cassette would potentially enhance an immune response to this polyvalent vaccine.

ACKNOWLEDGEMENTS

Although this is a rather general overview article it results from an evolving awareness of the multiple facets of leprosy at the clinical, immunological and molecular level, many collaborators and colleagues have contributed to this evolution and I would like to acknowledge them: Drs Doug Russell, Steve Smith, Robin Anders in Papua New

Guinea; Drs Rabia Hussain, Thomas Chiang and Ruth Pfau in Pakistan; Dr Pat Rose in Guyana; Drs David Duggan, Harout Dersimonian, David Stollar, Robert Schwartz in Boston and Drs Hazel Dockrell, Neil Stoker, Mary Locniskar, David Mudd, David Isenberg, Ali Zumla, Warren Williams, Fawzia Rasheed, John Raynes, Steven Lee, Saroj Young, Diana Lockwood, Esther Race, Anthony Bryceson, Michael Waters and Sebastian Lucas in London.

REFERENCES

Ab B K, Kiessing R, Van Embden J D, et al 1990. Induction of antigen-specific CD4+HLA-DR-restricted cytotoxic T lymphocytes as well as nonspecific nonrestricted killer cells by the recombinant mycobacterial 65 kDa heat shock protein. European Journal of Immunology 20(2): 369-377

Abou-Zeid C, Smith I, Grange J, Steele J, Rook G 1986 Subdivision of daughter strains of Bacille Camette-Guerin (BCG) according to secreted protein patterns. Journal of General Microbiology 132: 3047-3053

Abou-Zeid C, Filley E, Steele J, Rook G A W 1987 A simple new method for using antigens separated by polyacrylamide gel electrophoresis to stimulate lymphocytes in vitro after converting to antigen bearing particles. Journal of Immunology Methods 98: 5-10

Anderson D C, van Schooten W C A, Barry M E, Janson A A M, Buchanan T M, de Vries R R P 1988 A *Mycobacterium leprae* specific T-cell epitope cross reactive with an HLA-DR2 peptide. Science 242: 258-260

Baussermann L L, Herbert P N, McAdam K P W J 1980 Heterogeneity of human serum amyloid A proteins. Journal of Experimental Medicine 152: 641-655

Bloom B R, Mehra V 1984 Immunological unresponsiveness in leprosy. Immunological Reviews 84: 5-28

Bloom B R 1989 New approaches to vaccine development. Reviews of Infectious Diseases 11: 5460-5466

Bloom B R, Jacobs W R Jr 1989 New strategies for leprosy and tuberculosis and for development of bacillus Calmette-Guerin into a multivaccine vehicle. Annals of the New York Academy of Sciences 569: 155-173

Boerrighter G, Ponnighaus J M 1986 Ten years leprosy control work in Malawi. 1. Methods and outcome after treatment. Leprosy Reviews 5: 199-219

Booth R J, Harris D P, Love J M, Watson J D 1988 Antigenic proteins of *M. leprae*. Complete sequence of the gene for the 18 kDa protein. Journal of Immunology 140: 597-601

Born W, Happ M P, Dallas A, et al 1990 Recognition of heat shock proteins and cell function. Immunology Today 11: 40-43

Brennan P J 1986 The carbohydrate containing antigens of *M. leprae*. Leprosy Reviews 57: 39-51

Brett S J, Draper P, Payne S N, Rees R J W 1983 Serological activity of characteristic phenolic glycolipid from *M. leprae* in sera from patients with leprosy and tuberculosis. Clinical and Experimental Immunology 52: 271-279

Brett S J, Paynes S N, Gigg J, Burgess P, Gigg R 1986 Use of synthetic glycoconjugates containing *M. leprae* specific and immunodominant epitope of phenolic glycolipid 1 in the serology of leprosy. Clinical and Experimental Immunology 64: 476-483

Chirmule N B, Chaturvedi R M, Deo M G 1988 Immunogenic subunit of the ICRC antileprosy vaccine. International Journal of Leprosy 56: 27-35

Cho S N, Fugiwara T, Hunter S W, Rea T H, Gelber R H, Brennan P J 1984 Use of an artificial antigen containing 3,6-di-O-methyl-beta-D-glycopyranosyl epitope for the serodiagnosis of leprosy. Journal of Infectious Diseases 150: 311-322

Clark-Curtiss J E, Jacobs W R, Docherty M A, Richie L R, Curtiss R 1985 Molecular analysis of DNA and construction of genomic libraries of *M. leprae*. Journal of Bacteriology 161: 1093-1102

Clark-Curtiss J E, Walsh J P 1989 Conservation of genomic sequences among isolates of *M. leprae*. Journal of Bacteriology 171: 4844-4851

Colston M J, Hilson G R F 1976 Growth of *Mycobacterium leprae* and *M. marinum* in congenitally athymic (nude) mice. Nature 262: 399-401

Convit J, Ulrich M, Aranzazu N, Castellanos P L, Pinardi M E, Reyes O 1986 The development of vaccination model using two micro-organisms and its application in leprosy and leishmaniasis. Leprosy Reviews 57 (Suppl 2): 263-273

Dersimonian H, McAdam K P W J, Mackworth-Young C, Stoller B D 1989 The recurrent expression of variable region segments in human IgM anti-DNA autoantibodies. Journal of Immunology 142: 4027-4033

De Vries R R P, Ottenhof T H M, Shughang L, Young R A 1986 HLA class II restricted helper and suppressor T-cell clones reactive with *Mycobacterium leprae*. Leprosy Reviews 57 (Suppl 2): 113-121

De Vries R R P, Ottenhof T H M, Van Schooten W C A 1988 Human leukocyte antigens (HLA) and mycobacterial disease. Springer Seminars of Immunopathology 10: 305-318

Dockrell H M, Stoker N G, Lee S P, et al 1989a T-cell recognition of the 18kDa antigen of *M. leprae*. Infection and Immunity 57: 1979-1983

Dockrell H M, McAdam K P W J 1989b Immunisation against leprosy in Zuckerman A J (ed) 'Recent Developments in Prophylactic Immunisation'. Kluwer Academic Publishers London pp 62-73

Draper P 1984 Wall biosynthesis: a possible site of action for new antimycobacterial drugs. International Journal of Leprosy 52: 527-532

Duggan D B, Mackworth-Young C, Kari-Lefvert A, et al 1988 Polyspecificity of human monoclonal antibodies reactive with *Mycobacterium leprae*, mitochondria, ssDNA, cytoskeletal proteins, and the acetylcholine receptor. Clinical Immunology and Immunopathology 49(3): 327-340

Ellard G A 1988 Chemotherapy of leprosy. British Medical Bulletin 44: 775-790

Engers H D, Houba V, Bennedsen J et al 1986 Results of a World Health Organisation sponsored workshop to characterise antigens recognised by mycobacteria specific monoclonal antibodies. Infection and Immunity 51: 718-720

Fine P E M 1982 Leprosy—the epidemiology of a slow bacterium. Epidemiological Reviews 4: 161-188

Fine P E M, Ponnighaus J, Burgess P et al 1988 Sero epidemiological studies of leprosy in Northern Malawi based on an enzyme immunosorbent assay using synthetic glycoconjugate antigen. International Journal of Leprosy 56: 243-254

Fine P E M, Rodrigues L C 1990 Modern Vaccines: Mycobacterial diseases. Lancet 1 1016-1020

Gaylord H, Brennan P J 1987 Leprosy and the leprosy bacillus: recent developments in characterisation of antigens and immunology of the disease. Annual Reviews of Microbiology 41: 645-675

Gelber R H, Brennan P J, Hunter S W et al 1990 Effective vaccination of mice against leprosy bacilli with subunits of *Mycobacterium leprae*. Infection and Immunity 53(3): 711-718

Godal T, Negassi K 1973 Subclinical infection in leprosy. British Medical Journal 3: 557-559

Goren M B 1988 Phagocyte lysosomes: interaction with infectious disease agents and experimental perturbations in function. Annual Reviews of Microbiology 31: 507-533

Hall R M, Routledge C 1987 Exochelin mediated iron acquisition by the leprosy bacillus. Journal of General Microbiology 133: 193-199

Hansen G H A 1874 Undersolgelser angraaende spedalskhedens aasger. Nork Magazin for Laegervindenskaben Suppl 4; 1-88

Hartskeeri R A, De Wit M Y, Klatser P R 1989 Polymerase chain reaction for the detection of *Mycobacterium leprae*. Journal of General Microbiology 135: 2357-2364

Haregewoin A, Godal T, Mustafa A S, Belehu A, Tabebe Y 1983 T-cell conditioned media reverse. T-cell unresponsiveness in lepromatous leprosy. Nature 303: 342-334

Hopwood D A, Keiser T, Colston M J, Lamb F I 1988 Molecular biology of Mycobacteria. British Medical Bulletin 44: 528-546

Hunter S W, Brennan P J 1981 A novel phenolic glycolipid from *Mycobacterium leprae* possibly involved in immunogenicity and pathogenicity. Journal of Bacteriology 147: 728-735

Ivanyi J, Bothamley G H, Jackett PS 1988 Immunodiagnostic assays for tuberculosis and leprosy. British Medical Bulletin 44: 635-649

Jacobs W R, Tuckman M, Bloom B R 1987 Introduction of foreign DNA into mycobacteria using a shuttle plasmid. Nature 327: 532-535

Job C K 1973 Mechanism of nerve destruction in tuberculoid—borderline leprosy. An electron microscope study. Journal of Neurological Science 20: 25-38

Kaufman S H E 1986 Mini Review. Immunology of leprosy: new findings, future perspectives. Microbial Pathogenesis 1: 107-114

Kaufman S H E 1988 CD8+ T lymphocytes in intracellular microbial infections. Immunology Today 9: 168-174

Keeler R J, Ryan M A 1980 The incidence of disabilities in leprosy after the commencement of chemotherapy. Leprosy Reviews 51: 149-154

Kiran K U, Stanley J M A, Pearson J M H 1985 The outpatient treatment of nerve damage in patients with borderline leprosy using a semi-standardised steroid regimen. Leprosy Reviews 56; 127-134

Kircheimer W F, Storrs E E 1971 Attempts to establish the Armadillo as a model for the study of leprosy: Report of lepromatoid leprosy in an experimentally infected armadillo. International Journal of Leprosy 39: 693-702

Klebanoff S J, Shepard C C 1984 Toxic effect of the peroxidase—hydrogen peroxide—halide antimicrobial system on *M. leprae*. Infection and Immunity 44: 534-536

Lamb J R, Ivanyi J, Rees A D M et al 1988 Mapping of T-cell epitopes using recombinant antigens and synthetic peptides. EMBO Journal 6: 1245-1249

Lamb F I, Singh N B, Colston M J 1990 The specific 18 kDa antigen of *M. leprae* is present in *M. habana* and functions as a heat shock protein. Journal of Immunology 144: 1922-1925

Lamb J R, Young D B In press 1989 T-cell recognition of stress proteins: a link between infections and autoimmune disease. Molecular Biology & Medicine

Launois P, Blum L, Dieye A, Millan J, Sarthou J L, Bach M A 1989 Phenolic glycolipid-1 from *M. leprae* inhibits oxygen free radical production by human mononuclear cells. Research in Immunology 140(9): 847-855

Lee S P, Stoker N G, Grant K A et al 1989 Cellular immune responses of leprosy to fractionated *Mycobacterium leprae* antigens. Infection and Immunology 57: 2475-2480

Lockwood D, McAdam K P W J 1990 Leprosy. In: Gorbach S, Bartlett (eds) Infectious Diseases in Medicine and Surgery. WB Saunders Co. In Press

Locniskar M, Zumia A, Mudd D W, Isenberg D A, Williams W., McAdam K P 1988 Human monoclonal antibodies to phenolic glycolipid-1 derived from patients with leprosy, and production of specific anti-idiotypes. Immunology 64(2): 245-251

Lowrie D B, Andrew P W 1988 Macrophage antimycobacterial mechanisms. British Medical Bulletin 44: 624-634

Lucas S B 1988 Histopathology of leprosy and tuberculosis—an overview. British Medical Bulletin 44: 584-599

McAdam K P W J, Anders R F, Smith S R, Russell D A, Price M A 1975 Association of amyloidosis with erythema nodosum leprosum reactions and recurrent neutrophil leucocytosis in leprosy. Lancet ii: 572-576

Mehra V, Brennan P J, Rada E, Convit J, Bloom B R 1984 Lymphocyte suppression in leprosy induced by a unique *M. leprae* glycolipid. Nature 308: 194-196

Miller R A, Shen J Y, Rea T H, Harnisch J P 1987 Treatment of chronic erythema nodosum leprosum with cyclosporine A produces clinical and immunohistologic remission. International Journal of Leprosy and Other Mycobacterial Diseases 55(3): 441-449

Mitchison D A, Ellard G A, Grosset J 1988 New antibacterial drugs for the treatment of mycobacterial disease in man. British Medical Bulletin 44: 757-774

Modlin R L, Kato H, Mehra V et al 1986a Genetically restricted suppressor T-cell clones derived from lepromatous leprosy lesions. Nature 322: 459-461

Modlin R L, Mehra V, Jordan R, Bloom B, Rea T H 1986b *In situ* and *in vitro* characterisation of the cellular immune response in erythema nodosum leprosum. Journal of Immunology 136: 883-886

Modlin R L, Pirmez C, Hofman F M et al 1989 Lymphocytes bearing antigen specific T-cell receptors accumulate in human infectious disease lesions. Nature 339: 544-548

Mohagheghpour N, Gelber R, Larrick J W, Sasaki D T, Brennan P J, Engleman E G 1985 Defective cell-mediated immunity in leprosy: Failure of T-cells from lepromatous leprosy patients to respond to *Mycobacterium leprae* is associated with defective expression of interleukin 2 receptors and is not reconstituted by interleukin 2. Journal of Immunology 135: 1443-149

Molloy A, Gaudernack G, Levis W R, Cohn Z A, Kaplan G 1990 Suppression of T-cell proliferation by *M. leprae* and its products; the role of lipo polysaccharide. Proceedings of the National Academy of Science (USA) 87: 973-977

Mustafa A S, Gill H K, Nerland A 1986 Human T-cell clones recognise a major *M. leprae* protein antigen expressed in *E. coli*. Nature 39: 63-66

Nath I 1983 Immunology of human leprosy: current status. Leprosy Reviews 315-455 (special issue)

Nathan C F, Kaplan G, Levis W R, et al 1986 Local and systemic effects of intradermal recombinant interferon gamma in patients with lepromatous leprosy. New England Journal of Medicine 315: 6-15

Neil M A, Klebanoff S J 1988 The effect of phenolic glycolipid 1 from *Mycobacterium leprae* on the antimicrobial activity of human macrophages. Journal of Experimental Medicine 167: 30-42

Nerland A H, Mustafa A S, Sweetser D, Godal T, Young R A 1988 A protein antigen of *Mycobacterium leprae* is related to a family of small heat shock proteins. Journal of Bacteriology 170: 5919-5921

Nogueira N, Kaplan G, Levy G 1983 Defective γ interferon production in leprosy reversal with antigen and interleukin 2. Journal of Experimental Medicine 158: 2165-2170

Ottenhoff T H M, Klatser P R, Ivanyi J, Elferink D G, De Wit M Y L, De Vries R R P 1986 *Mycobacterium leprae* specific protein antigens defined by cloned human helper T-cells. Nature 319: 66-68

Ponnighaus J M, Fine P E M, Bliss L 1987 Certainty levels in the diagnosis of leprosy. International Journal of Leprosy 55: 454-462

Qin S X, Cobbold S, Benjamin R, Waldman H 1989 Induction of classical transplantation tolerance in the adult. Journal of Experimental Medicine 169(3): 779-794

Rasheed F N, Locniskar M, McCloskey D J, et al 1989 Serum lymphocytotoxic activity in leprosy. Clinical and Experimental Immunology 76(3): 391-397

Rees A D M, Scoging A, Dobson N et al 1987 T-cell activation by anti idiotypic antibody; mechanism of interaction with antigen reactive T-cells. European Journal of Immunology 17: 197-201

Rees R J W 1988 Animal models in leprosy. British Medical Bulletin 44: 650-664

Ridley D S, Jopling W H 1966 Classification of leprosy according to immunity: A five group system. International Journal of Leprosy 34: 255-273

Ridley D S, Rea T H, McAdam K P W J 1981 The histology of erythema nodosum leprosum. Variant forms in New Guineans and other ethnic groups. Leprosy Reviews 52: 65-78

Ridley M J, Ridley D S 1983 The immunopathology of erythema nodosum leprosum: the role of extravascular complexes. Leprosy Reviews 54: 95-107

Ridley M J, Ridley D S, DeBeer F C, Pepys M B 1984 C-reactive protein and apoB containing lipoproteins are associated *Mycobacterium leprae* in lesions of human leprosy. Clinical Experimental Immunology 56: 545-552

Selinger M J, McAdam K P W J, Kaplan M M, Sipe J D, Vogel S N, Rosenstreich D L 1980 Monokine induced synthesis of serum amyloid A protein by hepatocytes. Nature 285: 498-500

Shepherd C C 1960 Acid fast bacilli in nasal secretions in leprosy and results of innoculation of mice. American Journal of Hygiene 71: 147-157

Sheskin J, Sagher F 1969 Trials with Thalidomide derivatives in leprosy reactions. Leprosy Reviews 39: 203-205

Shinnick T M, Sweetser D, Thole J, van Embden J, Young R A 1987 The etiologic agents of leprosy and tuberculosis share an immunoreactive protein antigen with the vaccine strain *M. bovis* BCG. Infection and Immunity 55: 1932-1935

Sibley L D, Franzblau S G, Drahenbuhl J L 1987 Intracellular fate of *Mycobacterium leprae* in normal and activated mouse macrophages. Infection and Immunity 55: 680-685

Skamene E 1989 Genetic control of susceptibility to mycobacterial infections. Reviews of Infectious Diseases 11: S394-S399

Snapper S B, Lugosi L, Jekkel A, et al 1988 Lysogeny and transformation in mycobacteria. Stable expression of foreign genes. Proceedings of the National Academy of Sciences (USA) 85: 6987-6991

Stoker N G, Grant K A, Dockrell H M, Howard C R, Jouy N F, McAdam K P W J 1989 High level expression of genes cloned in phage gt11. Gene 78: 93-99

Theuvenet V. Personal communication.

Thompson J, Stoker N et al Ordered DNA library of *M. leprae* (in preparation)

Vachino G, Heck L W, Gelfland J A et al 1988 Inhibition of human neutrophil and Pseudomonas elestases by the amyloid P-component: a constituent of elastic fibres and amyloid deposits. Journal of Leukocyte Biology 44(6): 529-534

Van Eden W, Thole J E R, Van der Zee R, et al 1988 Cloning of the mycobacterial epitope recognised by T-cells in adjuvant arthritis. Nature 331: 171-173

Van Embden W, De Vries R R P 1984 Occasional Review—HLA and leprosy—a re-evaluation. Leprosy Reviews 55: 89-104

Van Schooten W C A, Ottenhoff T H M, Klatser P R, Tirole J, de Vries R R P, Kolk A H J 1988 T-cell epitopes on the 36 kDa and 65 kDa *M. leprae* antigens defined by human T-cell clones. European Journal of Immunology 18: 849-854

Vega-Lopez F, Stoker N G, Locniskar M F, Dockrell H M, Grant K A, McAdam K P W J 1988 Recognition of mycobacterial antigens by sera from patients with leprosy. Journal of Clinical Microbiology 26: 2474-2479

Watson S, Bullock W, Nelson K 1984 Interleukin 1 production by peripheral blood mononuclear cells from leprosy patients. Infection and Immunity 45: 787-789

Watson J D 1989 Leprosy: Understanding protective immunity. Immunology Today 10: 218-221

Wemambu S N G, Turk J L, Waters M F R, Rees R J W 1969 Erythema nodosum leprosum: a clinical manifestation of the arthus phenomenon. Lancet ii: 933-935

Wheeler P R 1984 Metabolism in *Mycobacterium leprae*: its relation to other research on *M. leprae* and to aspects of metabolism in other mycobacteria and intracellular parasites. International Journal of Leprosy 52: 208-230

Wheeler P R, Routledge C 1988 Metabolism in *Mycobacterium leprae*, *M. tuberculosis* and other pathogenic mycobacteria. British Medical Bulletin 44: 547-561

WHO Technical Report Series 675: 1982 Chemotherapy of leprosy for control programmes: report of a WHO study group

WHO Technical Report Series 716: 1985 Epidemiology of leprosy in relation to control: report of a WHO study group

237

WHO Technical Report Series 768: 1988 WHO Expert Committee on leprosy; 6th Report

Williams D L, Gillis T P 1989 A study of the relatedness of *Mycobacterium leprae* isolates using restriction fragment polymorphism analysis. Acta Leprologica (Geneva) 7 (Suppl 1): 226-230

Wolf R N, Gormus B J, Martin L N, et al 1986 Experimental transmission of *Mycobacterium leprae* to primates. Science 227: 529-531

Young D B, Dissanayake S, Miller R A et al 1984 Humans respond predominantly with IgM immunoglobulin to the species specific glycolipid of *Mycobacterium leprae*. Journal of Infectious Diseases 149: 870-873

Young R A, Mehra V, Sweetster D, et al 1985 Genes for the major protein antigens of the leprosy parasite *Mycobacterium leprae*. Nature 316: 450-452

Young D B, Lamb J R 1986 T lymphocytes respond to solid phase antigen: a novel approach to the molecular analysis of cellular immunity. Immunology 59: 167-171

Young D B, Ivanyi J, Cox J H, Lamb J R 1989 The 65 kDa antigen of mycobacteria - a common bacterial protein? Immunology Today 8: 215-219

Young D B 1990 Stress proteins as antigens during infection. In: Rice Evans C, Winrow V, Blake D, Burdon R, (eds) Stress proteins and Inflammation. Richlieu Press pp 155-168

Zaheer S A, Talwar G P, Walia R, Mukherjee R 1988 Results of one year of phase II/III trials with the candidate antileprosy vaccine *Mycobacterium W*. Health Co-operation Papers 9: 245

Zumla A, Williams W, Shall S, et al 1988 Human monoclonal antibodies to phenolic glycolipid-1 from leprosy patients cross react with poly (ADP-ribose), polynucleotides and tissue bound antigens. Autoimmunity 1: 183-195

Discussion of paper presented by K. P. W. J. McAdam

Reported by K. P. W. J. McAdam

The mechanism whereby *Mycobacterium leprae* invade Schwann cells was discussed. There is no known receptor for *M. leprae*, however, some immunochemical studies (Ridley 1984) have demonstrated various proteins surrounding *M. leprae* within phagocytic cells. These proteins include apolipoprotein B, C-reactive protein (CRP) and serum amyloid P component (SAP). Although these studies have not been repeated by others they perhaps suggest that organisms might be surrounded by these proteins and use conventional receptors to enter cells. Formal demonstration of the receptor for penetration has not been described, partly because live *M. leprae* are only obtainable from tissue extracts; the process of extraction from tissue utilises 'Triton', a solvent which strips off the lipid capsule of *M. leprae*. Presumably penetration of cells by the bacillus involves an interaction between the phenolic glycolipid and the cell surface receptor.

Although many people are exposed to *M. leprae* fewer and fewer people develop manifestations of clinical disease. Workers from Scandinavia who went out to work on leprosy in Ethopia were originally studied by Godal and his group; within a year of arriving in Africa these volunteers responded to antigens from *M. leprae* , although they were non-responsive on first arriving in Ethiopia. In Papua New Guinea, Anders described a few children who were lepromin skin test negative despite being close contacts of index cases of lepromatous disease—it was these children who went on to develop lepromatous leprosy. In this situation antibodies to phenolic glycolipid are useful in predicting those who develop multi-bacillary disease. People who develop indeterminate leprosy often have a positive lepromin skin test and go on to self cure.

Lagrange commented that there were several studies in New Caledonia, India and Africa, showing that the risk of developing lepromatous leprosy is 20 times higher in those who do not respond to lepromin and who have a high level of antibody against PGO1. Thus we now have the capacity to detect those who are lepromin non-responsive and it may be that it is appropriate to give chemoprophylaxis to these people. If these individuals are followed and PGO1 titres increased, there is a strong likelihood of their developing lepromatous disease.

Further discussion centred on the immunological defect of patients with lepromatous leprosy. One experimental model shows that the *bcg* gene in mice regulates the first contact with mycobacteria. In the resistant mice mycobacteria are unable to multiply within macrophages, whilst susceptible mice permit mulitiplication of intracellular organisms. After this initial contact there is the development of a specific T-lymphocyte mediated immunity to *M. leprae* . Some individuals are not able to respond at all, having a gap in their T-cell repertoire. Other individuals possess macrophages or T-cells able to suppress *M. leprae* responses. Others are unable to produce Interleukin-2 or gamma interferon, while yet others might have highly activated macrophages producing soluble suppression factors such as PGE2. Thus, lepromatous leprosy is likely to represent several sub-populations of patients whose underlying immunological defects are different.

Suppressive mechanisms may also be generated if antigens are first presented via the gut. There is increasing evidence that presentation of antigens by non-professional presenting cells, such as Schwann cells, can lead to the induction of suppression.

There were various comments about the relationship of mycobacterial infection to autoimmune diseases and Crohn's disease. This has been a topical subject over the last few years and has centred on the similarity between heat shock proteins produced by mycobacteria and analogous proteins made by humans following stress reactions. An immune response against the mycobacterial heat shock proteins and in particular the hsp65 (65,000 dalton heat shock protein) may lead to autoimmune responses. This topic is further discussed by Irun Cohen. A longstanding speculation that Crohn's disease is caused by *M. pseudotuberculosis* antigen remains unproven, but there is growing interest in the possibility of mycobacterial-triggered immune responses to heat shock proteins, when these proteins are homologous to human proteins.

The difficulty of working with armadillo for immunological studies has led to the development of new models for leprosy. The best of these is the monkey, which develops a longstanding neuritic disease as well as the lepromatus nodules found in other animals.

Although dogma suggest that patients with lepromatous leprosy have a persisting immunological defect, making them unable to respond to *M. leprae* skin tests or in lymphocyte proliferation assays, Waters et al have recent evidence that patients who have completed treatment for lepromatous leprosy eventually recover their lepromin sensitivity. These data strongly suggest an induced immune defect in lepromatus leprosy rather than a genetic susceptibility. Although phenolic glycolipid seems the most likely inducer of immune suppression, several laboratories have been unable to repeat the findings of Mehra et al. Watson et al have injected mice with phenolic glycolipid at the same time as other antigens and were unable to demonstrate any suppressive effects. However, it is unclear what phenolic glycolipid might do to antigen-presenting cell functions in terms of interfering with co-stimulators and intergrins. The possibility that phenolic glycolipid might prevent switching of B cell responses from IgM to IgG was also raised.

Finally, it was noted that the epidemic of leprosy in Norway had disappeared over the last 50 years. It was assumed that this related to improved living standards, lack of crowding and contact with environmental mycobacteria which might lead to an altered secondary response to *M. leprae* when it is first encountered.

Section V:
Intracellular mechanisms

Chairman: S. R. Norrby

14. The intracellular pharmacokinetics and activity of antibiotics

P. M. Tulkens

INTRODUCTION

Most antibiotics available so far have been designed and/or screened primarily for their activity against bacteria in acellular systems. Thus, compounds with increasingly greater intrinsic activity, chemical stability and resistance to bacterial inactivating mechanisms have been obtained for already established, as well as for new classes of antimicrobials. This, however, does not necessarily result in an improved efficacy in vivo, since the overall activity of an antibiotic is the result of many factors which are only partly taken into account in the above approach. Intracellular pharmacokinetics and activity are often neglected, except for those rare compounds primarily designed to treat intracellular infection. Actually, intracellular infection is too often viewed as being of importance only for specific, obligatory intracellular parasites. Whereas this is correct for diseases such as legionellosis, chlamydiosis, or leprosy, it is now becoming more evident that intracellular survival, or even multiplication of many other bacteria, referred to as facultative intracellular parasites, play a significant role in the pathogeny of the disease they cause. This is particularly evident for infections caused by *Salmonella* or *Listeria* (for a review see Moulder 1985), but is also seen for more common pathogens such as *Staphylococcus aureus* (Craven & Anderson 1979). Intracellular infection is also responsible for many of the difficulties encountered in controlling and eradicating those infections (Baillie 1984, Tulkens 1985, van den Broek 1989). Increasing attention, therefore, needs to be focused on intracellular pharmacokinetics and pharmacodynamics of antibiotics, as a complement to the evaluation of their properties in acellular systems.

This paper reviews present knowledge in this field. First, the uptake and subcellular localization of the main classes of antibiotics are examined. Then data on their activities are critically reviewed and quantitative results obtained in a selected model of *S. aureus*-infected J774 macrophage model are studied as an example of a potentially rational approach in the evaluation of available or new agents.

UPTAKE AND SUBCELLULAR LOCALIZATION

Most studies on the uptake and subcellular localization of antibiotics have been conducted in cells maintained or grown in vitro since these provide a much easier experimental set-up than in vivo models. Whereas the use of such models is understandable, it must be remembered that they do not necessarily describe the in vivo situation. Given this caveat, however, much basic information has been obtained in that way, which proved of clinical importance.

Aminoglycoside antibiotics

Many authors have claimed that aminoglycosides do not accumulate in cells. Whereas this is indeed a common observation for polymorphonuclear leukocytes or macrophages maintained in culture for short periods of time (Johnson et al 1980, Prokesh & Hand 1982), it is probably not true for cells maintained for several days in the presence of these drugs. Thus, Bonventre & Imhoff (1970) and Tulkens & Trouet (1978) observed that mouse peritoneal macrophages or rat fibroblasts exposed to aminoglycosides for 4 days accumulate them to an apparent intracellular concentration 2- to 4-fold larger than the extracellular concentration. The intracellular drugs remained potentially bioactive (i.e. they could be recovered in a microbiologically active form), which is in line with the lack of metabolism of aminoglycosides in mammals. Further studies disclosed that intracellular aminoglycosides are not homogeneously distributed within cells, but localize largely (if not exclusively) within lysosomes, as established by cell fractionation techniques (Fig. 14.1). Thus, the concentration of aminoglycosides in lysosomes was estimated to reach values at least 10 to 20-fold larger than in the extracellular fluid.

Extension of these findings to the in vivo situation has not been established with respect to phagocytic cells, even though there is evidence for activity of intraphagocytic aminoglycosides on intracellular bacteria if exposure of phagocytic cells to these antibiotics is made for a sufficient long time and/or at high enough doses (see later). Conversely, the observation that intracellular aminoglycosides localize in lysosomes has given a rational explanation to the known lysosomal toxicity exhibited by these drugs in proximal tubular cells of kidney (Kosek et al 1974, for review see Tulkens 1989). Eventually, this lysosomal localization was confirmed for kidney (Silverblatt & Kuehn 1979, Giurgea-Marion et al 1986). It also helped in understanding the mechanism of cell uptake of aminoglycosides, which most likely appears to be endocytosis (see discussion in Aubert-Tulkens et al 1979). Endocytosis of aminoglycosides is of the fluid type in fibroblasts and macrophages, which explains why it is relatively slow and leads to only moderate accumulation. In kidney, it is probably of the adsorbtive type (Silverblatt & Kuehn 1979, Giuliano et al 1986), and therefore proceeds with a much larger efficacy (see discussions in Jacques 1969, Silverstein et al 1977, Morin & Fillastre 1982).

β-lactam antibiotics

As for aminoglycosides, many authors have reported a lack of accumulation of β-lactams in phagocytic cells exposed for a few hours to these antibiotics (Brown & Percival 1978, Johnson et al 1980, Prokesh & Hand 1982, Forsgren & Bellahsène 1985). Contrary to aminoglycosides, however, this lack of accumulation (i.e. an apparent intracellular concentration lower than the extracellular concentration) is genuine and is observed even if cells are maintained in the presence of β-lactams for several days. Yet, erroneously, most authors have concluded that β-lactams do not penetrate into cells. Actually, these antibiotics diffuse through membranes, as

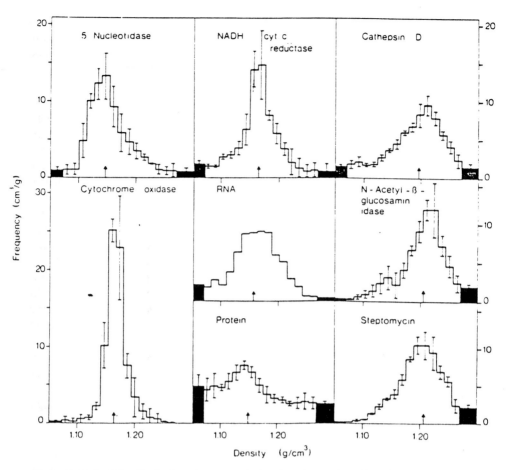

Figure 14.1 Subcellular distribution of streptomycin in cultured rat embryo fibroblasts. Cells were incubated for 4 days in the presence of 100 mg/l of streptomycin, collected, homogenized and a post-nuclear supernate fractionated by isopycnic banding in sucrose gradients. The diagrams show the distribution of the antibiotic in comparison with those of markers of the main cytoplasmic components, namely lysosomes (cathepsin D, *N*-acetyl-β-glucosaminidase), endoplasmic reticulum (NADH: cytochrome c reductase RNA), mitochondria (cytochrome c oxidase) and plasma membrane (5′ nucleotidase). A distribution similar to that of streptomycin was found for four other aminoglycosides (dihydrostreptomycin, amikacin, gentamicin and kanamycin A). (Reproduced from Tulkens & Trouet 1978.)

evidenced by their volume of distribution in vivo, which is considerably larger than the volume of extracellular water, and by the fact that most of them are absorbed, albeit to variable extents, after oral administration. This behaviour is in sharp contrast with that of aminoglycosides which indeed do not diffuse through membranes. The low amounts of β-lactams which become associated with cells incubated in their presence are distributed in the cytosol and quickly released upon transfer in fresh medium (Trouet et al 1981, Renard et al 1987).

Studies using a basic derivative of penicillin G, namely *N*-(3-dimethylaminopropyl)benzylpenicillinamide (ABP), have suggested why β-lactams are largely excluded from cells, even though they can penetrate them. ABP accumulates in cells to a much larger extent than penicillin G (or penicillin V) and

J

partly localizes in lysosomes (Fig. 14.2); yet, its membrane diffusion properties are not markedly different from those of the parent compound. The key difference between these substances lies in their acid/base properties. Thus, penicillin G like all β-lactams carry a free acid group (carboxyl in penicillins, cephalosporins and related compounds; sulphonic in monobactams), and therefore should be considered as an organic acid. As known for many drugs, this would cause the concentration of the ionized species to be considerably lower in acidic compartments surrounded by

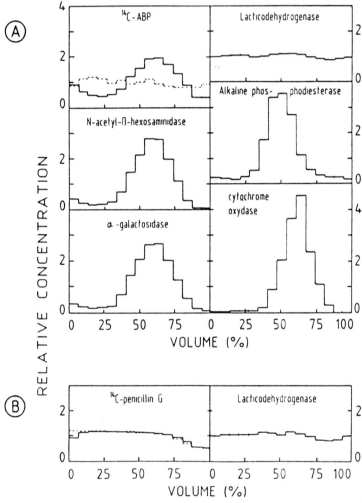

Figure 14.2 Subcellular distribution of N-(3-dimethylaminopropyl) benzylpenicillinamide (^{14}C-ABP; A) and penicillin G (B) in cultured J774 macrophages. Cells were incubated for 60 min in the presence of either drug at a concentration of 3 mM, collected, homogenized, and post-nuclear supernates were fractionated by isopycnic banding in Percoll® gradients. In this type of experiment, the sample is homogeneously distributed in the tube, and the organelles move to their buoyant position, displaying an enrichment of their markers in the corresponding fractions, whereas soluble constituents remain at almost the same concentration throughout. N-acetyl-β-hexosaminidase and, α-galactosidase are markers of lysosomes, cytochrome oxidase of mitochondria; alkaline phosphodiesterase of pericellular membrane, and lacticodehydrogenase of the cytosol (soluble enzyme). (Reproduced from Renard et al 1987.)

semipermeable membranes such as phospholipid bilayers (i.e. more permeable to the unionized species than to the ionized one), compared with serum (see Milne et al 1958 and de Duve et al 1974). The cytoplasmic pH is approximately 0.2-0.5 units lower than serum (Waddell & Bates 1969) but still much higher than the pK_a of the acidic group of β-lactams. The predominant form of the drug on both sides of the pericellular membrane is therefore the ionized species. Thus, there will be an overall lack of accumulation of β-lactams in cells, even though these antibiotics easily diffuse through membranes in their unionized form with which they are in constant equilibrium. Conversely, ABP, which is an organic base, will accumulate in cytosol, and still more in lysosomes because of a more acidic pH, which is around 2 units lower in these organelles compared with serum (Renard et al (1987); see also the review by de Duve et al (1974)).

Lincosaminides
Lincosaminide antibiotics such as clindamycin have been shown to accumulate in phagocytes (Klempner & Stirt 1981, Prokesh & Hand 1982). Experimental results have been presented suggesting that clindamycin uses the membrane transport system for nucleosides (Steinberg & Hand 1984). This mechanism, however, does not explain why lincomycin, which closely resembles clindamycin, is not accumulated by phagocytes. It also fails to provide an explanation for the observation (Zenebergh, Carlier and Tulkens, unpublished) that cell-associated lincosaminides (clindamycin, lincomycin or pirlimycin) are found partly in cytosol and partly in lysosomes, irrespective of their level of cellular accumulation. Finally, one would expect the uptake of lincosaminides to show saturation if it were transported by a carrier-mediated system, but this was not observed. Thus, at the present stage, it is fair to say that we have no clear explanation as to the mechanism of accumulation of lincosaminides. Yet, lincosaminides being all organic bases, non-ionic diffusion/segregation could account for their accumulation and subcellular distribution, as described earlier for ABP, and below for macrolides.

Macrolides
A marked intracellular accumulation of macrolide antibiotics has been observed in several types of cultured cells. Thus, polymorphonuclear leukocytes, macrophages and various cells in culture were shown to concentrate erythromycin 2 to 10-fold over the extracellular concentration (Hand et 1985, Martin et al 1985, Carlier et al 1987b). As for lincosaminides, marked differences are observed among apparently closely related derivatives, and, usually, new molecules such as roxithromycin show (or have been selected for ?) a larger accumulation (Carlier et al 1987a). Accumulation of macrolides is severely decreased upon incubation in acid pH. Conversely, it is considerably larger in activated macrophages, namely those collected by broncho-alveolar lavage of smokers (Hand et al 1985, Carlier et al 1987a).

Uptake of macrolides is usually rapid, but so is efflux (half-life of approximately 15-20 minutes, at most). A marked, recent exception is azithromycin (Gladue et al 1989) the intracellular concentration of which does not reach a plateau even after 24 hours incubation. Moreover, azithromycin leaks out remarkably slowly (half-life approximately 5-6 hours) from either polymorphonuclear neutrophils or macrophages. Cell fractionation studies have shown that, at equilibrium, cell-associated macrolides distribute almost equally between the cell soluble fraction and the lysosomes (Fig. 14.3). The latter association is stable to the extent that lysosomes are kept intact during the homogenization and fractionation procedures. A similar fast uptake, along with a dual distribution in lysosomes and cell cytosol, and a fast egress were also found for erythromycin and roxithromycin in cultured rat hepatocytes (Villa et al 1988a) and fibroblasts (unpublished), suggesting that these are general properties of macrolides. Moreover, recent studies showed that PMN cytoplasts, which do not contain granules, accumulate only half the amount of roxithromycin compared to intact PMNs (Hand & King-Thompson 1990). Since lysosomes represent only a small fraction of the whole cell volume, the *actual* amounts of drug associated with either cytosol and lysosomes can be similar, even though their *concentrations* are very different (for discussion see de Duve et al 1974, Renard et al 1987). Being highly diffusible, however, the localization of macrolides in cytosol (and perhaps also lysosomes?) does not prevent them from having access to other cell structures such as endoplasmic reticulum where they may undergo metabolism (Villa et al 1988b).

Altogether, the pharmacokinetic and distribution properties of macrolides strongly suggest that their uptake and disposition in phagocytes occur by non-ionic diffusion and segregation of the ionized species of the antibiotic in the acidic compartments of the cell. Physicochemical studies, comparing series of macrolides with different uptake and release rates, and accumulation levels, are, however, required before this proposal can be further substantiated. As for lincosaminides, uptake of macrolides is non-saturable, which argues against specific transport system(s).

Fluoroquinolones

Easmon & Crane (1985), Carlier et al (1987b) and Pascual et al (1989), among others, have reported that fluoroquinolones such as pefloxacin or ciprofloxacin accumulate in phagocytic cells. This observation has been extended to non-phagocytic cells, such as fibroblasts. Non-nucleated cells such as erythrocytes, however, do not accumulate fluoroquinolones (Carlier et al in press). Uptake of fluoroquinolones, as for macrolides, is rapid. The cell-associated drugs are also quickly released when cells are transferred to drug-free medium. Intracellular accumulation is similar to that of erythromycin (approximately 2 to 8-fold), and therefore lower than that of new macrolides like roxithromycin. In contrast to macrolides, accumulation of fluoroquinolones is slightly enhanced by incubation in acidic medium. No influence of the activation of macrophages has been observed. So far, no major differences have been observed among available fluoroquinolones with respect to cell accumulation. Recent studies (Carlier et al 1989, submitted), however, suggest that new compounds could offer possibilities in this respect. A most intriguing observation has been that the 'accumulation' of fluoroquinolones does not require cell viability and, actually, is enhanced by exposure of cells to formaldehyde or preincubation at 56°C (Easmon & Crane 1985, Scorneaux, Zenebergh and Tulkens unpublished). Nevertheless, fluoroquinolones that become cell-associated under these conditions retain full biological activity, i.e. no significant difference was seen between results of determinations using either radiolabelled drugs or microbiological assay of cell lysates.

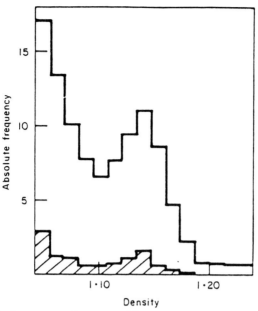

Figure 14.3 Distribution patterns of two macrolides, roxithromycin (open histogram) and erythromycin (hatched histogram) after isopycnic centrifugation of homogenates from J774 macrophages incubated with either drug for 30 min at 10 mg/l. The gradients were made of sucrose in water, and samples were deposited on the top of them. Thus, soluble material tends to remain in the first fractions, whereas organelles migrate into the gradient (from left to right) up to their position of buoyant density. In this system, lysosomes equilibrate at densities around 1.15-1.16 (data not shown, but see Fig. 14.4 and data in Renard et al 1987), i.e. in the same fractions as those displaying the second peak of macrolide. (Reproduced from Carlier et al 1987.)

The subcellular localization of fluoroquinolones is not known for certain. Thus, cell fraction studies (Carlier et al 1987b, 1988, submitted, in press) have failed to reveal significant association of accumulated fluoroquinolones to specific subcellular organelles. Rather, as shown in Figure 14.4, the drugs are almost entirely recovered in the so-called 'soluble fractions', suggesting that they are either truly free, and not even protein-bound in the cytosol, or that they elute very quickly and completely from their storage compartment. Yet, there is no indication as to what this compartment could be.

A lack of specific subcellular distribution and rapid efflux of fluoroquinolones were observed both in non-infected and *S. aureus*-infected macrophages, indicating that these properties are not dependent on the state of activation of the cells. Yet, recently, Carlier et al (in press) reported that in *Legionella*-infected guinea pig macrophages, pefloxacin exhibits partial retention upon exposure of cells to drug-free medium. Most interestingly, the tightly associated drug (approximately 30% of the total amount accumulated) showed a distribution suggestive of its association to intracellular *Legionella* and/or to *Legionella*-containing vacuoles. These findings need further confirmation with other fluoroquinolones and intracellular bacteria.

Ansamycins

Ansamycins, and rifampicin in particular, have been reported to accumulate in phagocytes. Interestingly enough, however, the actual accumulation ratios measured

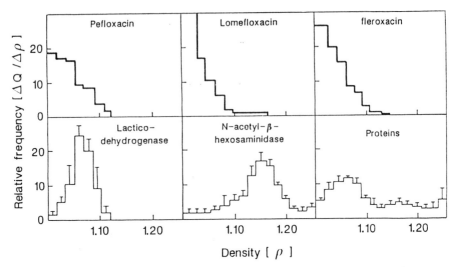

Figure 14.4 Distribution patterns of three fluoroquinolones after isopycnic centrifugation of homogenates from J774 macrophages incubated for 30 min with the corresponding drug at 10 mg/l. The technique used is similar to that described in Fig. 14.3. The lower panels show the distribution patterns of enzymes from the cytosol (lacticodehydrogenase) and the lysosomes (*N*-acetyl-β-hexosaminidase), respectively, along with that of total protein. The slight migration of lacticodehydrogenase in the gradient is consistent to its molecular weight (approx. 130 kDa) and our conditions of centrifugation (see Lopez-Saura et al 1978 for discussion). Fluoroquinolones are almost entirely collected in the first fractions corresponding to the samples deposited on the top of the gradients.

in several cell types are relatively low (of the order of 2 to 3; see for example Johnson et al 1980), indicating that liposolubility per se is not necessarily a favourable property for intracellular *accumulation*, even though it certainly plays a major role in determining the rate of *uptake*. Little is known about the subcellular distribution of ansamycins in cells. Trouet et al (1980) reported that rifampicin is distributed in the cytosol of fibroblasts, but, as for fluoroquinolones, this does not preclude loose association with other subcellular organelles from which the drug would be eluted during fractionation.

Other antibiotics
Information on uptake and distribution of other antibiotics in phagocytes is scanty. Tetracyclines and chloramphenicol were reported to accumulate in cells to moderate extents. Trimethoprin accumulates only transiently. Pleuromutilins (a class of antichlamydial agents) accumulate to a large extent. Nitroimidazoles diffuse easily through membranes (and need actually to be metabolized in sensitive bacteria and parasites to express their activity: Müller 1983), but do not accumulate in cells. Polypeptidic and glycopeptidic antibiotics show no, or only very low, accumulation.

ACTIVITY OF INTRACELLULAR ANTIBIOTICS

Activity of antibiotics against intracellular bacteria has been examined in a very large number of studies, both in vitro and in vivo, with many apparent conflicting results (see van den Broek 1989 for review). One of the main issues is to distinguish clearly between a true action of the antibiotic under study, and a stimulation or modulation of the host cell's bactericidal capabilities. Moreover, the determination of the antibiotic activity against intracellular organisms is often associated with methodological problems, especially when dealing with species that can grow both extra- and intracellularly. For instance, conflicting views have been expressed as to whether agents such as lysostaphin which are used to destroy extracellular *S. aureus* would not also affect intracellular bacteria (van den Broek et al 1982, Sanchez et al 1986). Mechanical washings and other approaches may be fraught with even larger difficulties. Another problem which concerns both facultative and obligatory intracellular parasites is related to the quiescent character of many intracellular bacteria, which often prevents antibiotics from expressing their activity.

Yet, in spite of these difficulties, it is now largely agreed that β-lactams and aminoglycosides are ineffective in controlling the growth, not to mention eradicating intracellular bacteria, unless given in large doses and for sufficient periods of time. The latter consideration is of importance if one wishes to understand the reasons for the many conflicting reports in this area. Thus, it is clear that ampicillin can be used to treat listeriosis, or that aminoglycosides are effective against tuberculosis, while there is strong evidence that both diseases are characterized by an important intracellular component. Actually, the intracellular pharmacokinetic data of β-lactams indicate that these drugs have access, albeit to a limited extent, to intracellular cell compartments. Therefore, it may be understood that large extracellular concentrations, maintained long enough, will eventually allow the intracellular concentration to reach the necessary threshold value (i.e. higher than MICs) to become efficacious. In addition, β-lactams and penicillins in particular may trigger the production of bactericidal substances by monocytes (van den Broek et al 1986). With respect to aminoglycosides, activity should in principle be observed if the intracellular drug can overcome two major defeating effects, namely its almost exclusive localization in lysosomes and its consequent exposure to acid pH. Thus, one can predict that aminoglycosides will be very poorly effective against organisms that stay away from lysosomes; in addition, the concentrations in lysosomes needed to impair bacterial growth may be up to 2 to 3 orders of magnitude greater than those measured in broth (see Tulkens & Trouet 1978). In most short-term experiments, the latter condition is not met in view of the slow penetration of aminoglycosides (see earlier), and, therefore, results have been systematically negative. Conversely, in long-term experiments, or with high extracellular concentrations, aminoglycosides are effective against several sensitive bacteria (Suter 1952, Mackaness 1952, Mackaness & Smith 1953, Jeukin & Benaceraf 1960, Chang 1969). The direct relation between aminoglycoside concentration and their bactericidal effect towards extracellular bacteria has been recently stressed by the use of pharmacodynamic models (Bläser et al 1985) and confirmed by clinical studies (Moore et al 1987). Thus, it was shown that activity was primarily correlated with peak levels/MIC ratios. These studies could be extended to intracellular bacteria, to the condition that the concentration of the drug and its apparent MIC towards the offending organism in the infected compartment are known. It is likely that many of the conflicting results reported concerning the efficacy of aminoglycosides would be amenable to a rational explanation on that basis.

The activity of intracellular lincosaminides is also subject to much controversy. Thus, Jacobs & Wilson (1983) reported that clindamycin was effective in reducing the bacterial density in PMN from children suffering from chronic granulomatous disease and infected with *S. aureus*. In their model, however, normal PMN were able to reduce partly the bacterial inoculum without antibiotic, even though clindamycin gave some increase to that effect. Conversely, Hand & King-Thompson (1986) and Sanchez et al (1986) reported that clindamycin was ineffective in reducing *S. aureus* counts in either human or bovine polymorphonuclear leukocytes (PMNs). As we shall see later, we ourselves found some activity of clindamycin towards *S. aureus* ingested by macrophages, but to a much lower extent than could be surmised from its intracellular concentration. So, somehow, the activity of clindamycin appears defeated intracellularly.

Suggestions have been made that PMNs which take up large amounts of clindamycin could actually deliver this drug at their site of migration, for example in abcesses. In our opinion, these considerations are of limited interest in view of the rapid efflux of clindamycin from PMNs, which will result in these cells arriving in tissues almost completely deprived of antibiotic, unless the extracellular concentration is maintained throughout. This is to say that cells will maintain a gradient, not an actual concentration.

Activity of macrolides and of fluoroquinolones is less subject to controversy. First, macrolides, and now more recently, fluoroquinolones, have been shown to be effective agents in the control of typical obligatory intracellular pathogens such as *Legionella* (Horwitz & Silverstein 1983, Fitzgeorge et al 1985, Dournon et al 1986, Vildé et al 1986) or *Chlamydia*. Moreover, both types of drug were shown to be effective in macrophages against *S. aureus* (Easmon et al 1986, and results shown later) and, for fluoroquinolones, against *Salmonella* (Chang, Pechère, Mondain & Tulkens unpublished). Sanchez et al (1986) and Hand & King-Thompson (1986), however, observed no activity of erythromycin against *S. aureus* in PMNs. The activities of these two classes of agents undoubtedly relate to their capacity to enter cells, and not to suffer too much defeating activity intracellularly. As will be shown later, however, differences in intrinsic intracellular activity exist between the two types of drugs, suggesting commensurate differences in their bioavailability or in the way they are influenced by the environment.

Compared with all antibiotics discussed so far, the 'golden standard' for intracellular activity is rifampicin, which in all studies constantly showed a large efficacy against all sensitive bacteria (van den Broek 1989) even under conditions in which drugs such as erythromycin are ineffective (see Sanchez et al 1986). As we explained earlier, efficacy of rifampicin does not primarily result from a higher accumulation of this drug, compared with other antibiotics. An attractive hypothesis is that the activity of rifampicin is somehow enhanced by the intracellular physicochemical conditions prevailing at the site of infection.

A QUANTITATIVE MODEL TO ASSESS INTRACELLULAR ACTIVITY OF ANTIBIOTICS

The development of new antibiotics (or new forms thereof) to act on intracellular bacteria can rely on either in vivo or in vitro models. In vivo models are attractive, in that they provide a response which, if positive, allows for immediate conclusions. Thus, a large body of literature has dealt with such in vivo models, using either liposome-entrapped drugs (see Popescu et al 1987 for review) or antibiotics associated with various particulate carriers (see for example Fattal et al 1989). However, these models do not sufficiently separate and analyse the various cellular (uptake, expression of activity) and extracellular (organ distribution, pharmacokinetics, metabolism) factors involved in the overall efficacy (or lack thereof) of the new compounds.

Conversely, in vitro models offer the unique possibility of addressing the very basic questions of penetration of the drug, and its relation to activity, so that a compound can be selected on the basis of its greater *intrinsic* activity towards intracellular infection. In this connection, we designed a model of J774 macrophages that can be infected by *S. aureus*. These cells were chosen since we already knew much about antibiotic uptake and distribution in them, and they allow for rapid growth of *S. aureus*, apparently because of their low, or hampered bactericidal mechanisms. J774 macrophages are derived from a mouse reticulosarcoma (Ralph et al 1975, Snyderman et al 1977).

The techniques of infection we used for this model are derived from those described by Easmon & Crane (1985) and Sanchez et al (1986) and will be described in full in a forthcoming publication. A critical aspect is that we could rule out a significant contribution of extracellular *S. aureus* to the variation of bacterial inoculum, as evidenced by experiments in which macrophages were transiently, but repeatedly exposed to lysostaphin. Interestingly also, we showed that the bactericidal mechanisms of these cells are not enhanced by phagocytosis (as judged from the results of experiments using antibiotic-resistant organisms) and that effects on bacterial growth are strictly limited to the periods of time during which cells keep the intracellular antibiotic.

This model has enabled us to draw several conclusions from key data summarized in Table 14.1. First, it is clear that clindamycin is effective, whereas lincomycin is not, in controlling intracellular growth of *S. aureus*. This is in spite of the fact that, by manipulating the extracellular concentration, it is possible to obtain intracellular concentrations of lincomycin that exceed 100-fold its MIC. Yet, compared with macrolides, or even still more fluoroquinolones, clindamycin remains only moderately efficacious in eradicating the bacteria.

For the purpose of comparing drugs, we used our model to determine their *intrinsic intracellular* activity (Scorneaux et al 1989a). This is defined as the potency of the antibiotic to reduce the intracellular inoculum divided by its intracellular/extracellular accumulation ratio. Actually, the intrinsic activity of each drug studied *increases* with increasing drug concentration, suggestive of threshold effects. Within the class of macrolides, and at a given extracellular concentration, activity is correlated with the degree of accumulation. Thus, the intrinsic activities of erythromycin and roxithromycin are similar, but for all practical purposes, roxithromycin will offer an advantage because of its greater accumulation (Scorneaux et al 1989b). A similar effect is seen with other macrolides (see Scorneaux & Tulkens 1989).

As shown in Table 14.1 the intrinsic activity of fluoroquinolones is greater—at the same intracellular/extracellular concentration ratio—than that of macrolides

Table 14.1 Correlation between accumulation and effectiveness of antibiotics in *Staphylococcus aureus*-infected J774 macrophages. Cells were allowed to phagocytoze opsonized *S. aureus* (from a bovine clinical isolate), washed with lysostaphin and then reincubated for 24 h at 37°C in the absence (control) or the presence of ^{14}C-labelled antibiotics. See Renard et al 1987 for other procedures. (Reproduced from Scorneaux et al 1989a,b and unpublished data of Scorneaux, Zenebergh & Tulkens.)

Drug	Extracellular concentration[a] (mg/l)	Intracellular concentration[b] (mg/l)	Variation from original inoculum[c] (%)	Intrinsic intracellular activity[d]
None (controls)			8722 ± 48	
Lincomycin	10 (10)	23.5 ± 3.2	13750 ± 267	-910
	50 (50)	118.7 ± 8.1	8769 ± 185	-792
Clindamycin	2.5 (10)	19.5 ± 2.4	110 ± 7	-5.2
	5.0 (20)	49.2 ± 1.4	60 ± 2	22.6
Erythromycin	0.5 (1)	4.2 ± 0.1	81 ± 4	11.5
	5.0 (10)	50.9 ± 1.7	43 ± 2	35.9
Roxithromycin	0.5 (1)	8.7 ± 1.3	64 ± 2	11.1
	5.0 (10)	107.8 ± 18.2	23 ± 2	30.4
Pefloxacin	1 (1)	10.9 ± 0.2	37 ± 3	53.6
	10 (10)	109.5 ± 10.2	19 ± 3	85.3
Ciprofloxacin	0.5 (1)	3.9 ± 0.2	22 ± 2	80.0
	5.0 (10)	45.2 ± 6.5	3 ± 2	140.0

[a] Figures in parentheses show the value in multiples of the MIC determined in broth against the strain of *S. aureus* used.

[b] Calculated concentration, based on the measurement of antibiotic/cellular protein ratio and assuming the drug is homogenously distributed in the cell (see Renard et al 1987 and discussion in Carlier et al submitted).

[c] The original inoculum amounted to approx. 1-2 bacteria/cell. Cells incubated in the presence of oxacillin or gentamicin (10 times the MIC) did not show significant difference from cells incubated without drug.

[d] Intrinsic intracellular activity is defined as the effectiveness of the drug divided by its level of accumulation. The unit used is: (log (CFU at time=0/CFU at time 24h) / Ci/Ce) $\times$ 10^3, where CFU is the number of viable bacteria per mg of cell protein, Ce the extracellular concentration, and Ci the calculated intracellular concentration.

(compare for example ciprofloxacin with erythromycin). Thus, one can anticipate that fluoroquinolones that would exhibit a larger accumulation than presently available ones, would offer a definite advantage, since they may combine both pharmacodynamic (intrinsic intracellular activity) and pharmacokinetic (accumulation) advantages. We also observe differences of intrinsic intracellular activity within the class of fluoroquinolones. Yet, we do not know so far how great and significant those differences can be. For each antibiotic, also, environmental factors can be tested in this system. For instance, we recently showed that acidic pH would decrease the *intrinsic* intracellular activity of macrolides (i.e. activity is lower than expected only on the basis of reduction of accumulation), whereas it increases the intrinsic intracellular activity of fluoroquinolones (Carlier et al in press). Interesting lines of research would be the elucidation of the mechanisms involved in the variations of intrinsic activity of antibiotics and how this activity can be increased.

PERSPECTIVES

The present review has tried to establish some link between intracellular pharmacokinetic parameters of antibiotics and their efficacy against intracellular bacteria. Determining which of these are critical is probably of primary importance in the rational development of new strategies aimed at a better control of bacterial infection. Table 14.2 lists some of the parameters we believe warrant study. Drug-related parameters obviously are of critical importance in the early steps of choosing or designing appropriate compounds. Prodrugs may allow for cellular delivery of diffusible but otherwise non-accumulated substances. The same could be done by coupling antibiotics to appropriate non-diffusile carriers. Great chemical and biological expertise, however, is needed to design modifications that would not lead to irreversible loss of activity (see for example Trouet et al 1982, Bounkhala et al 1988). The cellular and subcellular fate of prodrugs and carrier-coupled drugs will also be different, and the successful strategy will need first to establish where and how the drug is to be targeted.

Cellular parameters will be crucial to determine which are the drugs of choice among those available, and what are the potential target cells. Whereas it is clear that cell accumulation per se is not essential for activity, it is probably fair to say that it will definitely help. So will be the capability of the drug to remain cell-associated (as such or as a bioactive metabolite) so as to offer sustained protection. Toxicological considerations, however, may need to be put in the balance. Subcellular parameters are probably also of critical importance. Yet, to put it in a nutshell, and contrary to what we and others have often claimed (de Duve et al 1974, Trouet & Tulkens 1981, Baillie 1984), it now becomes increasingly clear that a specific subcellular localization may not necessarily be the first best thing for an antimicrobial, given the necessity to track down bacteria in different subcellular compartments. We do not know if this is the reason for the greater activity of fluoroquinolones compared with macrolides. Yet, two key parameters related to intracellular disposition certainly remain crucial, and those are the capability of the drug to reach the target and to act in that environment.

There is little we can do with the available antibiotics concerning the microorganism-related parameters, except to record whether the organisms are sensitive and accessible. Yet, recognition of these parameters may already provide us with more rational choices. Perhaps really new strategies may involve compounds

Table 14.2 Parameters involved in the activity of antimicrobial drugs against intracellular microorganisms

---

Drug-related
  Chemical stability and resistance to cellular enzymes
  Activity at acid pH
  Acid/base properties
  Possibilities to develop prodrugs or to reversibly associate to carriers

Cellular
  Uptake rate (and uptake mechanism)
  Accumulation level
  Efflux (vs retention of a bioactive compound)

Subcellular
  Subcellular localization, with respect to the infected compartment
  Capability of the drug to reach, even if not to accumulate in, infected compartments
  Physicochemical environment where drug has to act

Microorganism-related
  Metabolic state of the organism and/or acquired resistance to environment
  Subcellular localization (infectious vs non-infectious particles)

---

tailored for acting on the bacteria 'as they are', i.e. based on molecular pharmaco-dynamic considerations. Optimal cellular pharmacokinetic properties will then allow us to obtain definitely better agents.

ACKNOWLEDGEMENTS

The experimental work described in this paper was carried out with the collaboration of Drs A. Zenebergh and M. B. Carlier-Blouwer, and Mr B. Scorneaux, and supported by the Belgian *Fonds de la Recherche Scientifique Médicale* (grants no. 3.4516.79 and 3.4553.88 F) and *Services de la Programmation et de la Politique Scientifiques* (grant no. 88-93/122). I was Maître de Recherches of the Belgian *Fonds National de la Recherche Scientifique.*

REFERENCES

Aubert-Tulkens G, Van Hoof F, Tulkens P 1979 Gentamicin-induced lysosomal phospholipidosis in cultured rat fibroblasts. Laboratory Investigation 40: 481-493

Baillie A J 1984 Intracellular infection and drug targeting. Pharmacy International 5: 168-172

Bläser J, Stone B B, Zinner S H 1985 Efficacy of intermittent versus continuous administration of netilmicin in a two-compartment in vitro model. Antimicrobial Agents and Chemotherapy 27: 343-349

Bonventre P F, Imhoff J G 1970 Uptake of ^{3}H-dihydrostreptomycin by macrophages in culture. Infection and Immunity 2: 86-93

Bounkhala Z, Renard C, Baurain R, Ghosez L, Tulkens P M 1988 Coupling products of penicillin V and cephalothin with neutral and acidic aminoacids: synthesis, and susceptibility to carboxypeptidases and lysosomal enzymes. Journal of Medicinal Chemistry 31: 976-983

Brown K N, Percival A 1978 Penetration of antimicrobials into tissue culture cells and leucocytes. Scandinanian Journal of Infectious Diseases 14(suppl): 251-260

Carlier M B, Tulkens P M 1988 Uptake and subcellular localization of lomefloxacin (SC 47111) in phagocytic cells in comparison with pefloxacin and fleroxacin. In: 28th Interscience Conference on Antimicrobial Agents and Chemotherapy, Los Angeles, CA, Abstract 52

Carlier M B, Scorneaux B, Zenebergh A, Tulkens P M 1987a Uptake and subcellular distribution of 4 quinolones (Pefloxacin, Ciprofloxacin, Ofloxacin, RO-23-6240) in phagocytes. In: 27th Interscience Conference on Antimicrobial Agents and Chemotherapy, New York, Abstract 622

Carlier M B, Zenebergh A, Tulkens P M 1987b Cellular uptake and subcellular distribution of roxithromycin and erythromycin in phagocytic cells. Journal of Antimicrobial Chemotherapy 20(B): 47-56

Carlier M B, Scorneaux B, Maquet M, Tulkens P M 1989 Activity of 4 fluoroquinolones (pefloxacin, ciprofloxacin, BMY40062, and BMY40868) against intracellular *S. aureus* in J774 macrophages. In: 29th Interscience Conference on Antimicrobial Agents and Chemotherapy, Houston, TX, Abstract 159

Carlier M B, Faraji S, Tulkens P M in press Uptake and subcellular localization of sparfloxacin (AT4140; RP64206) in phagocytic cells. In: 30th Interscience Conference on Antimicrobial Agents and Chemotherapy, Atlanta, Ga,

Carlier M B, Scorneaux B, Desnottes J F, Tulkens P M in press Cellular uptake, localization and activity of fluoroquinolones in uninfected and infected macrophages. Journal of Antimicrobial Chemotherapy

Chang Y T 1969 Suppressive activity of streptomycin on the growth of *Mycobacterium lepraemurium* in macrophage cultures. Applied Microbiology 17: 750-754

Craven N, Anderson J C 1979 The location of *Staphylococcus aureus* in experimental chronic mastitis in the mouse and the effect on the action of sodium cloxacillin. British Journal of Experimental Pathology 60: 453-459

de Duve C, de Barsy Th, Poole B, Trouet A, Tulkens P, Van Hoof F 1974 Lysosomotropic agents. Biochemical Pharmacology 23: 2495-2531

Dournon E, Rajagopalan P, Vilde J L, Pocidalo J J 1986 Efficacy of pefloxacin in comparison with erythromycin in the treatment of experimental guinea pig legionellosis. Journal of Antimicrobial Chemotherapy 17: 41-48

Easmon C S F, Crane J P 1985 Uptake of ciprofloxacin by macrophages. Journal of Clinical Pathology 38: 442-444

Easmon C S F, Crane J P, Blowers A 1986 Effect of ciprofloxacin on intracellular organisms: in vitro and in vivo studies. Journal of Antimicrobial Chemotherapy 18(D): 43-48

Fattal E, Youssef M, Couvreur P, Andremont A 1989 Treatment of experimental salmonellosis in mice with ampicillin-bound nanoparticles. Antimicrobial Agents and Chemotherapy 33: 1540-1543

Fitzgerorge R B, Gibson D H, Jepras R, Baskerville A 1985 Studies on ciprofloxacin therapy of experimental Legionnaires' disease. Journal of Infection 10: 194-203

Forsgren A, Bellahsène A 1985 Antibiotic accumulation in human polymorphonuclear leucocytes and lymphocytes. Scandinavian Journal of Infectious Diseases 44(suppl): 16-23

Giuliano R A, Verpooten G A, Verbist L, Wedeen R, De Broe M E 1986 In vivo uptake kinetics of aminoglycosides in the kidney cortex of rats. Journal of Pharmacology and Experimental Therapeutics 236: 470-475

Giurgea-Marion L, Toubeau G, Laurent G, Heuson-Stiennon J, Tulkens P M 1986 Impairment of lysosome-pinocytic vesicle fusion in rat kidney proximal tubules after treatment with gentamicin at low doses. Toxicology and Applied Pharmacology 86: 271-285

Gladue R P, Bright G M, Isaacson R E, Newborg M F 1989 In vitro and in vivo uptake of azithromycine (CP-62, 993) in phagocytic cells: possible mechanism of delivery and release at sites of infection. Antimicrobial Agents and Chemotherapy 33: 277-282

Hand W L, King-Thompson N L 1986 Contrasts between phagocyte antibiotic uptake and subsequent intracellular bactericidal activity. Antimicrobial Agents and Chemotherapy 29: 135-140

Hand W L, King-Thompson N L, 1990 Uptake of antibiotics by human polymorphonuclear leukocytes and cytoplasts. Antimicrobial Agents and Chemotherapy 34: 1189-1193

Hand W L, Boozer R M, King-Thompson N L 1985 Antibiotic uptake by alveolar macrophages of smokers. Antimicrobial Agents and Chemotherapy 27: 42-45

Horwitz M A, Silverstein S C 1983 Intracellular multiplication of legionnaires' diseases bacteria (*Legionella pneumophila*) in human monocytes is reversibly inhibited by erythromycin and rifampin. Journal of Clinical Investigation 71: 15-26

Jacobs R F, Wilson C B 1983 Intracellular penetration and antimicrobial activity of antibiotics. Journal of Antimicrobial Chemotherapy 12(C): 13-20

Jacques P 1969 Endocytosis. In: Dingle J T, Fell H B (eds) Lysosomes in biology and pathology, Vol.2. Elsevier/North-Holland Biomedical Press, Amsterdam, pp 395-420

Jenkin C, Benacerraf B 1960 *In vitro* studies on the interaction between mouse peritoneal macrophages and strains of *Salmonella* and *Escherichia coli*. Journal of Experimental Medicine 112: 403-417

Johnson J D, Hand W L, Francis J B, King-Thompson N, Corwin R W 1980 Antibiotic uptake by alveolar macrophages. Journal of Laboratory and Clinical Medicine 95: 429-439

Klempner M S, Styrt B 1981 Clindamycin uptake by human neutrophils. Journal of Infectious Diseases 144: 472-479

Kosek J C, Mazze R I, Cousins M J 1974 Nephrotoxicity of gentamicin. Laboratory Investigation 30: 48-57

Lopez-Saura P, Trouet A, Tulkens P 1978 Analytical fractionation of cultured hepatoma cells (HTC cells). Biochimica et Biophysica Acta 543: 430-449

Mackaness G B 1952 The action of drugs on intracellular tubercle bacilli. Journal of Pathology and Bacteriology 64: 429-446

Mackaness G B, Smith N 1953 The bactericidal action of isoniazid, streptomycin and terramycin on extracellular and intracellular tubercle bacilli. American Journal of Tuberculosis 67: 322-340

Martin J R, Johnson P, Miller M F 1985 Uptake, accumulation and egress of erythromycin by tissue culture cells of human origin. Antimicrobial Agents and Chemotherapy 27: 314-319

Milne M D, Scribner B H, Crawford M A 1958 Non-ionic diffusion and the excretion of weak acids and bases. American Journal of Medicine 24: 709-729

Moore R D, Lietman P S, Smith C R 1987 Clinical response to aminoglycoside therapy: importance of the ratio of peak concentration to minimal inhibitory concentration. Journal of Infectious Diseases 155: 93-99

Morin J P, Fillastre J P 1982 Aminoglycoside-induced lysosomal dysfuntion in kidney. In Whelton A, Neu H C (eds) The aminoglycosides. Marcel Dekker, New York, pp 303-324

Moulder J W 1985 Comparative biology of intracellular parasitism. Microbiological Reviews 49: 298-337

Müller M 1983 Mode of action of metronidazole on anaerobic bacteria and protozoa. Surgery 93: 165-171

Pascual A, Garcia I, Perea E J 1989 Fluorometric measurement of ofloxacin uptake by human polymorphonuclear leukocytes. Antimicrobial Agents and Chemotherapy 33: 653-656

Popescu M C, Swenson C, Ginsberg S 1987 Liposome mediated treatment of viral, bacterial and protozoal infections. In: Ostro J (ed) Liposomes : from biophysics to therapeutics. Marcel Dekker, New York, pp 219-251

Prokesh R C, Hand W L 1982 Antibiotic entry into human polymorphonuclear leukocytes. Antimicrobial Agents and Chemotherapy 21: 373-380

Ralph P, Prichard J, Cohn M 1975 Reticulum cell sarcoma : an effector cell in antibody-dependent cell-mediated immunity. Journal of Immunology 114: 898-905

Renard C, Vanderhaeghe H G, Claes P J, Zenebergh A, Tulkens P M 1987 Influence of conversion of penicillin G into a basic derivative on its accumulation and subcellular localization in cultured macrophages. Antimicrobial Agents and Chemotherapy 31: 410-416

Sanchez M S, Ford C W, Yancey R J Jr 1986 Evaluation of antibacterial agents in a high-volume bovine polymorphonuclear neutrophil *Staphylococcus aureus* intracellular killing assay. Antimicrobial Agents and Chemotherapy 29: 634-638

Scorneaux B, Tulkens P M 1989 Comparative activity of erythromycin and 4 new macrolides (roxithromycin, dirithromycin, rokitamycin, midecamycin) against intracellular *S. aureus* in J774 macrophages. In: 29th Interscience Conference on Antimicrobial Agents and Chemotherapy, Houston, TX, Abstract 157

Scorneaux B, Zenebergh A, Tulkens P M 1989a Contrasting activities of ciprofloxacin, roxithromycin and clindamycin against intracellular *S. aureus* in J774 macrophages. Zeitschrift für Antimikrobielle Antineoplstische Chemotherapie (suppl) 1:144

Scorneaux B, Zenebergh A, Tulkens P M 1989b Activity of two macrolides (erythromycin, roxithromycin) that differ by their degree of cellular accumulation, against *S. aureus* phagocytozed by J774 macrophages. In: 16th International Congress of Chemotherapy, Jerusalem, Israel

Silverblatt F J, Kuehn C 1979 Autoradiography of gentamicin uptake by the rat proximal tubule cell. Kidney International 15: 335-345

Silverstein S C, Steinman R M, Cohn Z A 1977 Endocytosis. Annual Review of Biochemistry 46: 669-722

Snyderman R, Pike M C, Fischer D G, Koren H S 1977 Biologic and biochemical activities of continuous macrophage cell lines P 338 D1 and J 774 1. Journal of Immunology 119: 2060-2066

Steinberg T H, Hand W L 1984 Effects of phagocytosis on antibiotic and nucleoside uptake by human polymorphonuclear leukocytes. Journal of Infectious Diseases 149: 397-403

Suter E 1952 Multiplication of tubercle bacilli within phagocytes cultivated *in vitro*, and effect of streptomycin and isonicotinic acid hydrazide. American Review of Tuberculosis 65: 775-776

Trouet A, Tulkens P 1981 Intracellular penetration and distribution of antibiotics: the basis for an improved chemotherapy. In: Ninet L, Bost P E, Bouanchaud D H, Florent J (eds) The future of antibiotherapy and antibiotic research. Academic Press, London, pp 339-349

Trouet A, Tulkens P, Schneider Y-J 1980 Subcellular localization of infectious agents: pharmacological and pharmacokinetic implications. In: Vanden Bossche H (ed) The host invader interplay. Janssen Research Foundation, Elsevier/North-Holland Biomedical Press, Amsterdam, pp 31-44

Trouet A, Masquelier M, Baurain R, Deprez-De Campeneere D 1982 A covalent linkage between daunorubicin and proteins that is stable in serum and reversible by lysosomal hydrolases, as required for a lysosomotropic drug-carrier conjugate : in vitro and in vivo studies. Proceedings of the National Academy of Sciences (USA) 79: 626-629

Tulkens P, Trouet A 1978 The uptake and intracellular accumulation of aminoglycosides antibiotics in lysosomes of cultured fibroblasts. Biochemical Pharmacology 27: 415-424

Tulkens P M 1985 The design of antibiotics capable of an intracellular action : principles, problems and realization. In: Buri P, Gumma A (eds) Drug targeting. Elsevier Science Publishers, Amsterdam, pp 179-193

Tulkens P M 1989 Nephrotoxicity of aminoglycosides. Toxicology Letters 46: 107-123

van den Broek P J 1989 Antimicrobial drugs, microorganisms and phagocytes. Reviews of Infectious Diseases 11: 213-245

van den Broek P J, Dehue F A M, Leijh P C J, van den Barselaar M Th, van Furth R 1982 The use of lysostaphin in *in vitro* assays of phagocyte function: adherence to and penetration into granulocytes. Scandinavian Journal of Immunology 15: 467-473

van den Broek P J, Buys L F M, Mattie H, van Furth R 1986 The effect of penicillin G on *Staphylococcus aureus* phagocytosed by human monocytes. Journal of Infectious Diseases 153: 586-592

Vildé V L, Dournon E, Rajagopalan P 1986 Inhibition of *Legionella pneumophila* multiplication within human macrophages by antimicrobial agents. Antimicrobial Agents and Chemotherapy 30: 743-748

Villa P, Sassella D, Corada M, Bartosek I 1988a Toxicity, uptake, and subcellular distribution in rat hepatocytes of roxithromycin, a new semisynthetic macrolide, and erythromycin base. Antimicrobial Agents and Chemotherapy 32: 1541-1546

Villa P, Sassella D, Corada M, Bartosek I 1988b Effects of roxithromycin, a new semisynthetic macrolide, and two erythromycins on drug metabolizing-enzymes in rat liver. Journal of Antibiotics 41: 563-569

Waddell W J, Bates R G 1969 Intracellular pH. Physiological Reviews 49: 285-329

Discussion of paper presented by P. M. Tulkens

Discussed by W. Craig
Reported by S. R. Norrby

In discussing Tulkens paper, Craig pointed out that there is an increasing body of evidence that bacteria are also taken up by 'non-professional' phagocytes. The clinical importance of such an uptake can be illustrated by the fact that there are data in endocarditis suggesting that epithelial sequestration of bacteria may be one of the very first steps in the pathogenesis of the disease. Adequate antibiotic concentrations inside epithelial cells would then be a pre-requisite for successful prophylaxis and/or early treatment.

There is also increasing evidence that sequestration into non-professional phagocytes may be an important factor in persistent or relapsing infections. For these reasons one should not look just at antibiotic penetration into phagocytes, but also at non-professional phagocytes, which may be equally important.

Table 14.3 summarizes the data presented by Tulkens and also provides additional data on other drugs he did not discuss. The important thing is that intracellular penetration, whether we look at phagocytes or not, tends to show the same distribution. A problem with interpretation of the clinical relevance of intracellular accumulation of an antibiotic is that, with drugs that enter and leave cells by passive diffusion, accumulation will occur because the drug is either ionically trapped or bound to intracellular structures. The concentration of active drug would then be reflected adequately only by the extracellular concentration. On the other hand, if

Table 14.3 Degree of intracellular penetration; cellular/extracellular levels

Very High C/E > 10	High C/E 2-10	
Clindamycin	Chloramphenicol	Quinolones
Erythromycin	Ethambutol	Tetracycline
Other macrolides	Flucytosine	Trimethoprim
	Lincomycin	Rifampin

Intermediate C/E 0.8-1.5	Low C/E < 0.8	
Aminoglycosides (late)	Aminoglycosides (early)	
Isoniazid	Cephalosporins	
Metronidazole	Imipenem	
	Penicillins	

there is a transport system capable of concentrating the drug intracellularly, then the therapeutic importance would be more obvious.

Finally Craig emphasized the importance of the subcellular localization of intracellular antibiotics. Mycobacteria appear to be capable of evading the phagolysosomes and remain in the phagosomes. Thus, they are in an environment which is not acid and drugs such as aminoglycosides can be active. By using liposomal aminoglycosides it may then be possible to get enough drug into the cell to achieve sufficient concentrations in the phagosomes by intracellular diffusion. Another example of the importance of activity of antibiotics in phagosomes is erythromycin and legionella, an organism which locates in the phagosome where there is no risk of reduced erythromycin activity due to an acid pH.

In the general discussion of Tulken's presentation it was pointed out that the knowledge of the mechanisms responsible for active transport of antibiotics from a cell are incompletely studied. Some studies have indicated that both β-lactams and quinolones are removed from cells by an organic anion transport system, which should be blocked by probenecid. It was also emphasized, that in terms of intracellular drug penetration and distribution, very little information is available on the differences between normal macrophages and those macrophages that are infected or activated. Data are also lacking for the in vivo situation. In this context, it was pointed out that one problem—hitherto impossible to solve—is that the time lapse between tissue sampling and the analytic procedure is so long that considerable loss of intracellular antibiotic concentrations could be expected. This would be especially true if the antibiotic entered and left the cells by passive diffusion.

15. One microbial heat shock protein and two autoimmune diseases

I. R. Cohen

INTRODUCTION TO ANTIGENIC MIMICRY

The immune response of the host to a microbial invader can trigger an autoimmune response of the host to self-antigens; so many have concluded in noting acute rheumatic fever following infection with the group A streptococcus, reactive arthritis after infection with enteric bacteria, and ankylosing spondylitis associated with *Klebsiella* infection. One idea put forward to explain how microbial immunity can trigger autoimmunity has been molecular mimicry, that is, antigenic cross-reactivity between an epitope on a microbial antigen and a self-epitope of the host (Damian 1988). In responding to such a microbial epitope the host inadvertently responds to itself.

Despite its logic, the concept of molecular mimicry as a cause of autoimmune disease has relatively little experimental evidence in its favour.

Consultation of a library of amino acid sequences of proteins reveals that hosts and their parasites (be they viruses, bacteria or eukaryotes) express proteins with segments of identity or near identity. Chemical similarity can surely produce immunological similarity. Nevertheless, to blame molecular mimicry for an autoimmune disease, the tests of causality must be satisfied.

Postulates for incriminating an antigen as a cause of autoimmune disease are:

1. The disease, should it arise spontaneously, must be accompanied by an immune response to the specific epitope.
2. Premeditated immunization with the epitope should induce the disease.
3. T- or B-cells (antibodies) reactive to the epitope should transfer the disease to naive recipients.
4. Termination of the immune response to the epitope (immunological tolerance) should terminate the disease.

Until recently, few if any mimicking epitopes fulfilled all of these requirements. The experimental model coming closest to doing so has been the disease of rats called adjuvant arthritis (AA).

AA is a progressive, destructive inflammation of the joints of the extremities induced in genetically susceptible strains of rats by immunization to killed *Mycobacterium tuberculosis* (MT) (Pearson 1956). It has been suggested that AA may

263

serve as a model of some aspects of rheumatoid arthritis of humans (Pearson 1964). If AA is really an autoimmune disease induced by immunization to an epitope of MT, what is the nature of the molecular mimicry?

This article reviews investigations using a T-cell clone which have led to the discovery that the 65 kDa heat-shock protein (hsp65) of MT (MT-hsp65) is a candidate for the molecular mimicry between MT and joints. Also described are very recent experiments indicating that hsp65 may be the target antigen in the spontaneous autoimmune diabetes of the NOD strain of mice. Finally, some general questions arising from these observations regarding microbial immunity, autoimmunity and hsp65 are considered.

AUTOIMMUNE T-CELLS, AA AND HSP65

Our approach to the analysis and control of experimental autoimmune diseases has been to isolate in vitro lines and clones of autoimmune T-cells capable of causing particular organ-specific autoimmune diseases in rats and mice (Ben-Nun et al 1981a, Cohen 1986, 1988). Having the aetiological agents of autoimmune diseases in hand has made it possible to study pathogenesis—how the T-cells actually cause the disease. Moreover, we have been able to attenuate such autoimmune T-cells and use them as vaccines to induce resistance to the specific autoimmune process (Ben-Nun et al 1981b, Lider et al 1987, 1988, Cohen and Atlan 1989).

The use of the T-cell line approach to AA was initiated by Holoshitz et al (1983) who isolated line A2, a line of helper T-lymphocytes that could be used either to transfer AA or to vaccinate rats against AA induced by active immunization to MT. From line A2, Holoshitz et al (1984) isolated arthritogenic clone A2b. This clone, selected by its responsiveness to MT in vitro and for its ability to cause arthritis in vivo was used as a probe to answer the mimicry question: what does A2b see in MT and in joint tissue that can account for AA?

The question was studied by van Eden et al (1985) who discovered that A2b recognized crude preparations of protein from the cartilage proteoglycan of the rat joint. This led to the hypothesis that AA was caused by T-cells that responded to an epitope of MT antigenically cross-reactive with an epitope of the joint proteoglycan (Cohen et al 1985).

Turning to the MT organism itself, van Eden et al (1988) then discovered that clone A2b recognized the hsp65 molecule of MT (Thole et al 1985).

The hsp65 molecule, similar to other hsp molecules, is among the most conserved proteins in evolution with about 50% of the amino acid residues being identical for the hsp65 molecules of MT and humans (Jindal et al 1989). Hence, hsp65 should contain a treasury of cross-reactive epitopes between host and parasite.

Detailed analysis of the particular epitope led to identification of the nine amino acids comprising positions 180-188 in the sequence of MT-hsp65 (van Eden et al 1988). Surprisingly, this sequence is one of the variable parts of hsp65 and shows no homology between the bacterial and mammalian molecules (Jindal et al 1989). Thus it was not likely that the extensive mimicry between much of the MT and rat hsp65 molecules was related to AA.

Recall, however, that clone A2b was found to recognize an epitope in cartilage proteoglycan (van Eden et al 1985). Indeed, very weak homology was found between the 180-188 peptide and the link protein of the cartilage proteoglycan (van Eden et al 1988) giving rise to the hypothesis that this mimicry could explain AA (Cohen 1988). Subsequent work, however, has shown that clone A2b, at least in vitro does not respond to the particular link protein sequence (in preparation). So we are still without a meaningful mimicry to explain the association of MT-hsp65 with AA.

Moreover, the MT hsp65 molecule does not satisfy fully the tests of causality in AA. A2b, which recognizes MT-hsp65, can transfer AA and T-cell vaccination with attenuated A2b can be used to prevent or treat AA (Lider et al 1987), but immunization with MT hsp65 itself has not been shown to induce AA. In fact, such immunization only prevents AA (van Eden et al 1988). Strangely, treatment with MT-hsp65 has also been found to prevent arthritis induced by streptococcal cell walls (van den Broek et al 1989). Hence, it is conceivable that hsp65 and immunity to it might have some regulatory function in immunological arthritis beyond a simple antigenic mimicry (Lamb et al 1989).

HSP65 AND AUTOIMMUNE DIABETES

In contrast to AA, which is artificially induced by immunization, the autoimmune diabetes of NOD strain mice is a spontaneous disease (Rossini et al 1985). It begins with chronic inflammation of the pancreatic islets, insulitis, at about 4-5 weeks of age resulting in destruction of the insulin-producing β-cells. T-cells rather than autoantibodies probably cause the disease (Bendelac et al 1987). The loss of β-cells progresses until overt diabetes becomes clinically evident when the residual β-cells are no longer able to secrete sufficient insulin to maintain glucose homoeostatis. Female mice in most NOD colonies develop a much higher incidence of diabetes than do male mice.

While studying the autoimmune process of β-cell destruction, we chanced upon the observation that early insulitis at 1-2 months of age was accompanied by the appearance in the blood of affected mice of an antigen cross-reactive with MT-hsp65 (Elias et al 1990). Autoantibodies to this MT-hsp65 cross-reactive antigen developed several weeks after the antigen appeared in the blood.

It seemed reasonable to suppose that the MT-hsp65 cross-reactive antigen in the blood of the mice developing diabetes was mouse hsp65 that might have originated as a consequence of the stress of insulitis and β-cell destruction. However, to our surprise, further investigation led to the fulfilment of the postulates for incriminating the hsp65 cross-reactive antigen as a cause of autoimmune diabetes.
The following were observed:

1. Immunity to the antigen was associated with spontaneous diabetes; only mice that manifested reactivity went on to develop diabetes, mice that escaped diabetes did not respond to the hsp65 antigen.
2. Immunization of one-month-old prediabetic mice with the hsp65 antigen in adjuvant induced heightened insulitis and hyperglycaemia within two weeks.
3. T-cell clones specifically responsive to the hsp65 antigen transferred diabetes to prediabetic NOD mice.

4. Administration of hsp65 in a non-immunogenic form led to a decrease in spontaneous immune reactivity to the antigen and aborted the development of spontaneous diabetes.

Subsequent experiments (Elias et al in preparation) demonstrated that the key epitope recognized by the autoimmune effector T cells is primarily within the hsp65 molecule of the human or mouse; the MT-hsp65 molecule is only cross-reactive. Furthermore, a 12 amino acid peptide in the mammalian hsp65 sequence seems to comprise the epitope.

A most important question as yet unanswered is what immunity to the hsp65 molecule has to do with organ-specific damage to β-cells. We have detected a high spontaneous expression of the hsp65 molecule in normal β-cells (Elias et al in preparation) and the molecule or part of it may have a physiological function in healthy β-cells. In support of this hypothesis is our observation that immunization to human hsp65 of non-diabetic strains of mice such as C57BL/6 or C3H.eB can induce persistent diabetes (Elias et al in preparation). Thus the association of hsp65 with diabetes is not a genetic peculiarity of NOD mice.

ONE ANTIGEN AND TWO MIMICRIES

The above results indicate that two different experimental autoimmune diseases might be related in varying degrees to immunity to a bacterial hsp65 molecule: AA induced in rats and diabetes developing spontaneously in NOD mice. If these experimental diseases faithfully model clinical autoimmune disease of humans, such as rheumatoid arthritis or type I diabetes mellitus, then it is quite possible that anti-hsp65 immunity could play a role in these entities too. Indeed, rheumatoid arthritis patients have elevated T-cell reactivity to MT-hsp65 (Res et al 1988).

How can we explain two such different expressions of immunity to a single antigen? The simplest explanation appears to be multiple mimicries. The ability of MT-hsp65 to induce diabetes derives from its cross-reactivity with the mouse's own hsp65 molecule at the key epitope. In contrast, the association of the MT-hsp65 with AA may be related to the mimicry of an epitope of MT-hsp65, not with the mammalian hsp65 molecule, but rather with an epitope present on another molecule in cartilage (van Eden et al 1989). This mimicry and its function in the arthritic process must be clarified to prove the hypothesis.

The mimicry between MT-hsp65 and mouse hsp65 responsible for diabetes is clear, but the expression and function of hsp65 in the β-cell is unknown. Hence, this story too is yet incomplete. If and how these mimicries function in human autoimmune arthritis or diabetes is also an open question.

HSP65 AND MICROBIAL IMMUNITY

In addition to its association with two very different autoimmune diseases, immunity to hsp65 is a prominent feature of the immune response to bacteria (Young et al 1988). Around the time my colleagues and I were unwittingly led to hsp65 through our interest in autoimmunity, laboratories interested in the immunology of bacterial infection were identifying hsp65 as a dominant, common microbial antigen (Young et al 1987). Bacterial hsp65 is a common target for immune responses in individuals or animals infected or vaccinated with whole bacteria. Of all the bacterial macromolecules available for immune responses, hsp65 dominantly attracts the attention of the immune response. Indeed, it has been reported that 1 of every 5 mouse lymphocytes responding to antigens of mycobacteria is focused on the hsp65 molecule (Kaufmann et al 1987). It seems that dominant focus on hsp65 in infection does not usually trigger autoimmune disease. Nevertheless, AA and the diabetes of NOD mice teach us that an immune response to microbial hsp65 is not without such hazard. Why then does the immune system predictably choose to focus on this dangerous molecule?

Common sense suggests that self-like molecules, because of self-tolerance, should be very weakly immunogenic, if at all. Microbial hsp65 demonstrates the opposite; an overlap between the dominance of an antigen in autoimmunity and its dominance in infection.

The immune system has been fashioned by the selective pressures of surviving infection. Therefore, if the host's response to a particular microbial molecule is dominant in the host-parasite interaction, it is reasonable to suspect that the response to that antigen should serve the host. In other words we should consider the evolutionary advantages of having the microbial hsp65 molecule targeted by the host. Alternatively, it is conceivable that channelling the host response to hsp65 primarily serves the interests of the parasite. However, since the response to hsp65 is a common feature of the response to well-adapted mycobacteria and to usually benign enteric bacteria, it is likely that the response to hsp65 has evolved to serve both the host and microbial parasite in maintaining their equilibrium.

Another problem is to understand how the dominance of the hsp65 molecule as an antigen is encoded in the immune system (Cohen 1990). How does it attract so much attention by the system? Here too the definitive answers are lacking. The question, however, calls attention to the intimate relationship that must exist between the way the immune system views the microbe and the way it views the self (Shoenfeld & Cohen 1987). Hsp65 may hold a key to the balance between self-tolerance and microbial intolerance in a world in which it is becoming clear just how immunologically similar the host and parasite must be.

ACKNOWLEDGEMENTS

I thank Mrs Doris Ohayon for expert and dedicated help in preparing the manuscript. Parts of the research upon which this article is based were supported by the NIH (AR 32192), by the Juvenile Diabetes Foundation International, and by the Minerva Foundation. I am the encumbant of the Mauerberger Chair.

REFERENCES

Bendelac A, Carnaud C, Boitard C, Bach J F 1987 Syngeneic transfer of autoimmune diabetes from diabetic NOD mice to healthy neonates. Requirement for both L3T4⁺ and Lyt-2⁺ T cells. Journal of Experimental Medicine 166: 823-832

Ben-Nun A, Wekerle H, Cohen I R 1981a The rapid isolation of clonable antigen-specific T lymphocyte lines capable of mediating autoimmune encephalomyelitis. European Journal of Immunology 11: 195-199

Ben-Nun A, Wekerle H, Cohen I R 1981b Vaccination against autoimmune encephalomyelitis with T lymphocyte line cells reactive against myelin basic protein. Nature 292: 60-61

Cohen I R 1986 Regulation of autoimmune disease: physiological and therapeutic. Immunological Reviews 94: 5-21

Cohen I R 1988 The self, the world and autoimmunity. Scientific American 258: 52-60

Cohen I R 1990 Natural id-anti-id networks and the immunological homunculus. In: Atlan H, Cohen I R (eds) Theories of immune networks. Springer-Verlag, Berlin pp 6-12

Cohen I R, Atlan H 1989 Network regulation of autoimmunity: an automaton model. Journal of Autoimmunity 2: 613-625

Cohen I R, Holoshitz J, Van Eden W, Frenkel A 1985 T lymphocyte clones illuminate pathogenesis and effect therapy of experimental arthritis. Arthritis and Rheumatism 28: 841-845

Damian R T 1988 Parasites and molecular mimicry. In: Lernmark A, Dryberg T, Terenius L, Hokfelt B (eds) Molecular mimicry in health and disease. Elsevier, Amsterdam, pp 211-218

Elias D, Markovits D, Reshef T, Van der Zee R Cohen IR 1990 Induction and therapy of autoimmune diabetes in the non-obese diabetic (NOD/LT) mouse by a 65-kDa heat shock protein. Proceedings of the National Academy of Sciences (USA) 87: 1576-1580

Holoshitz J, Naparstek Y, Ben-Nun A, Cohen IR 1983 Lines of T lymphocytes induce or vaccinate against autoimmune arthritis. Science 219: 56-58

Holoshitz J, Matitiau A, Cohen I R 1984 Arthritis induced in rats by clones of T lymphocytes responsive to mycobacteria but not to Collagen type II. Journal of Clinical Investigation 73: 211-215

Jindal S, Dudani A K, Harley C B, Singh B, Gupta R S 1989 Primary structure of a human mitochondrial protein homologous to the bacterial and plant chaperonins and to the 65-kilodalton mycobacterial antigen. Molecular and Cellular Biology 9: 2279-2283

Kaufmann S H E, Vath U, Thole J E R, Van Embden J D A, Emmrich F 1987 Enumeration of T cells reactive with Mycobacterium tuberculosis organisms and specific for the recombinant mycobacterial 64 kilodalton protein. European Journal of Immunology 17: 351-357

Lamb J R, Bal V, Mendez-Samperio P et al 1989 Stress proteins may provide a link between the immune response to infection and autoimmunity. International Immunology 1: 191-196

Lider O, Karin N, Shinitzky M, Cohen I R 1987 Therapeutic vaccination against adjuvant arthritis using autoimmune T lymphocytes treated with hydrostatic pressure. Proceedings of the National Academy of Sciences (USA) 84: 4577-4580

Lider O, Reshef T, Beraud E, Ben-Nun A, Cohen I R 1988 Anti-idiotypic network induced by T cell vaccination against experimental autoimmune encephalomyelitis. Science 239: 181-183

Pearson C M 1956 Development of arthritis, periarthritis and periostitis in rats given adjuvant. Proceedings of the Society for Experimental Biology and Medicine 91: 95-101

Pearson C M 1964 Experimental models in rheumatoid disease. Arthritis and Rheumatism 7: 80-86

Res P C M, Schaar C G, Breedveld F C et al 1988 Synovial fluid T cell reactivity against 65KD heat shock protein of mycobacteria in early chronic arthritis. Lancet ii: 478-480

Rossini A A, Mordes J P, Like A A 1985 Immunology of insulin-dependent diabetes mellitus. Annual Review of Immunology 3: 289-321

Shoenfeld Y, Cohen I R 1987 Infection and autoimmunity. In: Sela M (ed) The antigens, vol vii. Academic Press, San Diego, pp 307-325

Thole J E R, Dauwerse H G, Das R K, Groothuis D G, Schouls L M, Van Embden J D A 1985 Cloning of Mycobacterium bovis BCG DNA and expression of antigens in E. coli. Infection and Immunity 50: 800-806

Van den Broek M F, Hogervorst E J M, Van Bruggen M C J, Van Eden W, Van der Zee, Van der Berg W B 1989 Protection against streptococcal cell wall-induced arthritis by pretreatment with the 65-kD mycobacterial heat shock protein. Journal of Experimental Medicine 170: 449-466

Van Eden W, Holoshitz J, Nevo Z, Frenkel A, Klajman A, Cohen I R 1985 Arthritis induced by a T lymphocyte clone that responds to Mycobacterium tuberculosis and to cartilage proteoglycans. Proceedings of the National Academy of Sciences (USA) 82: 5064-5067

Van Eden W, Thole J E R, Van Der Zee R et al 1988 Cloning of the mycobaterial epitope recognized by T lymphocytes in adjuvant arthritis. Nature 31: 171-173

Van Eden W, Hogervorst E J M, Van der Zee R, Van Embden J D A, Cohen I R 1989 A cartilage mimicking T cell epitope on a 65 kD mycobacterial heat-shock protein: adjuvant arthritis as a model for human rheumatoid arthritis. Current Topics in Microbiology and Immunology 145: 27-43

Young D B, Ivanyi J, Cox J H, Lamb J R 1987 The 65kDa antigen of mycobacteria: a common bacterial antigen. Immunology Today 8: 215-219

Young D, Lathigra R, Hendrix R, Sweetser D, Young R A 1988 Stress proteins as immune targets in leprosy and tuberculosis. Proceedings of the National Academy of Sciences 85: 4267-4270

268

Discussion of paper presented by I. R. Cohen

Discussed by R. M. Bernstein
Reported by S. R. Norrby

In his discussion of Cohen's paper, Bernstein emphasized the complexity of the immune reactions in rheumatoid diseases and diabetes. For example, the A2b clone of the hsp65 protein induces arthritis in rats while the A2c clone, which reacts with the same epitope of hsp65, prevents arthritis in the same model. In mice and humans there is recent work showing that an early sign of development of diabetes is emergence of antibodies to a 64 kDa protein of the β-cells. However, it is not known whether that protein is a heat shock protein.

In his own studies, Bernstein and co-workers have demonstrated antibodies against a 63 kDa protein from drosophila cell lines in patients with ankylosing spondylitis. This protein appeared to be a heat shock protein and reacted with a monoclonal against the mycobacterial hsp65 protein. However, although there was a prominent response to the drosophila protein in patients with ankylosing spondylitis, such response was found only rarely in patients with rheumatoid arthritis. Moreover, the antibody titres in ankylosing spondylitis patients were low; in addition the antibodies were mostly of the IgA class, as opposed to rheumatoid arthritis or lupus, where autoimmune antibodies are present in vast amounts and are of the IgG class. This seems to indicate that the IgA antibody levels in patients with ankylosing spondylitis, which correlate well with the total IgA levels, are controlled.

A concern expressed was that impurities in protein preparations may influence the experimental results. One example is that T-cells which were responsive to a 65 kDa protein from *M. leprae* responded much better to an *E. coli* hsp65 protein, and even more so to intact *E. coli* cells.

In the general discussion it was emphasized that the adjuvant arthritis animal is not always as simple as it may appear. If a mycobacterial preparation were to be injected intracutaneously at sites only 3 mm apart, in different animals of the same clone, the animals will develop either adjuvant arthritis or protection against adjuvant arthritis, dependent on the site of injection. There are also differences not only with respect to animal's sex, but also to the type and degree of bacterial colonization. Results in gnotobiotic animals also differ from those in non-gnotobiotic animals.

Section VI: Immunomodulators

Chairman: J. Verhoef

16. The interleukins and their use as therapeutic agents

C. S. Henney

INTRODUCTION

The immune response, and specifically the growth and differentiation of T- and B-lymphocytes, is regulated by a group of protein hormones collectively termed interleukins. Ten proteins of this group have been identified to date and the genes encoding them cloned. At least four of them, interleukin-1 (IL-1), interleukin-2 (IL-2), interleukin-4 (IL-4), and interleukin-7 (IL-7) have been shown to play a major role in lymphopoiesis and thus are of determining significance in controlling immune responsiveness. The others, and in particular interleukin-3 (IL-3), seem to function predominantly in the growth, differentiation or activation of non-lymphoid cells.

The interleukins are all single-chain polypeptides, but bear no structural homology to each other. There is therefore no interleukin gene family, as there is for example, among the interferons, and the classification of a given hormone as an interleukin is a rather tenuous one. Two features are shared by all the proteins classified to date as interleukins: (i) they are all growth or differentiation factors for leukocytes, and (ii) their activities are mediated by interaction with distinctive transmembrane proteins on the surface of target cells. Such proteins are termed interleukin receptors and they, in contrast to the ligands with which they interact, do have common structural features and appear to be members of a common ancestral gene family (Goodwin et al 1990).

There is no functional rationale for the numbering system among interleukins, rather it reflects, in a general sense, the order in which the proteins were initially described. Because of their broad activities on cells of the immune system, it has long been speculated that the interleukins might be useful therapeutically, to modulate and specifically to stimulate immune responsiveness. While IL-2 and IL-4 have indeed been studied clinically, their ability to potentiate the immune response has been little regarded. Rather, as will be discussed, most of the clinical emphasis has been placed on the ability of IL-2 to stimulate cytotoxic cells. More recently, IL-3, on account of its ability to stimulate the growth and differentiation of several leukocyte precursor populations, has also been explored clinically for its ability to stimulate haematopoiesis.

It is beyond the scope of this paper to review comprehensively the vast literature on the biochemistry of the interleukins, their receptors and all aspects of their clinical uses. Rather, attention will be focused on a limited number of recent observations, one set based on new structural and biological insights, the other on recent clinical studies. These observations have been selected because of the impact they have had on the field and because of the author's proximity to some of the studies. On the pre-clinical front, attention will be focused on IL-4 and IL-7 and the role that these proteins play in lymphocyte differentiation. The variability of the clinical effects of IL-2 as an adjunct to cellular therapy in cancer will be discussed.

To set these recent findings into our current understanding of the interleukins as a group, each of the proteins will be reviewed briefly and an attempt then made to integrate their activities in the context of immune responsiveness.

INTERLEUKINS AS REGULATORS OF IMMUNE RESPONSIVENESS

The biological activities attributed to *interleukin-1* (IL-1) are very broad and encompass the ability to initiate thymocyte and fibroblast proliferation; bone resorption (through osteoclast activation); acute-phase protein release from hepatocytes; and stimulation of neutrophil secretion (Dinarello 1984). IL-1 has two principal activities that relate to immune responsiveness: (i) the ability to stimulate IL-2 formation, which is the principal T-lymphocyte growth and differentiation factor, and (ii) the stimulation of pluripotent stem cells, making these cells susceptible to the action of both haemopoietic and, more specifically, lymphopoietic, growth factors.

Interestingly, and unique among the interleukins, there are two proteins that possess the full range of biological activities characteristic of IL-1 (March et al 1985). These proteins have been termed IL-1α and IL-1β and they are encoded by two distinct genes. IL-1α and IL-1β bear little structural homology (25% at the amino acid level), but bind to a common receptor, through which they manifest their activities (Dower et al 1986). The gene encoding this receptor has recently been cloned (Sims et al 1988).

Interleukin-2 was the first lymphokine to be chemically characterized and the gene encoding it was the first interleukin gene to be identified (Taniguchi et al 1983). The identification of IL-2 as the hormone controlling T-cell proliferation and differentiation has had an enormous impact on immunology (see for example Smith 1988). IL-2 is absolutely required for the production of fully differentiated T-cells, which function as the effector cells of the cell-mediated immune response. IL-2 also causes the proliferation of T-helper cells, that T-cell subset responsible for the production of the majority of cytokines (including the interleukins). Resting T-cells do not, however, make IL-2, nor do they respond to IL-2 when it is exogenously added. Further, IL-2 receptors are not detectable on the majority of freshly isolated T-cells. Antigen is the primary stimulus for both IL-2 production and for IL-2 receptor display. IL-2, acting via its specific receptor, acts in the late G_1 phase of the cell cycle, causing DNA synthesis in activated T-cells. The role of IL-2 in the differentiation of cytotoxic T-cells by acting on both cytotoxic precursor cells and the phenotypically distinctive lymphokine-producing cells is outlined in Figure 16.1.

In addition to its action on T-cells, IL-2 has also been shown to be capable of causing the proliferation and differentiation of antigen-activated B-cells, thereby

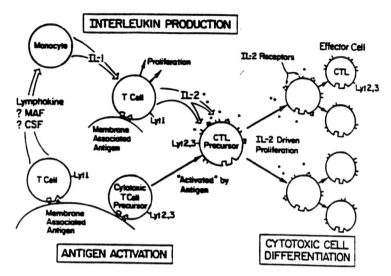

Figure 16.1 The role of interleukins-1 and -2 in cytotoxic T-cell differentiation (after Henney 1989b)

increasing antibody responses. Furthermore, IL-2 has effects on lymphoid precursor cells, which lack surface markers of mature T- and B-cells, inducing a portion of them to become cytotoxic. These cells have been termed lymphokine-activated killer (or LAK) cells and have, as will be discussed, been used, in conjunction with IL-2, to treat cancer patients (Rosenberg et al 1985).

Interleukin-3 appears not to be involved in lymphopoiesis, but is a powerful potentiator of haematopoiesis, functioning as a pluripotent growth factor, encouraging the proliferation of cells of the granulocytic, monocytic and megakaryocytic lineages (Fung et al 1984). Clinical trials using IL-3 to stimulate haematopoiesis began in 1988, but although there have been early reports of positive effects on the rate of platelet differentiation, the studies are yet too few to allow evaluation.

The protein termed *interleukin-4* was originally described as an activity which stimulated the proliferation of purified B-cell populations in the presence of anti-μ chain antisera (O'Garra et al 1986). It is thus viewed as the biological analogue of IL-2, but with B-cells rather than T-cells as its target. The human gene encoding IL-4 has been cloned (Lee et al 1986) and clinical trials aimed at evaluating the therapeutic efficacy of IL-4 have begun.

IL-4, although originally identified as a protein which causes the proliferation of activated B-cells has also been shown to enhance antibody synthesis, to promote immunoglobulin gene class switching from IgM to IgG_1, and to enhance the expression of class II MHC molecules on resting B-cells. Interestingly, IL-4 has also been shown to increase IgE production by LPS-activated B-cells (Coffman & Carty 1986).

Because IL-4 was originally purified and cloned by following its activity on B-cells, it was frequently referred to in the literature by names that alluded to this activity: B-cell stimulation factor (BSF-1) and B-cell growth factor (BCGF). It came as somewhat of a surprise, therefore, when it was observed that some T-cell lines also proliferated in the presence of IL-4, indicating that IL-4 had both T- and B-cell stimulatory activities (Widmer et al 1987).

In initial studies with a small number of T-cell clones, it appeared that IL-4 served primarily as a growth factor for CD8$^+$ (formerly Ly2$^+$; cytotoxic/suppressor phenotype) T cells, whereas so-called helper T-cell clones (CD4$^+$/CD8$^-$ phenotype) proliferated weakly, if at all, in the presence of IL-4. This stood in contrast to the proliferative effects of IL-2 on T-cells, which show no subclass specificity. Later, on analysis of a much larger set of both human and mouse T-cell clones, including those that are both antigen dependent and independent, the preference for cells of the CD8$^+$ phenotype was still apparent but was not absolute: CD4$^+$ T-cell clones can also proliferate in response to IL-4. An examination of the proliferative response to IL-2 and IL-4 of several cytotoxic T-lymphocyte (CTL) clones demonstrated that IL-4 responsive cells comprise a subset of cells which respond to IL-2.

Subsequently, Widmer et al (1987) have shown that IL-4 can act as a potent helper factor for the generation of cytotoxic T-cells in mixed lymphocyte culture (MLC) and, furthermore, that IL-4 shared with IL-2 the ability to induce cytolytic activity in 'memory' cell cultures, even in the absence of antigen.

Recently, these same investigators have shown that IL-4 and IL-2 are both produced in mixed lymphocyte reactions, but with different kinetics; IL-2 being produced early, IL-4 later. Both lymphokines appear to contribute independently to the differentiation of cytotoxic cells, for antibodies specific for IL-2 or IL-4 only partially suppress effector cell production, whereas mixtures of anti-IL-2 and anti-IL-4 antibodies are needed to arrest completely cytotoxic T-cell development.

IL-2, as was mentioned earlier, is characterized by its ability to generate directly a population of cytotoxic cells (termed lymphokine-activated killer or LAK cells) when cultured with normal, unstimulated, lymphocyte populations. IL-4 was found not to possess this ability directly, but appears to synergize with IL-2 in inducing these cells. The significance of this observation is unclear, but seems certain to be pursued by those interested in exploiting the potential antitumour effects of LAK cells.

The response to IL-2 and IL-4 of several functionally defined lymphoid cell types has recently been assessed at the individual responding cell level in limiting dilution cultures in which exogenous IL-2 or IL-4 was used to promote cellular activation and expansion (Widmer et al 1987). Splenic precursors that give rise to alloreactive cytotoxic T-cells in cultures supplemented with IL-2 were approximately three-fold more frequent than those detected with IL-4. Of special interest was the observation that cytolytic cultures arising in primary allogeneic cultures supplemented with IL-4 exhibited a greater degree of lytic specificity than did those arising in IL-2. This difference may be due to an inherently broader specificity of cytotoxic T-cells cultured in IL-2, but is more likely explained by a concomitant activation of CTL and LAK in individual IL-2 supplemented microcultures. In this regard, estimation of LAK-precursor frequencies in cultures established without an overt antigenic stimulus revealed that IL-2 activates a twenty-fold higher frequency of LAK precursors than does IL-4.

Interleukin-5 was originally described as a B-cell growth factor, stimulating the proliferation of the BCL$_1$ leukaemic cell line and of normal B-cells following their activation with dextran sulphate (Swain & Dutton 1982). Following the cloning of the mouse and human genes encoding for this protein, IL-5 was also shown to increase immunoglobulin (Ig) secretion by dextran sulphate activated murine B-cells, as well as initiating B-cell proliferation (Kishimoto & Hirano 1988). The immunoglobulin isotype most frequently enhanced by IL-5 in activated mouse B-cell populations is IgA. Murine IL-5 has also been shown to function as a B-cell maturation factor, inducing maturation of resting B-cells without proliferation.

Interestingly, while the effects of murine IL-5 on mouse B-cells have been readily demonstrable, the principal effects of the human analogue protein appear to be directed towards the eosinophil. IL-5 in man is a potent eosinophil differentiation factor. Whether, physiologically, it also plays a role in lymphopoiesis is, at this point, unknown.

Interleukin-6 is a protein factor produced by human T-cells which induces increased immunoglobulin production by plasmacytomas, hybridomas and lymphoblastoid cell lines. Because of this activity, the factor has also been referred to as B-cell differentiating factor (BCDF) and B-cell stimulatory factor-2 (BSF-2). The gene encoding IL-6 was first cloned from an HTLV-transformed T-cell line (Hirano et al 1986). Somewhat surprisingly, consideration of its nucleotide sequence revealed it to be identical to that of a gene previously described to encode β-2 interferon (Zilberstein et al 1986), a protein, which, like others of the interferon family was characterized by its virus-neutralizing properties. Recent studies have revealed that IL-6 is pleiomorphic, having stimulatory activities on both hepatocytes and nerve cells in addition to lymphocytes (Gauldie et al 1987). The precise role, if any, that IL-6 plays in B-cell differentiation awaits clarification. It has continued to be easy to demonstrate that IL-6 supports Ig secretion by lymphoblastoid cells and by hybridomas, but difficult to establish that it has a similar role with normal B-cell populations.

A major impediment to the study of lymphocyte development has been the difficulty associated with obtaining enriched populations of lymphoid precursor cells. One approach that has proven useful in this regard, however, was initially developed by Whitlock et al (1983) and employs an adherent (or 'feeder') layer of stromal-derived fibroblasts, macrophages and endothelial cells to support the growth of non-adherent lymphoid precursor cells. One population of cells from such cultures are characterized by their cytoplasmic display of μ antigen (but absence of surface μ) in the absence of cytoplasmic light-chain. These cells are believed to be pre-B-cells, the immediate precursors of mature functional pluripotent B-cells. A factor derived from murine bone marrow stromal cells supported the proliferation of these pre-B-cells and, as this activity could not be duplicated by other known soluble factors (including interleukins-1-6), it was considered to be the property of a unique factor, which was termed *interleukin-7* (IL-7).

By preparation of a clonal cell line from the stromal elements of a long-term mouse bone marrow culture, a reproducible source of IL-7 was obtained and, following purification to homogeneity of the protein from these cells (Namen et al 1988a), a strategy was developed (shown in Fig. 16.2) which led Namen et al (1988b) to succeed in cloning the gene encoding murine IL-7. Cross-hybridization led to the isolation of a human cDNA encoding the human IL-7 protein.

As was expected from its original activity in bone marrow cultures, IL-7 was shown to support the proliferation of B-cell precursors but showed no activity whatsoever against B-cells or plasma cells. It was further found that on fractionation of the cells

K

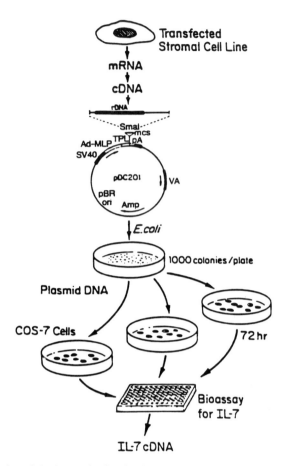

Figure 16.2 Overview of cloning murine interleukin-7 cDNA (after Namen et al 1988b)

present in long-term bone marrow cultures on the basis of B220 antigen display, into B220⁻ cells (which are pro-B-cells, the precursor of pre-B-cells) and the B220⁺ pre-B-cells, both cell populations proliferated in the presence of IL-7, but not in the presence of other known lymphokines. Thus, the pro-B-cell, which lacks cytoplasmic μ, like the pre-B-cell (in which the immunoglobulin heavy-chain gene has been rearranged and expressed in the cytoplasm) are both IL-7 responsive. Furthermore, clonal cell lines that are IL-7 dependent have been derived, suggesting that the stimulus exerted by IL-7 is a direct action on the responding cell. How early in B-cell development IL-7 acts, awaits precise definition, but recent reports that non-adherent cells from long-term bone marrow cultures have the ability to reconstitute both B-cell and T-cell compartments in vivo suggest the possibility that IL-7 is active on a lymphoid stem cell.

These suggestions led to the examination of the effects of IL-7 on cells of the T-cell lineage. Resting spleen cells did not respond to IL-7, but Con A blasts did; although to a lesser extent than their responses to IL-2 or IL-4 (Namen, Widmer & Grabstein, unpublished observations). Interestingly, the earliest (CD4⁻, CD8⁻) thymocytes respond to IL-7 but both CD4⁺ and DC8⁺ cell populations respond to IL-7 only in the presence of a 'second signal' (antigen or mitogen). Most, but not all, antigen-activated T-cell clones respond to IL-7, leading to the suggestion that IL-7 responsive T-cells are a subset of IL-2 responsive cells. As antibodies against IL-2 and IL-4 failed to neutralize the IL-7 induced proliferation of T-cell clones, it appears that IL-7 is directly mitogenic. Thus, IL-7 is a growth factor for both early B- and early T-cells, has no effect on mature B-cells (whether or not 'second signals' are present) and acts on mature T-cells only in the presence of antigen or mitogen. These effects are summarized in Figure 16.3 (from Henney 1989a).

Interleukin-8, also known as neutrophil-activating protein, was first identified as a 72-amino acid polypeptide secreted by monocytes in response to bacterial lipopolysaccharide, with the properties of activating and attracting polymorphonuclear leukocytes in vitro (Bagglioni et al 1989). Subsequently, it was shown that IL-8 was produced in response to IL-1 in a number of cell types, notably endothelial cells. Sequence data have shown that IL-8 has homology to a group of peptides which include platelet basic protein and macrophage inflammatory protein 2. The effects of IL-8 on lymphopoiesis and immune responsiveness are unknown.

It is becoming increasingly apparent that lymphokines originally isolated on the basis of their activity towards a given lymphocyte lineage have a broader cellular activity than was previously supposed. This is summarized in an outline of the role lymphokines plays in lymphocyte differentiation shown in Figure 16.4 (from Henney 1989b). Thus, IL-2, the prototypical T-cell growth factor, has been shown to have diverse effects on B-cell differentiation. In contrast, two B-cell growth factors, IL-4 and IL-7 have been shown to have significant effects on T-cell maturation. The recent cloning of the genes encoding these various growth and differentiation factors has provided access to homogeneous proteins in unlimited quantities and will be invaluable in dissecting to a greater extent the regulatory pathways involved in B- and

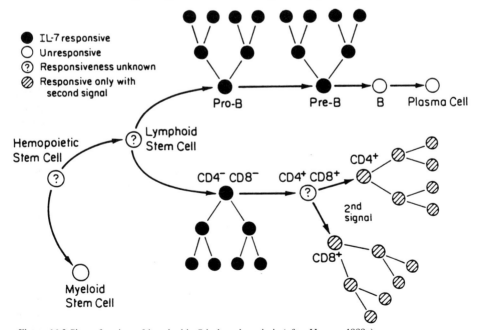

Figure 16.3 Sites of action of interleukin-7 in lymphopoiesis (after Henney 1989a)

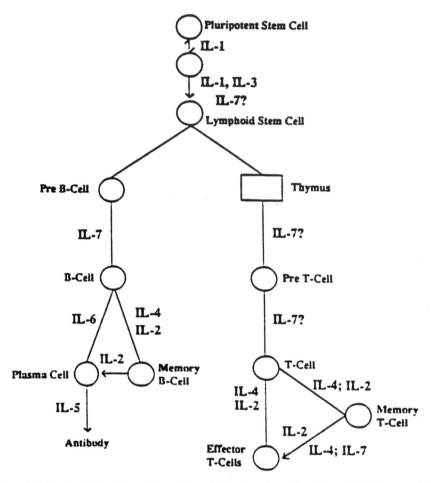

Figure 16.4 Outline of the role of the interleukins in lymphopoiesis (after Henney 1989b)

T-cell lymphogenesis. The principal gaps in our current understanding lie in the earliest stages of lymphopoiesis; it is only within the last two years that it has been possible to isolate the self-renewing, pluripotent haematopoietic progenitor cell, and so far still only in the mouse (Spangrude et al 1988). With access to such cells and to the interleukins which modulate their growth, a full description of the development biology of the haematolymphoid system is at last within our grasp.

INTERLEUKINS AS ADJUNCTS TO CELLULAR THERAPY IN CANCER

As mentioned earlier, IL-2, in addition to inducing T-cell proliferation, can activate lymphocyte precursor cells to become cytotoxic. These cells, termed lymphokine-activated killer (or LAK) cells, have the peculiar ability to lyse neoplastic cells preferentially. In general, cells of normal phenotype are not targets for LAK cells. The molecular basis of the recognition process leading to cell lysis is not known, but the presence of unique glycolipids on transformed cells has been implicated by some.

280

The powerful and selective antineoplastic activities of LAK cells (Grimm et al 1983) led Rosenberg to propose the use of these cells for the destruction of solid neoplasms. As LAK cells display IL-2 receptors, Rosenberg introduced IL-2 along with LAK cells, hoping to cause the proliferation of the cells in vivo or, minimally, to prolong LAK cell survival. There is a large body of cogent experimental evidence to support the addition of IL-2 to cytotoxic cell populations, largely pioneered by Greenberg, Cheever and their collaborators at the University of Washington. Cheever et al (1982) have conclusively shown that the efficacy of cytotoxic cells to treat leukaemia in the mouse is markedly increased by the administration of exogenous IL-2. In the absence of IL-2, cytotoxic cells do not survive long on transfer and are only weakly antineoplastic.

Rosenberg et al (1985) in their initial LAK cell protocols for the treatment of cancer in man employed the continuous infusion of very large doses of IL-2 following a bolus administration of LAK cells. In an initial group of 55 patients with a wide variety of advanced cancers, the results of such combined administration were remarkable: almost half (21/55) of the patients had at least 50% reduction in tumour size. These responses occurred most notably in patients with melanoma, colorectal, kidney and lung cancer and in B-cell lymphoma. Five patients showed complete disappearance of widespread cancer (Rosenberg et al 1985).

These results elicited enormous excitement in the clinical and lay communities alike and a huge increase worldwide in the number of cancer patients receiving IL-2. It is estimated that in the period 1986-1990 more than 5000 patients received IL-2, either together with LAK cells, as in Rosenberg's original studies, or alone. While successes following such therapy have been noted, none of the studies has come close to repeating the incidence of remission observed in the initial studies. In some cancers, however, notably renal cell carcinoma and melanoma, significant effects of IL-2 have been repeatedly seen.

The greatest amount of positive data assembled to date concerns the use of IL-2 in metastatic renal cell carcinoma (Hamblin 1989). The median survival in this condition is 8 months; there is no effective treatment. Spontaneous remissions have been reported in <1% of patients, and these are usually short lived. To date, data are available for evaluation in 506 patients treated with IL-2. Twenty-six studies ranked in terms of dose and schedule intensity have demonstrated increasing responses with increasing dose, an optimum dose has however probably been reached. In eight trials in which doses near to this optimum have been used, responses of between 20 and 30% were achieved, with 8-9% complete remissions. Responses have proved durable; with a median duration of 10.8 months. More than half of the complete responders have yet to relapse. The longest response so far is 30 months. In some patients who achieved a partial response, later examination at a time when no further treatment had been given, showed that patients had proceeded to a complete response. The responses translate into a survival advantage. In the treated group, median survival is 14.5 months compared with 8 months in historical controls; 85% of complete responders and 67% of partial responders are still alive.

In Rosenberg's own extended trials (Rosenberg et al 1987) involving more than 150 patients, 8/72 patients with renal cell carcinoma showed complete remission and an additional 17 patients showed partial remission.

From the outset, the clinical results were obtained at a considerable price.

Unexpectedly, considering its important physiological role, IL-2 administered exogenously has proved to be extremely toxic. Chills and fever immediately following IL-2 administration were controllable clinically by administration of meperidine, but other side-effects could be controlled only by removal of the drug. The most significant side-effect of IL-2 administration was fluid retention, the majority of patients gaining more than 10% of their body weight. Fluid retention also often resulted in interstitial oedema in the lungs, causing breathing difficulties. Rosenberg's initial protocols have been repeatedly modified and, of late, studies initiated by Oldham, West and their collaborators, have led to the use of much lower IL-2 doses with consequently lowered toxicity, but comparable clinical effects.

Of some considerable surprise, examination of all of the trials suggests that it is not necessary to give LAK cells with IL-2 to achieve this response, nor does it matter whether the IL-2 is given by bolus injection or intravenous infusion.

The findings that IL-2 alone was as effective as IL-2/LAK protocols, first observed in studies with renal cell carcinoma, have shown to hold in other cancer settings. Consequently, the mechanism by which tumours are reduced, previously assumed to be by the direct lytic action of LAK cells, has been questioned. It has recently been suggested (Parmiani 1990) that IL-2 functions by stimulating cytotoxic T-cell precursors in vivo and that it is these cells rather than LAK cells that are responsible for the tumour reduction. The fact that cytotoxic T-cells harvested from solid tumours (called TIL for tumour-infiltrating lymphocytes) have been shown to be more efficacious than LAK cells in causing tumour reduction is viewed as support for this hypothesis (Rosenberg et al 1988).

Where do these studies leave us? IL-2 is clearly a potent biological agent that has shown to be an effective antineoplastic agent in some settings. Indeed, it has recently been approved as a therapeutic agent for the treatment of renal cell carcinoma in approximately ten European countries, but not yet in the United States.

Unfortunately, the successes are less frequent and are applicable to less tumours than had been hoped following Rosenberg's early studies. Further, IL-2, when given intravenously, is still markedly toxic, considerably limiting its usefulness as a therapeutic agent. Renal cell carcinoma is, however, a uniformly fatal disease and IL-2 has proved to be an effective, sometimes an extremely effective, therapeutic agent in this condition. It also seems likely that IL-2 will also prove to be a useful treatment for melanoma and perhaps other solid tumours. Many trials (as high as 100 by one count) are still in progress and seem certain to continue for at least 2-3 more years.

One aspect of interleukin therapeutic development to date continues to puzzle many: why the emphasis on antineoplastic effects? IL-2 is the most potent potentiator of T-cell growth yet described, but it has not yet been extensively tested in settings where this, its primary physiological role, might be exploited. It seems natural to expect that IL-2 would be a potent agent with which to treat immunosuppression or to potentiate immune responses to infectious agents or vaccines. In animal models from mouse to cattle, IL-2 has been shown to boost immune responses. It is more than 10 years since Gillis et al (1979) showed that congenitally immunodeficient nu^+/nu^+ mice could be restored to immune responsiveness by treatment with IL-2. It seems surprising that such observations have not yet lead to the treatment of immune unresponsiveness either congenital, or acquired, in man. Rather, it appears that those charged with the commercial development of IL-2 have been so overwhelmed by Rosenberg's early observations in the treatment of cancer that they have let all other potential uses of the molecule fall by the wayside. It is to be hoped that this is only a temporary distraction and that when the antineoplastic effects of IL-2 have been fully exploited, it will be looked at in other settings.

Several such studies are indeed beginning to emerge: Meuer and his colleagues in Heidelberg (Meuer et al 1989) have recently shown that low doses of IL-2 can augment systemic immune responses against hepatitis B vaccine, even in immunodeficient individuals who are non-responders to the vaccine with the absence of IL-2 (Fig. 16.5). These findings suggest that IL-2 can be an efficient means of inducing systemic antigen-specific immune responses in immunodeficient subjects. Hopefully, other investigators will take advantage of these findings in other clinical settings.

All of the interleukins so far identified are now available in amounts that will permit their clinical usefulness to be fully explored. This is a remarkable achievement given that a decade ago none of them had been defined in any biochemically

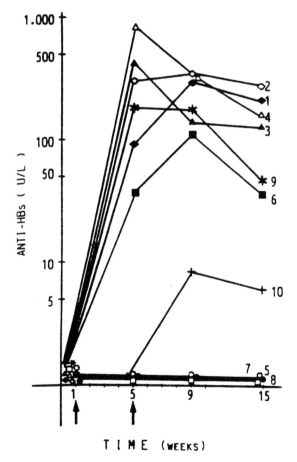

Figure 16.5 Serum antibody levels in patients who were previous non-responders to hepatitis B vaccination after combined injection with vaccine and interleukin-2 (after Meuer et al 1989)

meaningful way. Hopefully, as our understanding of the role of these molecules in the integration of the immune response reveals itself, the next decade will see individual interleukins added to the physician's armamentarium, and with it the ability to modulate successfully immune responsiveness.

ACKNOWLEDGEMENT

I am grateful to my former colleagues at Immunex for their many contributions to the experimental work reported.

REFERENCES

Bagglioni M, Walz A, Kunkel S L 1989 Neutrophil-activating peptide−1/interleukin−8, a novel cytokine that activates neutrophils. Journal of Clinical Investigation 84: 1045-1049

Cheever M A, Greenberg P D, Fefer A, Gillis S 1982 Augmentation of the anti-tumour therapeutic efficacy of long-term cultured T−lymphocytes by in vivo administration of purified interleukin−2. Journal of Experimental Medicine 155: 968-980

Coffman R L, Carty J 1986 T-cell activity that enhances polyclonal IgE production and it's inhibition by interferon-gamma. Journal of Immunology 136: 949-954

Dinarello C A 1984 Interleukin−1 and the pathogenesis of the acute-phase response. New England Journal of Medicine 311: 1413-1418

Dower S K, Kronheim S R, Hopp T P et al 1986 The cell surface receptors for interleukin−1 alpha and interleukin−1 beta are identical. Nature 324: 266-268

Fung M C, Happel A V, Ymer S et al 1984 Molecular cloning of cDNA for murine interleukin−3. Nature 307: 233-237

Gauldie J, Richards C, Harnish D, Landsdorp P, Baumann H 1987 Interferon beta 2/B−cell stimulatory factor type 2 shares identity with monocyte-derived hepatocyte-stimulating factor and regulates the major acute phase protein response in liver cells. Proceedings of the National Academy of Sciences (USA) 84: 7251-7255

Gillis S, Union N A, Baker P E, Smith K A 1979 The in vitro generation and sustained culture of nude mouse cytolytic T−lymphocytes. Journal of Experimental Medicine 149: 1460-1476

Goodwin G G, Friend D, Ziegler S F et al 1990 Cloning of the human and murine interleukin−2 receptors: Demonstration of a soluble form and homology to a new receptor superfamily. Cell 60: 941-951

Grimm E A, Ramsay K M, Nazumder A, Wilson D J, Djeu J Y, Rosenberg S A 1983 Lymphokine-activated killer cell phenomenon. II. Precursor phenotype is serologically distinct from peripheral T−lymphocytes, memory cytotoxic thymus-derived lymphocytes, and natural killer cells. Journal of Experimental Medicine 157: 844-897

Hamblin T 1989 In: Clinical impact of the interleukins. Royal College of Physicians Proceedings (abstract). London April 10/11

Henney C S 1989a Interleukin−7: effects on early events in lymphopoiesis. Immunology Today 10: 170-173

Henney C S 1989b The Interleukins as lymphocyte growth factors. Transplantation Proceedings 21: 22-25

Hirano T, Yasukawa K, Harada H et al 1986 Complementary DNA for a novel human interleukin (BSF-2) that induces B-lymphocytes to produce immunoglobulin. Nature 324: 73-76

Kishimoto T, Hirano T 1988 Molecular regulation of B-lymphocyte response. Annual Reviews of Immunology 6: 485-512

Lee F, Yokota T, Otsuka T et al 1986 Isolation and characterization of a mouse interleukin cDNA clone that expresses B−cell stimulatory factor 1 activities and T−cell and mast-cell-stimulating activites. Proceedings of the National Academy of Sciences (USA) 83: 2061-2065

March C M, Mosley B, Larsen A et al 1985 Cloning, sequence and expression of two distinct human interleukin−1 complementary DNAs. Nature 315: 641-647

Meuer S C, Dumann H, Zum Buschenfelde K H, Kohler H 1989 Low-dose interleukin−2 induces systemic immune responses against HBs Ag in immunodeficient non-responders to hepatitis B vaccination. Lancet i: 15-18

Namen A E, Schmierer A E, March C J et al 1988a B—cell precursor growth-promoting activity. Purification and characterization of a growth factor active on lymphocyte precursors. Journal of Experimental Medicine 167: 988-1002

Namen A E, Lupton S, Hjerrild K et al 1988b Stimulation of B—cell progenitors by cloned murine interleukin−7. Nature 333: 571-573

O'Garra A O, Warren D J, Holman M, Popham A M, Sanderson C J, Kalus G G B 1986 Interleukin 4 (B-cell growth factor II/eosinophil differentiation factor) is a mitogen and differentiation factor for preactivated murine B-lymphocytes. Proceedings of the National Academy of Sciences (USA) 83: 5228-5232

Parmiani G 1990 An explanation of the variable clinical response to interleukin−2 and LAK cells. Immunology Today 11: 113-115

Rosenberg S A, Lotze M T, Muul L M et al 1985 Observations on the systemic administration of autologous lymphokine-activated killer cells and recombinant interleukin−2 to patients with metastatic cancer. New England Journal of Medicine 313: 1485-1492

Rosenberg S A, Lotze M T, Muul L M et al 1987 A progress report on the treatment of 157 patients with advanced cancer using lymphokine-activated killer cells and interleukin−2 or high-dose interleukin−2 alone. New England Journal of Medicine 316: 889-897

Rosenberg S A, Lotze M T, Muul L M et al 1988 New England Jounral of Medicine 319: 1676-

Sims J E, March C J, Cosman D et al 1988 cDNA expression cloning of the IL−1 receptor, a member of the immunoglobulin superfamily. Science 241: 585-589

Smith K A 1988 Interleukin−2: inception, impact and implications. Science 240: 1169-1176

Spangrude G J, Heimfield S, Weissman I L 1988 Purification and characterization of mouse hematopoietic stem cells. Science 241: 58-62

Swain S K, Dutton R W 1982 Production of a B—cell growth promoting activity, (DL)BCGE, from a cloned T—cell line and its assay on the BCL1B cell tumor. Journal of Experimental Medicine 156: 1821-1834

Taniguchi T, Matsui H, Fujiti T et al 1983 Structure and expression of a cloned cDNA for human interleukin−2. Nature 302: 305-310

Whitlock C A, Zeigler S F, Truman L J, Statford J L, Witte O N 1983 Differentiation of cloned populations of immature B—cells after transformation with Abelson murine leukemia virus. Cell 32: 903-911

Widmer M B, Acres R B, Sassenfield H M, Grabstein K H 1987 Regulation of cytolytic cell populations from human peripheral blood by B—cell stimulatory factor 1 (interleukin−4). Journal of Experimental Medicine 166: 1447-1455

Zilberstein A, Ruggieri R, Korn J H, Revel M 1986 Structure and expression of cDNA and genes for human interferon-beta-2, a distinct species inducible by growth-stimulatory cytokines. European Molecular Biology Organisation Journal 5: 2529-2537

L

Discussion of paper presented by C. Henney

Discussed by P. Kaye
Reported by H. C. Neu

It is clear that in vivo lymphokines have not yet really fulfilled the expectations that were raised after the in vitro findings. In particular, in the field of infection, the value of these agents has yet to be established. Initially cytokines were considered for use as single effector molecules. For example, in the treatment of infections caused by intracellular pathogens, one method of choice might be to directly stimulate macrophage function by a macrophage activating factor. However, it has now become increasingly clear that cytokines have important secondary actions, particularly on the qualitative regulation of the immune system. In addition there is a complex interplay between the different cytokines which is complicated by the fact that cytokines produced by different T–cell populations can give rise to different immune responses.

One possibility for the use of cytokines, poorly considered to date, is to overcome the state of unresponsiveness which is often seen in chronic infections such as leprosy or leishmaniasis. Interferon-gamma for example, is a potent macrophage activating factor but its release is associated with the production of numerous other cytokines. In murine leishmaniasis resistance to infection and activation of macrophages was optimal when interferon-gamma was used in the presence of IL–2, IL–4 or GM–CSF. However, it was found that the synergism between these cytokines only took place when a large number of actively dividing parasites were present. In the situation where parasites are only just beginning to transform into their normal intracellular multiplying forms, IL–4 or IL–3 inhibits the macrophages activating effects of interferon.

To complicate matters further, it is not only the stage of the parasite within the macrophage which determines the outcome but possibly also the biological state of the macrophage population we are dealing with. If macrophage populations are treated with any of the colony stimulating factors their responses to many of the different cytokine permutations change dramatically. However, one must remember that the behaviour of macrophages in vitro is unlikely to be the same as in the intact animal. In an in vivo situation therefore, do we need to know how many cytokines are present, what the status of the cytokine receptors on different macrophage populations, and which specific macrophage population is harbouring the parasite in question?

One example of how complex the situation is in vivo, and how difficult comparisons between in vivo and in vitro effects are, is in the case of chronic visceral leishmaniasis in which a state of T−cell unresponsiveness occurs; here defined as an inability of T−cells to produce interferon-gamma in vitro.

It has been known for many years that the ability to reduce parasite numbers in vivo is directly correlated with the ability to produce interferon in vitro. It was thought possible therefore, to use co-stimulator molecules to increase the activity of T−cells to produce interferon in vitro, which would in vivo give a reduction in the number of parasites. Unfortunately this does not happen.

When animals are given in vivo recombinant IL−1α, the lymphocytes of these animals produce much more interferon-gamma. However, when the levels of parsites in these animals are measured no change is observed. This takes us back to what Dr Henney described as the multiple effects of IL−1. Although these T−cells can produce interferon-gamma after stimulation by IL−1 they still do not clear the parasites.

Another approach in the elucidation of the function of each cytokine is to study the effects of monoclonal antibodies. These could be monoclonal antibodies against the lymphokine itself or potentially against the lymphokine receptor. Preliminary evidence suggests that anti IL−4 can alter the response to leishmaniasis in the murine model.

Overall the situation is complex and certainly more cytokines will be discovered. Potentially cytokines could be used to influence other cytokines, and a great deal more information is needed on down regulation. Knowledge of receptor antagonists at the membrane level may, in the end, provide a way for better regulation of interleukins and for prevention of their deleterious effects.

17. The role of the colony-stimulating factors in the treatment of infections

D. Metcalf

INTRODUCTION

Cellular immunologists and haematologists would confidently identify four types of white cells as being involved in resistance to infections—neutrophilic granulocytes (hereafter referred to simply as granulocytes), monocytes and their derivative macrophages, T-lymphocytes and B-lymphocytes. These cells have each been assigned unequivocal functions, such as antibody production by B-lymphocytes or phagocytosis and destruction of bacteria by granulocytes or macrophages, but in no single infectious disease is the exact role of each of the four cell types completely established nor does it seem possible to generalize with much confidence regarding the relative roles of these cells in specific classes of infections, e.g. viral versus bacterial.

These uncertainties are no longer of merely academic interest because the development of regulatory molecules specific for various cell types now permits the selective stimulation and/or functional activation of precise subsets of candidate resistance cells. With clinical trials in progress on these agents, it could be argued that in time the clinical data will indicate well enough which types of infection are benefited, for example by stimulation of granulocytes. However, this is a somewhat circular argument. If traditional views suggest, for example, that granulocytes are not of much relevance for resistance to viral infections, there is a risk that granulocyte-stimulating factors may never be tested clinically in this role and opportunities be lost or delayed in the introduction into clinical practice of a valuable agent.

A large body of clinical data indicate clearly that susceptibility to infections increases sharply when granulocyte levels fall below 1000 per mm^3 (Bodey et al 1966). This situation occurs in some rare disorders such as cyclic neutropenia and congenital neutropenia but is seen most often in hospital medicine as a complication arising from the cytotoxic therapy of cancer.

The discussion to follow will be concerned only with granulocytes and monocyte-macrophages. This is because of the existence of a large body of information concerning the regulation of these populations, the availability of the relevant regulators in recombinant form and the fact that extensive clinical trials are now in progress on these agents. This discussion will review the basic experimental findings and in vivo data on this subject, indicate where further information is required and point out opportunities that may exist for a broader use of these agents.

COLONY-STIMULATING FACTORS (CSFs)

The introduction in the mid-1960s of high-efficiency clonal culture techniques permitted the growth of colonies of differentiating granulocytes and/or macrophages from their specific precursor cells in the marrow or spleen (Bradley & Metcalf 1966, Pluznik & Sachs 1966). Early work on these cultures made it evident that the precursors of granulocytes and macrophages cannot divide spontaneously. As is now known to be true for all haemopoietic populations, every cell division requires stimulation by adequate concentrations of one or a combination of specific growth-stimulating factors. The use of clonal cultures allowed these growth factors to be recognized and served as bioassay systems during the subsequent purification of the molecules (Metcalf 1984, 1988). These were demanding projects in separative protein chemistry because of the high specific activity of the molecules (typically 10^8 units/mg protein) and the correspondingly minute concentrations of them present in any tissue source. Indeed, fold purifications in the range of 0.5-1×10^6 were required for some before material of sequence-grade purity was obtained.

For granulocytic and macrophage populations, this work led to the discovery and characterization of four distinct glycoproteins involved in regulating the production of these cells (Metcalf 1988). These were given the operational name colony-stimulating factors (CSFs), since this was the method used initially for monitoring their biological activity. Table 17.1 lists the four murine CSFs together with the corresponding molecules in man. Subsequent studies have identified several other haemopoietic growth factors as also having some actions on granulocytic and macrophage cells—interleukin-6 (Suda et al 1988, Metcalf 1989a), interleukin-4 (Lee et al 1988) and interleukin-1 (Moore & Warren 1987)—but these are believed to contribute in a relatively minor manner to the normal growth control of granulocytes and macrophages.

Certain generalizations can be made regarding the CSFs. All are glycoproteins: the carbohydrate content of the molecules varies widely and is not required for receptor binding or biological action of the molecules either in vitro or in vivo. Three of the

Table 17.1 The colony-stimulating factors

Species	Factor	Molecular weight (glycosylated)	Molecular weight (polypeptide)	Chromosomal location of gene
Murine	GM-CSF	18-25 000	14 400	11 A5-B1
	G-CSF	25 000	19 100	11 D-E1
	M-CSF	45-90 000	21 000, 18 000	3 F3
	Multi-CSF (IL-3)	18-30 000	16 200	11 A5-B1
Human	GM-CSF	18-30 000	14 700	5q23-31
	G-CSF	20 000	18 600	17q11.2-21
	M-CSF	45-90 000	21 000, 18 000	5q33.1
	Multi-CSF (IL-3)	15-30 000	15 400	5q23-31

CSFs are monomeric proteins and the fourth (M-CSF) is a homodimer of two identical polypeptide chains. In each, mandatory disulphide bridges maintain the molecules in a necessary three-dimensional configuration and multiple portions of the molecule contribute to the active binding site.

Amino acid sequencing of the CSFs and the deduction of the full amino acid sequence of the molecules from subsequently cloned cDNAs revealed the surprising finding that the four CSFs share no sequence homology or likely common secondary structure. Confirming this unrelatedness, is the existence of unique, non-cross-reactive, membrane receptors for each CSF on responding cells (for review, see Nicola 1989).

The original common name of 'CSFs' applied to these molecules did assume a relatedness between them and while this was not substantiated by their amino acid sequence, other evidence validates the original concept. The unique genes encoding the CSFs exhibit an intriguing clustering, e.g. for GM-CSF, Multi-CSF with the genes for IL-4 and IL-5 on chromosome 5 in man and on chromosome 11 in the mouse (Metcalf 1987); a number of the CSF receptors, e.g. for GM-CSF, Multi-CSF and G-CSF, have homologous regions in their extracelluar domains (Gearing et al 1989) and transmodulation of other CSF receptors occurs on the membrane of responding cells during the action of individual CSFs (Walker et al 1985).

The receptor for M-CSF (the product of c-fms) is a prototype transmembrane tyrosine kinase glycoprotein (Sherr et al 1985) whereas the receptors for the other three CSFs are members of a novel class of glycoprotein transmembrane receptors that lack a tyrosine kinase domain and must therefore initiate signalling by a different mechanism.

With all four CSFs, the number of receptors on responding cells is remarkably small (a few hundred per cell) and biological responses can be initiated by occupancy of approximately 10% of these receptors (Nicola 1989). This highly efficient signalling system also has a novel aspect in that individual precursor cells usually co-express receptors for more than one, and often all four, of the CSFs. This permits different CSFs to act in concert in eliciting amplified responses and, on occasion, even to exhibit antagonistic or competitive effects (Metcalf 1989b).

The population of committed progenitors generating granulocytes and macrophages is quite heterogeneous, some being capable only of forming granulocyte progeny, some only macrophage progeny and many (a majority in the mouse) being bipotential. In their interactions with these heterogeneous progenitors, the CSFs display certain distinctive differences. G-CSF is a relatively selective stimulus for granulocytic formation while M-CSF is strongly biased to the selective stimulation of macrophage formation. GM-CSF and Multi-CSF have an ability to stimulate most progenitors leading to the production of both granulocytes and macrophages (Metcalf 1987). Some CSFs can exhibit actions on a broader range of haemopoietic populations. GM-CSF, at progressively higher concentrations, can stimulate in sequence the formation of eosinophils, megakaryocytes then erythroid cells (Metcalf et al 1986). Multi-CSF has a particularly broad range of actions being the only CSF able to stimulate the formation of mast cells and also having the capacity to stimulate the formation of eosinophils, megakaryocytes and erythroid cells (Metcalf et al 1987).

There is increasing evidence, whose implications remain somewhat unclear, that some CSFs can have actions on non-haemopoietic cells. For example, G-CSF and GM-CSF have been reported to stimulate endothelial cell migration and proliferation (Bussolino et al 1989) while GM-CSF and M-CSF can stimulate the function of placental trophoblasts (Athanassakis et al 1987). In this context, the CSFs show to a limited degree the polyfunctionality seen in extreme form with some other haemopoietic growth factors, most notably interleukin-6 (Kishimoto 1989) and leukaemia inhibitory factor (LIF) (Gough et al 1989).

When acting on granulocyte macrophage populations, each CSF displays multiple biological actions, all of which presumably can be initiated by signalling from the single class of receptor involved (for review, see Metcalf 1987). The primary action of the CSFs is to act as mandatory proliferative stimuli for these cells. The presence of CSF is required for a major portion, and possibly the entire duration, of the cell cycle. The concentration of CSF determines the length of the cell cycle and the total number of progeny generated in a given time interval. In addition, the CSFs are necessary for maintaining viability and the integrity of membrane transport of responding cells. The CSFs can also initiate differentiation commitment, i.e. the decision whether to form granulocytic or macrophage progeny and the subsequent initiation of maturation in granulocytes and macrophages (Metcalf 1989b). From the point of view of infections, an action of major importance of the CSFs is their ability to enhance the functional activity of the mature cells. This can be monitored by a wide range of parameters such as phagocytosis, cytotoxicity, production of superoxide or other pharmacologically active agents such as prostaglandin E, γ-interferon or tumour necrosis factor. The CSFs can also elicit the increased transcription and production of other CSFs, allowing the possibility of escalating responses in terms of CSF production.

In general, the CSFs can be produced by multiple cell types and certain cells such as T-lymphocytes, fibroblasts and endothelial cells can simultaneously produce more than one type of CSF (Metcalf 1984, 1987). In considering the biology of infections, the nature and location of these CSF producing cells are highly relevant. Cell types known to produce CSF include endothelial cells, fibroblasts, stromal cells, macrophages and T-lymphocytes. These cells are widely distributed in the body and likely to make early contact with the products of invading microorganisms. It remains possible that most cell types in the body have some potential for CSF production if primed by suitable inductive stimuli. Typically, the constitutive production of CSF by known CSF-producing cells is low or undetectable. However, these cells have a marked ability to be rapidly induced to produce CSF by appropriate inducing signals, one of the strongest of which is endotoxin—acting either directly or indirectly by first inducing IL-1 production (Metcalf 1984, 1988). This type of induction is probably of most relevance for endothelial and stromal cells. T-lymphocyte induction occurs following contact with lectins, antisera to the T-cell receptor or by exposure to antigens (Kelso & Metcalf in press). Recent studies in this laboratory suggest that anoxia or tissue damage may be another powerful inducing stimulus for some tissues (Brown & Metcalf 1990).

In general, the CSF system is highly labile. Levels of production and plasma CSF levels are able to be elevated up to 1000-fold within hours. The CSFs have short plasma half-lives of at most a few hours and, following cessation of increased production, elevated levels of CSF in the serum rapidly return to normal levels.

The CSF system is, in principle, ideally suited to mediate ultrarapid responses to invading microorganisms since the rises in CSFs are extremely rapid and, if the CSFs are able to enhance the functional activity of existing mature granulocytes and macrophages within minutes or hours as indicated from in vitro studies, the whole system is geared to respond extremely rapidly on challenge. Similarly the system is designed to unwind promptly with the elimination of the inducing signal such as microorganisms. It needs to be emphasized, however, that in sustained infections, elevated CSF levels can be maintained for prolonged periods of days or weeks and in this situation the ability of the CSFs to stimulate the formation of additional mature cells becomes of progressively greater importance.

IN VIVO EFFECTS OF THE CSFs

The in vitro studies suggested that the CSFs must be important in the regulation of granulocyte and macrophage formation and the sites and inducibility of CSF production appeared to be ideally designed to provide a mechanism mediating early responses to any infection where functionally active granulocytes and monocytes were desirable. Indirect evidence that the CSFs were indeed involved in such responses came from the demonstration of serum CSF rises in patients with acute infections and in experimental animals injected either with endotoxin or infectious agents. Conversely, in germ-free or pathogen-free animals serum CSF levels were low or undetectable (for reviews see Metcalf 1984, 1988).

Direct confirmation of the in vivo actions of the CSFs only became feasible with the production of purified recombinant CSFs and the initial studies in this laboratory were performed in mice. Injection of GM-CSF, Multi-CSF or G-CSF in a dose range of 2-200 ng three times daily elicited obvious dose-related elevations in granulocyte or monocyte levels and these responses followed expectations from in vitro studies, at least with respect to the type of cells responding. Thus the injection of G-CSF induced rises in granulocytes but not monocytes, the injection of GM-CSF elevated levels of macrophages, granulocytes and eosinophils while the injection of Multi-CSF elevated these three cell types together with the induction of marked rises in mast cells (Metcalf 1988). In each instance, the induced rises in cell numbers were consistent with an increased production of cells since several days were required before responses became obvious.

There were, however, several unexpected aspects of the observed responses to the injection of the CSFs. The first was a discrepancy between in vitro and in vivo responses in the magnitude of the changes observed with the different CSFs. G-CSF was expected to elicit relatively weak responses because of its ability in vitro only to stimulate the formation of small numbers of very small granulocyte colonies. Total granulocyte numbers in colonies stimulated in vitro either by GM-CSF or Multi-CSF far exceed those stimulated by G-CSF. The opposite occurred in vivo, for G-CSF was clearly superior to GM-CSF or Multi-CSF in its ability to elevate blood granulocyte levels. With G-CSF, it was possible to induce levels of granulocytes in excess of 100 000 per mm^3 versus the normal level of 1000 per mm^3, whereas the injection of comparable doses of GM-CSF or Multi-CSF elevated levels at most two- to three-fold. Subsequent studies with mice engrafted with haemopoietic cells producing either GM-CSF or Multi-CSF have shown that both agents can elevate granulocyte levels beyond 100 000 per mm^3 but in this situation CSF concentrations are extremely high (Chang et al 1989a, Johnson et al 1989).

Anomalous responses were also observed, the most striking of which was seen in mice injected with G-CSF where erythropoiesis switched location from the marrow to the spleen. This response is so far unexplained since G-CSF has no direct action on erythroid cell proliferation in vitro.

Possibly the most important phenomenon encountered was that of a discrepancy between circulating and local cellular responses. This requires some comment since it introduces an important concept into the biology of granulocytic and macrophage populations. If CSFs are injected intraperitoneally, an opportunity exists to compare systemic (blood and bone marrow) responses with purely local responses at the site of injection. The CSFs differ markedly in the changes they induce in these parameters. The injection of G-CSF induces the largest responses as monitored by blood levels or percentage of granulocytic and monocytic populations in the marrow, whereas the changes induced at the local site of injection are relatively small in magnitude (Fig. 17.1). In sharp contrast, the injection of GM-CSF at the same doses

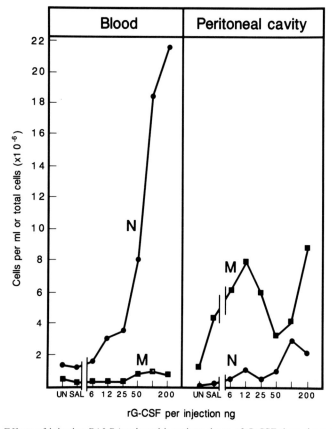

Figure 17.1 Effects of injecting BALB/c mice with various doses of G-CSF three times daily for six days. Note large rise in blood neutrophils (N) and little change in monocytes (M). In contrast the rises in local cellularity in the peritoneal cavity are small compared with levels in uninjected (UN) or FCS/saline (SAL) injected control mice.

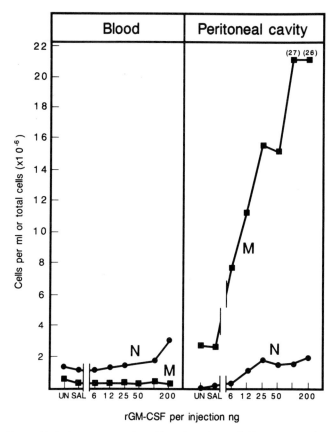

Figure 17.2 Effects of injecting BALB/c mice with various doses of GM-CSF three times daily for six days. Note failure of GM-CSF at these doses to elevate blood neutrophil levels significantly but the ability of GM-CSF to induce large rises in peritoneal macrophage numbers. Symbols as for Fig 17.1.

induces little change in blood or marrow granulocytic and monocytic populations but a massive rise in the total numbers of macrophages at the site of injection (Fig. 17.2). Multi-CSF is intermediate in the response pattern it induces.

Subsequent studies with transgenic mice have emphasized the divergence that can exist between systemic and local responses (Lang et al 1987, Metcalf & Moore 1988). In GM-CSF transgenic mice with constitutive elevations of 100-fold in plasma GM-CSF levels, levels of granulocytes and monocytes in the blood are normal, as is the cellularity and composition of the bone marrow. In marked contrast, peritoneal and pleural cellularity are massively increased, with levels of up to 200 million cells per peritoneal cavity versus a normal number of 1-4 million (Fig. 17.3).

The lesson emerging from these observations is that granulocyte and macrophage responses either to injected CSF or in real-life perturbations during infections cannot be evaluated with any completeness simply by sampling blood or marrow populations. Such measurements monitor the 'systemic type' of response and are not necessarily capable of following crucial events occurring locally. This presents an obvious problem in the clinic where the only practicable observations are on blood or bone marrow. The consequences of this limitation are that, in many situations, no

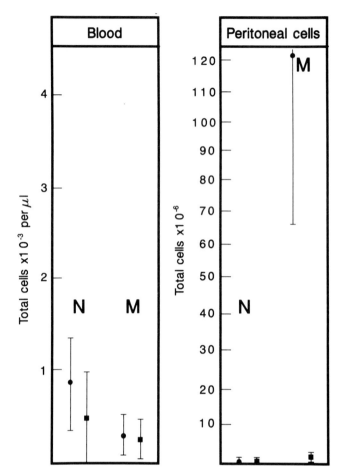

Figure 17.3 Levels of neutrophils (N) and monocyte-macrophages (M) in adult GM-CSF transgenic mice (●) and littermate control mice (■). Note the normal levels of these cells in the blood of transgenic mice but the extreme rise in peritoneal macrophages in transgenic mice. Mean values ± standard deviations from groups of 12 mice.

estimate at all is possible of important local granulocyte-macrophage responses or agents preferentially regulating responses of this type.

This is reflected in the current clinical view that G-CSF is superior to GM-CSF in its actions, based on the exclusive observation of blood and marrow responses. This restricted view of the biology of granulocytes and macrophages is potentially fallacious and there is therefore a need to monitor very carefully the actual induced resistance to infections in man as a probably more relevant parameter, since it need not necessarily be true in all infections that systemic responses of granulocytes and monocytes correlate with resistance.

Subsequent studies in primates and patients have essentially confirmed the pattern of responses observed in mice. Injection of G-CSF has proved superior to that of GM-CSF or Multi-CSF in eliciting rises in blood granulocyte levels (Groopman et al 1987, Gabrilove et al 1988, Morstyn et al 1988, Lieschke et al 1989). An early rise in granulocyte levels after the injection of CSF probably indicates release of pre-existing cells from the marrow but this is followed by a larger sustained rise based on increased cell production in the bone marrow. Elevated levels of granulocytes following the injection of G-CSF or of granulocytes, monocytes and eosinophils following the injection of GM-CSF can be sustained for as long as injections are continued, with the levels of these cells then declining within days of cessation of injections. Similar rises can be elicited in patients with subnormal marrow haemopoietic populations but are predictably of somewhat lesser magnitude.

Fewer studies have been performed on the functional status of granulocytes and monocytes from animals or patients following the injection of CSF but, where these have been performed, activation has been observed as measured by phagocyte activity, superoxide production or other parameters.

These studies have documented that the CSFs can regulate granulocyte and monocyte production in vivo. They can also induce increased levels of mature cells even in patients with cytotoxic drug-induced leukopenia or marrow aplasia where it might have been postulated that regulatory controls should have become activated and have been stimulating maximal possible regeneration. An important conclusion from these observations is that while few patients are likely to exhibit an absolute inability to produce CSF on demand, it cannot be assumed that this elicits maximal possible responses since the injection of additional CSF can clearly further increase the formation of granulocytes and monocytes. The most useful analogy is probably that with adrenal corticosteroids. Again, few patients have an inability to produce such steroids yet there are many situations where the administration of additional corticosteroids accelerates resolution of disease or provides symptomatic relief.

ROLE OF THE CSFs IN RESISTANCE TO INFECTIONS

The known correlation between leukopenia and heightened susceptibility to infections leads to the expectation that elevation of the numbers and/or functional activity of granulocytes and macrophages should increase resistance significantly and be evident as the reduction in either the frequency or severity of infections. This proposition is now able to be tested either experimentally or by clinical studies.

The effects have been determined of injected CSF on many model infections in animals but to date few of these studies have passed from company documents to scientific publications. One such study is that of Matsumoto et al (1987) where mice, rendered hypersusceptible by injection of the cytotoxic drug cyclophosphamide, were then challenged with lethal doses of organisms of clinical relevance ranging from *Pseudomonas* to *Candida*. Pre-injection of G-CSF dramatically increased the resistance (1000-fold) to these infections as monitored by survival. Supporting data also come from studies on survival from whole-body irradiation or cyclophosphamide where deaths are normally based on secondary microbial infections (Talmadge et al 1989, Uckun et al 1990). In such mice, injections of G-CSF or GM-CSF significantly reduced subsequent mortality to otherwise lethal doses of whole-body irradiation or cyclophosphamide.

Clinical data have been more difficult to accumulate because most such studies have involved cancer patients of a heterogeneous type with wide differences in previously administered cytotoxic therapy. In such patients, mortality from infections is relatively low and a dramatic change in resistance is therefore hard to document in terms of reduced mortality. There are, however, consistent reports of significant reduction in mucositis and associated infections following CSF treatment and there are many anecdotal examples of resolution of infections previously resistant to antibiotics (Antman et al 1988, Gabrilove et al 1988). The accumulation of such data is being pursued actively in current trials but some time must elapse before clear data emerge.

One patient group where a favourable outcome has already been achieved by CSF administration is the group of patients with cyclic neutropenia, a disease associated with cyclic variations in CSF levels and matching cycles of neutropenia at 21 day intervals that are accompanied by cyclical attacks of infections of multiple types and severity. Patients with cyclic neutropenia have now been maintained on G-CSF injections for more than a year with essentially complete suppression of such recurrent infections and no evidence of either induced antibody production or diminished responsiveness to G-CSF in terms of elevated neutrophil levels (Hammond et al 1989). Curiously, these patients tend to maintain a cyclical fluctuation in neutrophil levels now with a periodicity of 14 days, but these fluctuations occur at a level above those leading to susceptibility to infections.

Less advanced studies are documenting a similar useful result in congenital neutropenia where administration of G-CSF or GM-CSF has achieved significantly elevated neutrophil levels sufficient to provide protection from infections (Bonilla et al 1989, Vadhan-Raj et al 1990).

FUTURE LABORATORY STUDIES

One of the most vexing questions concerning the biology of the CSFs is their cellular source. Is the ability to produce CSF restricted to the few cell types so far available for testing—fibroblasts, endothelial cells, stromal cells, macrophages and lymphocytes—or is this capacity latent in many cell types and expressed after inductive signalling?

Analysis of the CSF content of tissue extracts does not identify the cell types responsible and may merely detect stored CSF, thereby giving no useful information if secretion is rapid and intracellular storage minimal. Measurement of levels of CSF mRNA can be quite misleading if there is post-transcriptional regulation blocking the synthesis of CSF protein. In situ hybridization can detect CSF mRNA transcripts in cell lines producing large amounts of CSF but, as presently performed, the technique is far too insensitive to detect the low levels being produced in vivo in normal tissues. Estimates of a tissue's ability to produce bio-assayable CSF in vitro tell little about the activity of that tissue in vivo because of the frequent occurrence of a major induction of mRNA transcription after transfer of the tissue to the culture dish. Even the use of radioimmunoassays to establish serum CSF levels is a potentially fallacious technique if the material being detected has intact antigenic epitopes but is biologically inactive.

A wide range of in vitro studies indicates that co-stimulation by pairs of CSFs or more complex combinations leads to strong enhancement of proliferative responses but, oddly enough, no comparable studies have explored whether functional activation is similarly enhanced. The question of the net consequence of functional enhancement—particularly of macrophages—needs much further exploration. It is quite possible that phagocytosis of organisms may be enhanced without any corresponding enhancement of intracellular killing, a situation which for some microorganisms that preferentially reside intracellularly might exacerbate an infection rather than enhance its suppression.

This question has arisen in AIDS infections where stimulation of monocytes by M-CSF or GM-CSF actually enhanced production of retrovirus by the cells whereas stimulation by G-CSF had no such effect (Koyanagi et al 1988). This type of study suggests that it may be unwise to use a macrophage-stimulating CSF when using CSF therapy to enhance resistance to secondary infections in AIDS patients.

It was recognized that if the CSFs stimulate mature cells to exhibit heightened functional activity, some of the products of the activated cells might be toxic and cause either tissue damage or disease in vivo. This possibility applied to macrophages because of the demonstration that CSF stimulation could enhance the production of a variety of potentially toxic products such as prostaglandin E, γ-interferon, tumour necrosis factor, fibroblast growth factor, interleukin-1 or plasminogen activator. The likely involvement of granulocytes in the development of acute respiratory distress syndrome suggested that granulocyte stimulation might also have some hazards.

These questions need further experimental analysis but already several experimental models in which chronically elevated CSF levels can be induced have indicated that this situation can result in severe tissue damage. Thus transgenic GM-CSF mice die prematurely with a wasting syndrome including blindness, polymyositis in skeletal and cardiac muscle, fibrotic nodules in the peritoneal and pleural cavities and bowel damage (Lang et al 1987; Metcalf & Moore 1988). The evidence suggests that CSF-activated macrophages play a central role in the genesis of these lesions. Similar lesions develop in mice engrafted with GM-CSF-producing marrow cells (Johnson et al 1989). In contrast, in mice engrafted with G-CSF-producing marrow cells, little evidence of tissue damage was observed despite the presence of extremely elevated CSF levels and very high numbers of granulocytes in the blood and haemopoietic tissues (Chang et al 1989b).

These murine studies have been paralleled by clinical observations indicating no serious toxicity for G-CSF but a definite dose-limiting toxicity for GM-CSF associated with myocarditis and a capillary leak syndrome.

FUTURE CLINICAL STUDIES

Existing clinical trials have already established effective dose levels, at least for G-CSF and GM-CSF and future clinical trials can be expected to define most of the situations in hospital medicine in which the CSFs can be used with advantage. Trials on M-CSF and Multi-CSF have yet to reach this stage but these studies are in active progress.

From the studies in mice, combinations of CSFs are capable of eliciting enhanced responses without eliminating the special features of responses to individual CSFs and there is an obvious need to commence comparable studies in patients.

It can never be regarded as wholly satisfactory to use agents clinically with no adequate information on pre-existing levels in the body. There is almost no precise information on levels of all four CSFs in the serum or tissues in any infection. Minimal information would relate to serum levels but ideally levels in marrow tissue (the production site for granulocytes and macrophages) and in local lesions (the site of effector responses) would also be very useful. So far only one study of *Listeria monocytogenes* in mice has addressed levels of the four different CSFs in the circulation and the results indicate the complexity of the CSF responses (Cheers et al 1988).

It would be very valuable to extend such studies to humans with various infections. Here it might be assumed that such data would be easy to collect but there are suggestions that the type of data obtained might be quite misleading. What, for example, happens to CSF levels during a simple attack of mumps or measles? The answer is almost impossible to obtain simply because the typical case never reaches hospital. Patients who become hospitalized are those who have developed complications and such patients might in fact be exhibiting quite atypical responses as part of the reason for their complex clinical progress. An early study of serum CSF levels in Swedish Army personnel with mononucleosis did indeed show that an initial failure to exhibit elevated serum CSF levels during the acute phase of the illness was associated with a longer duration of fever and a more complex clinical course (Metcalf & Wahren 1968).

No data have been produced for tropical infections such as malaria, leishmaniasis or leprosy where macrophage responses are prominent and can be assumed to be of importance.

With the potential availability of methods for correcting neutropenia by what amounts to replacement therapy, there is merit in investigating the frequency of neutropenia in various population groups. If there are population groups, e.g. US Blacks with relatively low neutrophil levels, are there subsets of these in which neutropenia is so severe as to constitute a significant potential hazard following surgical procedures or during epidemic viral infections?

There are three factors that will determine to a large degree the future scope for the use of CSFs in clinical infections: (i) the toxicity of the CSFs, (ii) the antigenicity of the CSFs, and (iii) the cost of the CSFs.

The possible toxic consequences of CSF administration have been referred to earlier. As with all therapy, some toxic consequences must be anticipated and, as for other drugs, a decision whether or not to use the CSFs will need a balanced judgement of potential gain versus potential toxicity.

To a degree, the same considerations apply should some forms of recombinant CSF prove to be antigenic and elicit antibodies that either inactivate injected recombinant material or, worse, cross-inhibit native CSF. Information is sparse on the antigenicity of recombinant CSFs but one report has described the development of antibodies to recombinant GM-CSF (Gribben et al 1990), a phenomenon possibly related to the ability of GM-CSF to enhance antigen presentation by macrophages.

Where an infection is life-threatening and the situation critical, considerations of toxicity or antigenicity become of lesser importance but they are issues of relevance if the infection proposed for CSF therapy is chronic and not life-threatening e.g. chronic renal infections.

The cost of CSF therapy has yet to be revealed but is likely to be largely at the whim of the pharmaceutical companies concerned. It can be assumed that the cost will be inflated far above true production costs on the usual general grounds of covering research and development. It is arguable whether this attitude should be allowed to persist for agents that were discovered and characterized in basic scientific institutes. The question is not trivial because the cost of an agent determines very much the scope of its potential clinical use.

Assuming the CSFs to be expensive drugs when licensed for general use, their application in dramatic life-threatening illness is still acceptable on grounds of preventing mortality and even as cost-effective hospital procedures. However, the use of expensive CSFs will tend not to be envisaged in less dramatic infections. This will be an unfortunate circumstance that may even prevent clinical trials on such infections.

Candidate infections in this latter category are numerous and include chronic renal tract infections, prophylactic use of CSFs in abdominal and prostate surgery where complicating infections are not uncommon. Also possibly in this category is the prophylactic use of CSFs in epidemics of influenza in certain patient categories at risk of secondary infections and possibly even the use of CSFs in patients with chronic infections such as otitis media or chronic leg ulceration.

The future clinical uses of the CSFs in infectious disease therefore depend not only on whether or not they prove to be biologically effective agents in particular infections and on the usual considerations of toxicity and continued effectiveness, but also on the novel aspect of the pricing structure chosen to offset pharmaceutical costs.

REFERENCES

Antman K S, Griffin J D, Elias A et al 1988 Effect of recombinant human granulocyte-macrophage colony-stimulating factor on chemotherapy-induced myelosuppression. New England Journal of Medicine 319: 593-598

Athanassakis I, Bleackley C R, Paetkau V, Guilbert L, Barr P J, Wegmann T G 1987 The immunostimulatory effect of T cells and T cell lymphokines on murine fetally derived placental cells. Journal of Immunology 138: 37-44

Bodey G P, Buckley M, Sathe Y S, Freireich E J 1966 Quantitative relationship between circulating leukocytes and infections in patients with leukaemia. Annals of Internal Medicine 64: 328-340

Bonilla M A, Gillio A P, Ruggeiro M et al 1989 Effects of recombinant human granulocyte colony-stimulating factor on neutropenia in patients with congenital agranulocytosis. New England Journal of Medicine 320: 1574-1580

Bradley T R, Metcalf D 1966 The growth of mouse bone marrow cells in vitro. Australian Journal of Experimental Biology and Medical Science 44: 287-300

Brown M, Metcalf D 1990 Unpublished data

Bussolino F, Wang J M, De Filippi P et al 1989 Granulocyte- and granulocyte-macrophage colony stimulating factors induce endothelial cells to migrate and proliferate. Nature 337: 471-473

Chang J M, Metcalf D, Lang R A, Gonda T J, Johnson G R 1989a Nonneoplastic haematopoietic myeloproliferative syndrome induced by dysregulated Multi-CSF (IL-3) expression. Blood 73: 1487-1497

Chang J M, Metcalf D, Gonda T J, Johnson G R 1989b Long-term exposure to retrovirally-expressed G-CSF induces a non-neoplastic granulocytic and progenitor cell hyperplasia without tissue damage in mice. Journal of Laboratory and Clinical Investigation 84: 1488-1496

Cheers C, Haigh A M, Kelso A, Metcalf D, Stanley E R, Young A M 1988 Production of colony-stimulating factors (CSFs) during infection: Separate determinations of macrophage-, granulocyte-, granulocyte-macrophage-, and Multi-CSFs. Infection and Immunity 56: 247-251

Gabrilove J L, Jakubowski A, Scher H et al 1988 Effect of granulocyte colony-stimulating factor on neutropenia and associated morbidity due to chemotherapy for transitional cell carcinoma of the urothelium. New England Journal of Medicine 318: 1414-1422

Gearing D P, King J A, Gough N M, Nicola N A 1989 Expression cloning of a receptor for human granulocyte-macrophage colony-stimulating factor. EMBO Journal 8: 3667-3676

Gough N M, Williams R L, Hilton D J et al 1989 LIF: A molecule with divergent actions on myeloid leukaemic cells and embryonic stem cells. Reproduction, Fertility and Development 1: 281-288

Gribben J G, Devereux S, Thomas N S B et al 1990 Development of antibodies to unprotected glycosylation sites on recombinant human GM-CSF. Lancet 335: 434-437

Groopman J E, Mitsuyasu R T, De Leo M J, Oette D H, Golde D W 1987 Effects of recombinant human granulocyte-macrophage colony-stimulating factor on myelopoiesis in the acquired immunodeficiency syndrome. New England Journal of Medicine 317: 593-598

Hammond W P, Price T H, Souza L M, Dale D C 1989 Treatment of cyclic neutropenia with granulocyte colony-stimulating factor. New England Journal of Medicine 320: 1306-1311

Johnson G R, Gonda T J, Metcalf D, Hariharan I K, Cory S 1989 A lethal myeloproliferative syndrome in mice transplanted with bone marrow cells infected with a retrovirus expressing granulocyte-macrophage colony stimulating factor. EMBO Journal 8: 441-448

Kelso A, Metcalf D in press The T-lymphocyte-derived colony stimulating factors. Advances in Immunology

Kishimoto T 1989 the biology of interleukin-6. Blood 74: 1-10

Koyanagi Y, O'Brien W A, Zhao J Q, Golde D W, Gasson J C, Chen I S Y 1988 Cytokines alter production of HIV-1 from primary mononuclear phagocytes. Science 241: 1673-1675

Lang R A, Metcalf D, Cuthbertson R A et al 1987 Transgenic mice expressing a hemopoietic growth factor gene (GM-CSF) develop accumulations of macrophages, blindness and a fatal syndrome of tissue damage. Cell 51: 675-686

Lee F, Yokota T, Chiu C P et al 1988 The molecular cloning of interleukins 4 and 6: Multifunctional hemopoietic growth factors. Behring Institute Mitteilungen 83: 8-14

Lieschke G S, Maher D, Cebon J et al 1989 Effects of subcutaneously administered bacterially-synthesized recombinant human granulocyte-macrophage colony-stimulating factor in patients with advanced malignancy. Annals of Internal Medicine 110: 357-364

Matsumoto M, Matsubara S, Matsuno T et al 1987 Protective effect of human granulocyte colony-stimulating factor on microbial infection in neutropenic mice. Infection and Immunity 55: 2715-2720

Metcalf D 1984 The hemopoietic colony stimulating factors. Elsevier, Amsterdam

Metcalf D 1987 The molecular control of normal and leukaemic granulocytes and macrophages. Proceedings of the Royal Society, London B 230: 389-423

Metcalf D 1988 The molecular control of blood cells. Harvard University Press, Boston, USA

Metcalf D 1989a Actions and interactions of G-CSF, LIF and IL-6 on normal and leukemic murine cells. Leukemia 3: 349-355

Metcalf D 1989b The molecular control of cell division, differentiation commitment and maturation in haemopoietic cells. Nature (London) 339: 27-30

Metcalf D, Moore J G 1988 Divergent disease patterns in granulocyte-macrophage colony-stimulating factor transgenic mice associated with different transgene insertion sites. Proceedings of the National Academy of Science (USA) 85: 7767-7771

Metcalf D, Wahren B 1968 Bone marrow colony stimulating activity of sera in infectious mononucleosis. British Medical Journal 3: 99-101

Metcalf D, Burgess A W, Johnson G R et al 1986 In vitro actions on hemopoietic cells of recombinant murine GM-CSF purified after production in *Escherichia coli*: Comparison with purified native GM-CSF. Journal of Cellular Physiology 128: 421-431

Metcalf D, Begley C G, Nicola N A, Johnson G R 1987 Quantitative responsiveness of murine hemopoietic populations in vitro and in vivo to recombinant Multi-CSF (IL-3). Experimental Haematology 15: 288-295

Moore M A S, Warren D J 1987 Synergy of interleukin-1 and granulocyte colony stimulating factor: In vivo stimulation of stem cell recovery and haematopoietic regeneration following 5-fluorouracil treatment of mice. Proceedings of the National Academy of Science (USA) 84: 7134-7138

Morstyn G, Campbell L, Souza L M et al 1988 Effect of granulocyte colony-stimulating factor on neutropenia induced by cytotoxic chemotherapy. Lancet i: 667-672

Nicola N A 1989 Hemopoietic cell growth factors and their receptors. Annual Review of Biochemistry 58: 45-77

Pluznik D H, Sachs L 1966 The induction of clones of normal mast cells by a substance from conditioned medium. Experimental Cell Research 43: 553-563

Sherr C J, Rettenmier C W, Sacca R, Roussel M F, Look A T, Stanley E R 1985 The c-fms proto-oncogene product is related to the receptor for the mononuclear phagocyte growth factor, CSF-1. Cell 41: 665-676

Suda T, Yamaguchi Y, Suda J, Miura Y, Okana A, Akiyama Y 1988 Effect of interleukin-6 (IL-6) on the differentiation and proliferation of murine and human hemopoietic progenitors. Experimental Hematology 16: 891-895

Talmadge J F, Tribble H, Pennington R et al 1989 Protective, restorative and therapeutic properties of recombinant colony stimulating factors. Blood 73: 2093-2103

Uckun F M, Souza L, Waddick K G, Wick M, Song C W 1990 In vivo radioprotective effects of recombinant human granulocyte colony-stimulating factor in lethally irradiated mice. Blood 75: 638-645

Vadhan-Raj S, Jeha S S, Buescher S et al 1990 Stimulation of myelopoiesis in a patient with congenital neutropenia: Biology and nature of response to recombinant human granulocyte-macrophage colony-stimulating factor. Blood 75: 858-864

Walker F, Nicola N A, Metcalf D, Burgess A W 1985 Hierarchical down-modulation of hemopoietic growth factor receptors. Cell 43: 269-276

Discussion of paper presented by D. Metcalf

Discussed by P. H. Lagrange
Reported by H. C. Neu

In contrast to many other immunomodulators where in vitro findings often contradict in vivo results, the preliminary data with CSFs in hmans confirm what has been demonstrated in vitro. CSFs, therefore offer the real possibility to treat or to prevent infections under certain conditions.

When we study the effect of the various CSFs on the host defense systems, we must determine their independent effect on polymorphonuclear leukocytes, or on macrophages. It is also important to know whether the effect on cells in different parts of the body is the same. As discussed, CSFs are able to increase the blood levels of the polymorphonuclear leukocytes. However, very few of these cells enter the peritoneal cavity when G–CSF is given. Gm–CSF on the other hand induces a marked increase in local cellularity in the peritoneal or pleural cavities. It is important to know which factors dictate entry into these areas in the body; in other words we need to study both the central and peripheral effects of CSF. It is also important to study transmodulation: the network of all the glycoproteins. For example, we know that Gm–CSF is able to increase IL–1 and TNF levels, and TNF by itself is able to increase CSF production. One way to determine the specific activity and biological effects might be to produce analogues of each CSF.

With regard to the therapeutic indications of the CSFs, we still do not know the proper dosage that will be adequate to produce a favourable risk-benefit ratio. As far as toxicity is concerned it has become clear that subcutaneous injections produce fewer side-effects than IV injections. It now appears that toxicity seems to be related to modulation of expression of the family of adhesins on the surface of the cell, but it is also possible that the production of TNF after Gm–CSF administration is responsible for toxicity. The use of anti-TFN monoclonal antibodies might diminish toxicity, as a similar approach has been shown to reduce IL–2 toxicity in mice. More studies are needed to evaluate possible long term toxicity particularly the risk of renal failure.

A further important question relating to biological toxicity is the possibility that use in the pre-leukemic patient might cause transformation of cells. Extensive work has shown that this does not happen, as excessive stimulation of cells alone, without the presence of co-factors, does not lead to transformation. As an extension of this would we feel comfortable using CSFs to treat patients with myeloid leukemia who have become neutropenic? This is a complicated issue because all myeloid leukemic

304

cells depend on CSF for every cell division. The concentration required is exactly the same as in normal cells. One would think that this would be the last sort of patient who would benefit from CSF because it would stimulate the leukemic cells to divide. On the other hand, however, one of the other actions of the CSFs is induction of differentiation and commitment, and in fact a myeloid leukemic population is suppressed by inducing the cells to differentiate.

Ideally, if it was known in advance that the differentiation induction effect in a specified patient would be stronger than the proliferative effect, CSFs could be used with confidence. At present CSFs can only be recommended where the leukemic cells have been removed to the best of the ability of the clinician, for example following massive chemotherapy or in bone marrow transplants following chemotherapy and total body irradiation.

Overall there is great enthusiasm about the use of G−CSF and Gm−CSF in cancer patients with the hope that in the future, fine tuning of the action of these molecules or the use of cocktails or mixtures, might lead to major advances in the treatment of specified infections.

Index

307

310